Waking Up /
Fighting Back

Also by Roberta Altman

THE COMPLETE BOOK OF HOME ENVIRONMENTAL HAZARDS
THE PROSTATE ANSWER BOOK

with Michael J. Sarg

THE CANCER DICTIONARY

Waking Up / Fighting Back

The Politics of Breast Cancer

ROBERTA ALTMAN

LITTLE, BROWN AND COMPANY

BOSTON   NEW YORK   TORONTO   LONDON

First Edition

Library of Congress Cataloging-in-Publication Data

Altman, Roberta.
    Waking up, fighting back : the politics of breast cancer / Roberta
Altman.
        p.   cm.
    Includes bibliographical references.
    ISBN 0-316-03532-7
    1. Breast — Cancer — Social aspects — United States.   I. Title.
RC280.B8A444   1996
362.1'9699449 — dc20   95-25211

10 9 8 7 6 5 4 3 2 1

HAD

Published simultaneously in Canada
by Little, Brown & Company (Canada) Limited

Printed in the United States of America

To Rose Kushner, who, speaking out loudly for her own rights and the rights of all women at a time when the words "breast cancer" were not spoken in public, inspired me and thousands of other women. . . . She lost her life but won the undying respect, admiration, and gratitude of all who followed in her footsteps. And to the hundreds of thousands of courageous women who have fought valiantly and lost the battle and the women who today are fighting for their own lives as well as the lives of all women . . . their mothers, sisters, and daughters.

Contents

Acknowledgments

I am indebted and grateful to the many breast cancer survivors who willingly and graciously told me their stories, sent me materials (frequently unsolicited), and suggested others with whom I might be interested in talking. They include Rita Arditti, Elizabeth Belden, Zora Brown, Emma Lu Bullard, Nancy Cardwell, Coleen Chaney, Susan Claymon, Nancy Classer, Doris Erickson, Loretta Fields, Ellen Hobbs, Lana Jensen, Ester Johnson, Susan Kaplan, Mary Jo Kahn, Mary Katzke, Marlene Kessler, Jan Kutschinski, Betsy Lambert, Amy Langer, Susan Pringle, Congresswoman Marilyn Lloyd, Ann Marcou, Terry MacKinon, Ruth Mendoza, Melissa Miller, Lee Miller, Barbara Parker, Rebecca Parker, Janet Perkins, Joanne Rathgeb, Betty Reed, Judy Rodgers, Joyce Salzburg, Donna Sauer, Pat Skowronski, Virginia Soffa, Loretta Steen, Ricky Stouch, Lois Joy Thomi, Bettie Tuthill, Fran Visco, Congresswoman Barbara Vucanovich, Patricia Walsh, Sandy Warshaw, and Diane Zarafonetis.

Health professionals who took time out from busy schedules include Lou Fintor, Scott Frey, Annette Brown, M.D., Michael Sarg, M.D., Julia Rowland, Ph.D., George Raptis, M.D., Lisa Sclafani, M.D., Larry Norton, M.D., Karen Schmidt, R.N., Mary Rose Oakar, Harvey Kushner, Terry Castagno, David P. Rose, M.D., Ph.D., D.Sc., Roz Kleban, M.S.W., Nora Waters, R.N., Sharon Green, Alison Estabrook, M.D., Barbara Balaban, Harold Freeman, M.D., Irene

Card, Ellen Stovall, Deborah Ash, Joyce Ford, Kimberly Calder, Susan Love, M.D., Maryann Napoli, and Victor Vogel, M.D.

Numerous organizations supplied materials, including the National Cancer Institute, American Cancer Society, National Alliance of Breast Cancer Organizations (whose list of local organizations was especially helpful), *BMT Newsletter,* CAN ACT, Cancer Care, CPSC, FDA, Greenpeace, National Breast Cancer Coalition, Office of Women's Health, National Coalition for Cancer Survivorship, National Institute of Environmental Health Services, Center for Medical Consumers, Environmental Protection Agency, National Women's Health Network, Office of Alternative Medicine, Susan G. Komen Breast Cancer Foundation, Women's Environment and Development Organization, Ladies of Courage/Y-ME, Save Ourselves, Breast Cancer Action, Massachusetts Breast Cancer Coalition, "EXPRESSIONS" for Women, SHARE, Virginia Breast Cancer Foundation, and Victory in the Valley.

Special thanks to Bonny Redlich, Hilary Ziff, and Juanita Jones for their help in research and editing and their constant support. And to family and friends who put up with my breaking dates and being just "too busy" all the time.

Without the commitment and support of Jennifer Josephy, my editor, Abigail Wilentz, her assistant, senior copyeditor Betty Power, and Janis Vallely, my agent, this book would never have come to fruition. Thank you for your input and encouragement, especially during times when I did not see the light at the end of the tunnel.

Waking Up /
Fighting Back

Introduction

In 1976, when I was 34, I was diagnosed with breast cancer. I had discovered a small lump in my breast while showering. I was working in Washington, D.C., and called my gynecologist in New York immediately. The rest of the week, until my appointment, I checked my breast again and again and again. Maybe I had imagined it. Maybe it would just go away.

My gynecologist confirmed that I had a lump, "But," she said, "it is nothing to worry about. At some point you should probably have it removed, but there is no rush. Come back in six months." To me, her words were in no way reassuring. (To many women, those words *are* reassuring and they go home with a great sense of relief. Some of these women find out months or even years later that the lump was malignant and that their breast cancer is far more advanced than it had to be.) I told my gynecologist I wanted it out immediately. She repeated that it really wasn't necessary, but at my insistence agreed to get me into a hospital as soon as possible.

My boyfriend, Dave, suggested I go for a second opinion. "Why?" I asked. "It doesn't matter what anyone thinks — I am getting this out." But I acquiesced and went for a second opinion to a well-known Manhattan gynecologist. He said the lump moved and that if the lump was malignant it would not move. He told me a biopsy was not necessary and it was nothing to worry about. I knew I would continue to worry until the lump was removed.

I was in the hospital the following Friday for the biopsy. I asked why the biopsy couldn't be done under a local. Having general anesthesia frightened me. "It just can't be," I was told. I did not make a fuss. That night a doctor who identified himself as a "fellow" came into my room with a consent form for me to sign. The form gave permission to the surgeon to perform a mastectomy if cancer was found. I hadn't met the surgeon who would be doing the biopsy. I couldn't imagine letting someone I had never even met automatically remove my breast. Although the doctor tried to persuade me to sign the form, I refused. With a look of disgust he left the room.

Because of what I had been told by both doctors, I expected the lump to be benign. I was shocked when I found out that it was malignant. And I was terrified. I was also grateful that I had not followed the advice of the doctors who cavalierly told me it was "nothing," and that my own level of anxiety, which the doctors probably attributed to "neurotic female behavior," left me no choice but to have the lump removed.

At the hospital, while I was recovering from the biopsy, my friend Judy intervened, pleading with me to get a second opinion. "What's the point?" I asked. In my mind, if there was cancer in my breast that could kill me, I wanted to do anything I could to survive, and if that meant removing my breast, well, so be it. But I finally said okay, she could call her breast surgeon. (I didn't know at the time that there were breast surgeons.) The surgeon called me back in the hospital and told me that my only option was to have my breast removed. I had the mastectomy two days later. And my life was changed forever.

When I saw the surgeon a few days after the mastectomy, he told me there was a 20 percent chance the cancer would recur. My heart sank. Walking out of the office with me, Dave said, "but there is an 80 percent chance that it will not recur." I felt better, but only slightly.

The surgeon told me that one thing I could do for added insurance that the breast cancer would not come back would be to get radiation to the chest wall. I asked the question that is still asked by women. "What would you tell your wife to do?" I had the radiation treatments, which are no longer routinely done.

I also made an appointment with an oncologist to find out if I should have chemotherapy. I wanted to do everything that was needed. The oncologist said that it was not necessary, since the lymph nodes that had been removed during surgery had not contained cancer.

During my first visit to the oncologist who eventually saved my life, Michael Sarg, M.D., at St. Vincent's Hospital in New York, I told him my well-thought-out plan. I would see him one month, the radiologist the following month, the surgeon the month after that, and then start all over. That way I would leave no stone unturned. Surely if I was checked by a doctor once a month, the cancer would be picked up immediately should it recur. Sarg explained to me that unfortunately it didn't work that way and that I'd be wasting my money and time as well as the time of the doctors I'd be seeing. I was shocked when I found out, in 1976, that there was no simple test that could tell if the cancer was back. As I write this nearly 20 years later, there still is none.

When I had the mastectomy, I was living with a man. I couldn't conceive of Dave's loving me any less because I had just one breast. I was right. He was supportive and loving, and on the day I got home carefully made love to me. That was reassuring, and our sexual life continued as usual. When we broke up several years later, I was no longer so confident that my having one breast would make me no less desirable. How did you tell someone? When did you tell someone? You couldn't just let him find out, could you?

I went out briefly with several different men and stopped seeing each before the issue came up. Finally, it was the moment of truth. I was with a man I'd seen a number of times and liked. I was sitting on his lap and we were getting more and more affectionate. I finally took a deep breath and said, "There's something I have to ask you. Do you know what a mastectomy is?"

He said, "Yes, it's when a woman has a breast removed."

I said, "Well, I had one."

He said, "So?" whereupon I burst into tears.

He looked at me and asked, "Did I say something wrong? I'm sorry, I didn't mean to."

He had no way of knowing that he was the first postmastectomy man I'd been with and that for months I'd been worrying what I'd say, how I'd say it, and what kind of response I'd get. As time passed and I had other relationships, I found that his reaction was typical. It seemed that my missing breast was more important to me than to the men I was seeing.

Another fear I had, in the beginning, was that someone would be able to see that I had just one breast. I was very self-conscious, constantly looking down to make sure the prosthesis and breast were even. I was also fearful that somehow the prosthesis would fall out. The first time I went into a store with an open dressing room, I went into a corner, opened the buttons of the blouse I wanted to try on, opened the buttons of the blouse I was wearing, and switched as quickly as possible. Knowing intellectually that none of the women around me hurriedly trying on clothes were the least bit interested in me, and that if they did look my way, it was virtually impossible to tell that one of the breasts in my bra was not real, was of no help emotionally. (It has taken me a long time but I have come a long way since 1976. Today, as in my premastectomy days, I hardly ever wear a bra. I will try clothes on in an open dressing room when I am not wearing a bra and prosthesis. One woman even came up to me and said, "Thank you.")

Things went relatively well for about four years. I'd get anxious when a doctor's visit was coming up. And whenever I had a pain anywhere, I'd become terrified that the cancer was back. Then, in early spring of 1981, I just wasn't feeling right. I was meeting a friend in Paris in June and decided to get my annual mammography early, before the trip, just to be sure. I didn't get to Paris that year.

My cancer had recurred in my lymph nodes, lung, and on my optic nerve. I was sure I was going to die. Riding a bus up Riverside Drive, I looked at the green trees and thought how beautiful they were and that I could be experiencing my last spring. I was more frightened than ever and I was also very angry. "If you're going to take my life," I kept thinking with teeth clenched, "you're going to have to fight for it." I was ready for battle. This time around I did things differently.

I was working at NBC and had the librarian do a computer search for me for the latest articles on breast cancer. I talked to anyone I could — from Rose Kushner, a breast cancer activist who had written a book about her experience, to a medical reporter at the *New York Times*. I even went to the National Cancer Institute in Bethesda, Maryland, to see about being treated there. In the end I went back to my own oncologist, whom I liked and trusted.

I had virtually all the side effects one could have from the chemotherapy. I ended up in the hospital when Cytoxan caused my bladder to shrink. The more your bladder shrinks, the more often you have to urinate. I lost control in my elevator. Riding in the taxi to the hospital, I didn't know how to tell the driver I'd left a little puddle on the seat. I gave him a very big tip. I took no more Cytoxan. I was totally humiliated. As a result of the vincristine, I would trip in the street and had trouble climbing the steps to get on buses. I didn't look sick so there was no reason for anyone to offer me a seat. I took no more vincristine. As a result of the prednisone I would wake at about three in the morning raring to go. I got a lot of closets cleaned that hadn't been touched in years. I lost a lot of weight because it was difficult for me to eat. I had sores in my mouth and the smell of food made me feel sick. Not one person said, "Gee, you've lost weight, you look great." The radiation treatment to my head to destroy the cancer on my optic nerve caused my hair to fall out.

I refused to cry uncle. At the time I was working as a radio reporter. I went to work every day. I scheduled my chemotherapy late in the day so that I was available to cover stories. I would frequently call in my reports from the doctor's office. Minimizing the impact of the cancer on my life was the only way I could deal with it and feel I had some control.

I had one other very distressing side effect, which was from the hormonal treatment tamoxifen. I became very dry and did not lubricate during sexual foreplay. Sexual intercourse became very painful. Nobody had warned me about this. I now had something else I had to tell a man, that I needed a lot of foreplay before sexual intercourse. The response was usually something like, "Relax, you're just tense, don't worry about it." That infuriated me. This was not a psychological problem, it was a physiological problem. I was far more affected by this than by the loss of a breast. I felt like less of a woman. I also had a revelation. I gained new compassion and understanding for men who at times "could not get it up." In the past, I'd said similar things to them to relieve their anxiety. "Don't worry about it. It's no big deal." For the first time I fully understood what a big deal it was.

My hair grew back and the side effects from the chemotherapy eventually went away. The side effects from the tamoxifen did not. Chemotherapy was not pleasant. Even with good medical coverage, which I had, the treatment was costly. If I had it to do over, would I? In a second. It saved my life.

Have things changed a lot since I was diagnosed with breast cancer in 1976? In some ways, yes. In too many ways, no.

It is a fact that many women do survive breast cancer. It is also a fact that the survival rate is way too low. I am one of the *very* lucky ones. I believe I survived because of three things: my attitude (I was very angry and determined to fight for my life as hard as I could); the state-of-the-art care I received, administered by a compassionate doctor; and luck. As far as I'm concerned, the most important factor in my survival was luck. And I do not think that any woman should have to be lucky to survive breast cancer.

I can also tell you that surviving is just the beginning of the battle. One woman, a teacher, told me she had to take off time from work for her surgery, her treatment, and for various medical complications that arose. She worked at a progressive, highly regarded private school in Manhattan. She was finally called in and told she could not be kept on. It was too disruptive to the students to have her out so much. She did not make a fuss or file a lawsuit because her child was attending the school. Another woman on the New York City police force was fired because she was "no longer able to perform her job as a result of the cancer." She had been back on the force for months when she got the pink slip in the mail. She fought and won her job back (along with back pay).

A woman in her mid-forties fighting metastatic breast cancer told me that she felt the stress on her job was a negative factor in her recovery, but she was afraid to quit. "I'd lose my medical coverage and my husband's coverage is minimal. If I didn't have this job, I wouldn't have been able to get the medical care I am now receiving." I, too, am one of many cancer survivors "locked" into a job because of the medical coverage it supplies. If I wanted to quit, I could not afford adequate health insurance on my own, and I know that despite anti-discrimination laws, my medical history would make it hard, if not impossible, for me to find another job.

How many women are locked into jobs they'd just as soon leave? How many women are fired? And how many women, after experiencing the trauma and cost of a life-threatening illness, have the emotional and financial resources it takes to wage another battle to fight discrimination?

There are many unanswered questions about breast cancer. For example, the main means of detecting early breast cancer, before it can be felt, is the mammogram, which is far from perfect. However, we still don't know whether women under 50 benefit from mammography, how often women should get a mammogram, how we can make sure that every woman who should be getting a mammogram gets one and can afford one, and how to make sure that every mammogram performed is of the highest possible quality.

As for treatment, once breast cancer is diagnosed, too many women are still needlessly losing breasts. There are still many doctors who will advise every woman diagnosed with breast cancer to get a mastectomy when she could get a breast-conserving lumpectomy. Today there is a wealth of data showing that a lumpectomy is as effective as a mastectomy in a great many cases.

Too many women are not getting state-of-the-art treatment. When I co-led a support group for women with metastatic breast cancer in 1990, it was primarily comprised of well-educated, professional women who worked and had medical coverage. One woman was a teacher who had just turned 50. She had widespread metastatic disease to the bone (a common and painful place for breast cancer to spread). When she described the treatment she had received, I was shocked, appalled, and greatly saddened. She was dying because she had not been given the tests she should have gotten, which could have picked up the metastatic disease before it had spread to so many parts of her body. Her metastatic disease should have been detected earlier and treated earlier, giving her a better chance at survival. I looked at this educated, intelligent woman, a typical middle-class working mother, and thought about the thousands of women in the United States who don't even have medical coverage, who can barely read (or are illiterate), who are certainly not educated about breast cancer, who cannot afford to get a mammogram — and if they do get a mammogram and there is a problem, cannot afford to get the proper treatment.

In the 1970s, when I was diagnosed with breast cancer, I was well aware that women faced discrimination. We were barred from top positions in companies, barred from all-male clubs where important networking took place, barred from job promotions, and barred from making the same wages as a man doing the same work we were doing. I did not know then that we were also barred from getting the same quality of medical care provided to men. It is well documented that men's diseases have consistently gotten more money for research; and women have consistently been closed out of clinical trials that might have benefited them.

In 1989 the National Institutes of Health (NIH) spent far more money on AIDS research than it did on breast cancer. From 1981 to the end of 1994, some 620,000 women died of breast cancer. During that same period approximately 270,000 people died of AIDS. AIDS can be prevented; breast cancer cannot.

Breast cancer is the most prevalent cancer in this country. It reached epidemic proportions years ago. In 1996, statistically one in eight women in this country will get breast cancer during her lifetime. Today, virtually every woman knows at least one woman with breast cancer, and many women know more than one. The lives of husbands, children, parents, and friends of women with breast cancer are all affected.

Breast cancer is finally getting media coverage. Network news shows have done series on breast cancer; television news magazine shows have done segments; in 1993 the staid *New York Times Sunday Magazine* ran a cover with a half-nude picture of a woman whose mastectomy was clearly visible.

Grassroots breast cancer support and advocacy groups have been springing up all over the country. The National Breast Cancer Coalition, founded in 1991, has made massive inroads into the war against breast cancer by substantially raising the amount of funding for research. While it is gratifying to tell a story of so many women finally waking up and fighting back, at the same time it is saddening to tell the story of the inadequate and unequal health care women have received for so many years, of the many poor women in the United States who die because they don't have access to good medical care, and how far we still have to go in our battle against this killer disease.

In writing this book, I had the opportunity to meet and talk with many courageous women who willingly, even eagerly, shared some of the worst moments of their lives with me. Some of the women I am still in touch with. Others have died. Why were they so willing to tell me their stories? Mostly they were angry and asking the same questions I was asking. Many of them had never been active in any organization, much less a political movement. They felt they had to speak out. They were well aware that what they were doing in all likelihood would be too late to benefit themselves. But they felt that as a result of their efforts, their children and grandchildren might not have to face the possibility of breast cancer, and that perhaps their children and grandchildren would be able to live the full, long lives of which they, themselves might be deprived.

The stories were not really new to me but were just more variations of stories I'd been hearing for years. I'd always been very open about having had breast cancer and over the years have frequently received calls from friends and acquaintances asking if I'd be willing to talk with a cousin, a colleague at work, a friend who had just been diagnosed with breast cancer. I never refused. I heard hair-raising stories that would make me furious, set off a crying jag when I hung up the phone, and give me nightmares at night.

I also got calls from my own fearful friends who had discovered a lump or had gone for a routine mammogram and been told that it looked suspicious. In four years three good friends were diagnosed with breast cancer.

I heard similar concerns and personal stories from women all over the United States. I talked with women who never thought it could happen to them; women who were told they had six weeks to live, or one year (and are still here); women who were patronized, humiliated, and dismissed by doctors; women who were treated rudely and insensitively by doctors; women who were misdiagnosed and mistreated; women who were told they should really be seeing a psychiatrist; women who were told the lump in their breast was benign and not to worry about it; women who were simply told, "You're too young to have breast cancer" (a phrase I heard repeatedly when I was diagnosed with breast cancer at the age of 34); women who found out that the insurance they counted on proved to be no insurance at all; and women who were fired because they had breast cancer.

When I visited a member of my metastatic breast cancer support group who was in the hospital dying, I met her mother and sister, who had flown in from California. Her sister said to me, "I was with a good friend when she died of breast cancer a year ago. Now it's my own sister. I said then I was going to do some kind of volunteer work and never got around to it. I have been reading about radical groups in San Francisco and I'm going to join with them. I've never been a demonstrator or shouter, but something has to be done."

The wrenching, horrendous, and infuriating stories of the women in this book, many in their own voices, may cause you some anxiety, discomfort, and fear, but I hope reading these terrible true stories within the context of the controversial issues that surround them will empower you to take action or at least recognize that it is up to each one of us to take responsibility for the care and control of our body.

Many friends, knowing my history, have asked how I could write this book; wouldn't the topic be stressful, depressing? My answer was, "How could I not?"

Part I

Waking Up

1

Health Care on the Back Burner

Women's health has risen to the public's consciousness in a way I never would have dreamed of.

Vivian Pinn, *director, Office of Research on Women's Health*[1]

As we focus on breast cancer, we know that was one part of a larger agenda in accomplishing the improvement of the health status of American women.

Senator Barbara A. Mikulski (D-Maryland)[2]

Women have been getting short shrift in health care for years. We have been left out of clinical trials and patronized by doctors who called our ills neurotic and psychosomatic. We've sat back and taken it, but we're not taking it anymore. At least some of us aren't.

In 1979, a study on the medical treatment of women versus men found that doctors treated men and women who complain of the same symptoms differently. Doctors were more likely to refer male patients for diagnostic tests and to attribute women's complaints to stress or hypochondria. Female patients were twice as likely as men to have the abnormal results of an exercise test blamed on "psychiatric or other noncardiac causes."

The study also showed that women were less likely than men to

- receive kidney transplants
- have coronary bypass surgery
- have their lung cancer diagnosed

Frequently, women simply did not receive the same quality of treatment as men. The study concluded, "There is evidence that physicians are more likely to perceive women's maladies than men's as the result of emotionality."[3]

A Louis Harris poll for the Commonwealth Fund in 1993 found 25 percent of the women questioned said they had been "talked down to" or treated like a child by a doctor compared to 12 percent of the men. And 17 percent of women compared to 7 percent of the men were told by the doctor that the condition they thought they had was "all in their head."[4] Speaking at a breast cancer conference in May 1994, former National Institutes of Health (NIH) director Bernadine Healy, M.D., said, "Women who have chest pains are not treated the same as men unless tests show they are having a heart attack."[5]

For years women's health concerns have been dismissed or just plain ignored. Women were told by (usually male) physicians that their complaints were hysterical or hypochondriacal. They were not taken seriously. An article in 1993 on women's experiences with the silicone breast implant is a prime example of how women are treated in a male-oriented medical society. The authors say, "The issue of having women's concerns about medical problems heard and respected is not new and persists in contemporary society." They found many similarities between the way the silicone breast implant problem and the Dalkon Shield (an IUD device) problem were handled. In both cases, it took widespread publicity to finally generate investigations. In the case of the Dalkon Shield, many women with that IUD who experienced serious health problems were frequently not taken seriously by physicians, and their symptoms were often not acknowledged by the manufacturer to be related to the IUD.[6] The eventual investigations into the Dalkon Shield, prompted by extensive media coverage, led to its removal from the American market. The silicone breast implant and Dalkon Shield are two of the most important medical device incidents of modern times. In both situations, if women's complaints had been listened to and taken seriously early on, the problems with these devices might have been found years sooner and many women would have been spared unnecessary suffering.

All-male studies have been the norm until only very recently. Former Congresswoman Mary Rose Oakar (D-Ohio) remembers her early years in Congress. "When I was a fairly new member, a 20-year study was done [by the National Institute on Aging] in Baltimore on aging diseases. They came before our committee to talk about the results of the aging process. I asked how many women were in the study. They said none. Twenty years and they couldn't find one woman." When I spoke with Oakar in the fall of 1993, she told me that in her opinion there was and still is a cultural bias against women's diseases. She said that when women went to get grants, "somehow they couldn't cut the mustard. There's tremendous prejudice out there. . . . There is a tremendous bias and it's so culturally inherent that it's honestly hard to even cut through."[7]

Another much-publicized all-male study was the Physicians' Health Study, in which 22,000 male doctors 40 years of age and older were randomly assigned to take an aspirin or placebo every other day. The results of the study were impressive. The men who took the aspirin had a 44 percent lower heart attack rate than the men who took the placebo. Women were intentionally left out of the study. For that reason, it is not known if women, in whom the greatest cause of death is heart disease, can reduce their risk by taking aspirin.[8]

Mary Ann Liebert, M.D., cites that study as being instrumental in her founding of the *Journal of Women's Health* in 1992. She says her interest in equality between men and women in health care goes back to the 1980s. Both she and her husband were Harvard Medical School graduates; her husband was invited to take part in the school's aspirin study and she wasn't. "I remarked to my husband that the study should include women, if only because we have some biological difference. And, in fact, that's why we were excluded."[9]

Rebecca Dresser, a bioethicist at Case Western Reserve University's medical school, wrote about the lack of women in medical trials and gave some examples:[10]

- The relationship between low-cholesterol diets and heart disease "has been almost exclusively studied in men."
- Evidence that aspirin can prevent some migraine headaches was pro-

duced in studies on men even though women suffer from migraines
up to three times more often than men.

- Studies of AIDS treatment frequently omit women, even though
women represent "the fastest-growing infected population."
- A study of the possible relationship between caffeine and heart
disease involved over 45,000 men and no women.

There is growing evidence that life-threatening illnesses manifest
themselves differently in men and women. For example, the treadmill
test that can identify men at risk for heart disease is not as accurate
when used on women. Chest pains and angina are more likely to be
warning signs of heart disease in men than in women. Because wom-
en's heart problems are diagnosed later than men's, women's heart
disease is frequently more advanced, and that results in women being
less likely to survive bypass surgery or a heart attack. As a result, says
Healy, "49 percent of women who have heart attacks die within one
year compared with 31 percent of men who have heart attacks."[11]

James Todd, M.D., an executive vice president of the American
Medical Association, acknowledges that health problems affecting only
women have not received the same serious attention given those affecting men, that there has been a history of neglect of women's
health. Why? Todd says there are several reasons. For years men dom-
inated the power end of the medical field — they were the doctors and
scientists. So they chose to study other men. Because there were so
few women doctors and scientists, there were few strong voices for
women. It was believed that conditions such as heart disease were rare
in women. There was a paternalistic attitude held by many doctors,
who sought to exclude women from trials in order to "protect" them.
One of the possible risks a woman had to be protected from was the
risk that should she be pregnant, the developing fetus might be
harmed. (That same risk has also kept women from getting jobs in
some businesses and industries.) And finally, women's female hormonal changes would complicate the studies.[12]

Whatever the reason, the result is that women have been and remain at a distinct disadvantage when it comes to their health. And this
is not something that was just brought to light.

In 1983, a Public Health Service Task Force on Women's Health
was established. In the first part of its report, published in 1985, a

wide variety of women's health issues were examined. The report concluded that research policies in the United States put women at a disadvantage. The task force made a number of recommendations, including one that said, "Biomedical and behavioral research should be expanded to ensure emphasis on conditions and diseases unique to, or more prevalent in, women in all age groups."[13]

In 1986, NIH put out a policy statement urging applicants for grants to include women and minorities in clinical trials or to have a good reason for excluding them.[14] It was the right direction, but unfortunately not many took that road.

In 1989, the Congressional Caucus for Women's Issues pointed out that women's health problems accounted for only 13.5 percent of spending by NIH and called on the General Accounting Office (GAO) to study the exclusion of women in medical research at NIH.[15] In June 1990, the GAO issued its report, which found that medical research was (still) mainly being done on men, and that NIH had been inconsistent in implementing its policy, which called for encouraging the inclusion of women in clinical trials.[16]

After release of that report, there were other reports of discrimination or "gender bias" at NIH. For example, it was reported that only three of NIH's two thousand researchers specialized in obstetrics and gynecology, and that not one division was devoted exclusively to that area. The NIH research center was spending less than 14 percent of its annual budget on women's health care.

In August 1993, a new, revised NIH *Guide for Grants and Contracts* was published.[17] It stipulated, among other things:

- The number of women included in a study would be proportional to their prevalence in the condition being studied.
- If the correct number of women were not included, the investigators' ability to answer the questions posed would be compromised, unless an appropriate justification were provided.
- There would be peer review of any justification given for not including women; if it was not considered appropriate, that would be factored into the final recommendation of approval or disapproval and the level of relative merit given to the proposal.
- Studies which exclude women would have to have compelling justification to do so to be awarded funding.

The last sentence in the guide says, "It is important to note that regardless of the program relevance of the proposed research, the NIH/ADAMHA funding components will not fund/award grants or contracts that do not comply with this policy."

At that time, the Office of Research on Women's Health (ORWH) noted the possible problems of including women of childbearing age in some studies. It requested a hearing by the Institute of Medicine (IOM) in 1991 to examine how to include that population of women in clinical trials while dealing with problems related to possible fetal harm, safety, and liability; where there should be guidelines to determine when clinical studies should be designed to evaluate gender differences; and how guidelines should be developed to determine when changes in drug metabolism during the menstrual cycle should be investigated.

In July 1990, Congresswoman Pat Schroeder (D-Colorado) and then congresswoman (now senator) Olympia Snowe (D-Maine), co-chairs of the Congressional Caucus for Women's Issues, introduced the Women's Health Equity Act (WHEA). The creation of an office on women's health research was included in the first WHEA in large part as a result of the GAO study released in June. The ORWH was created in September 1990 by NIH to "strengthen and enhance the efforts of NIH to improve the prevention, diagnosis, and treatment of illness in women and to enhance research related to diseases and conditions that affect women,"[18] or, to put it more simply, it was charged with making sure that women got their fair share. The ORWH identified breast cancer as one of its top priorities for the 1990s. Following are the ORWH guidelines for what it planned to accomplish:[19]

- Establish goals and policies throughout the NIH for research related to women's health.
- Develop a plan to increase support of research that is done by NIH and then implement the plan, monitor it, and evaluate it.
- Coordinate the activities of the NIH devoted to women's research.
- Provide advice and staff support to NIH staff regarding the overall direction of, and approaches to, NIH research programs related to women.
- Establish a liaison with the scientific and medical communities,

organizations with an interest in women's health, and other government agencies; keep them informed and involve them in efforts to expand and encourage women's health research.

- Develop special initiatives to boost participation of women in clinical trials being performed by investigators and institutions; the initiatives could take the form of regional or national meetings to raise awareness of the need for research on women's health, forums on women's health issues, and materials to help in obtaining funds/grants for this research.

When Bernadine Healy, M.D., became the first woman to head the NIH In April 1991, she announced, within a week of her confirmation, preliminary plans for a huge, $500 million study of women's health problems. On April 19, at a hearing of the Senate Labor and Human Resources subcommittee on Aging, she described the Women's Health Initiative (WHI) as "the most definitive and far-reaching study of women's health ever undertaken in the United States, if not the whole world." At that hearing, Congresswoman Pat Schroeder commented on the fact that menopause had never really been looked at as a health issue. Unfortunately, said Schroeder, "there's still a notion in our society that men age and women rot." Senator Brock Adams (D-Washington) commented that "women receive second-class health care" as a result of "the lack of research, particularly on gender differences in aging and the development of disease."

In June 1991, Healy formally announced the Women's Health Initiative. Testifying about the WHI before a congressional subcommittee that December, she said that the enormity of the breast cancer problem among American women was "one of the compelling reasons why we embarked on a major interdisciplinary study of women's health."[20]

The WHI was formally launched in October of that year. The proposal, at that time, called for the participation of some 140,000 women aged 50 to 79 (postmenopausal) over a period of from 10 to 12 years. The participants would be followed for some nine years. Among the issues in women's health problems to be evaluated were the genetic, dietary, and other risk factors associated with breast cancer. The WHI was to be codirected by William Harlan, M.D., an associate director of the NIH Office of Disease Prevention. A House-Senate conference on NIH's budget agreed to give an initial $25 million to launch the project. At that time, the recruitment of women to the trial was scheduled to start the following year, in the fall of 1992.

In September 1992, the Fred Hutchinson Cancer Research Center in Seattle, Washington, was awarded a $140 million contract to serve as the Clinical Coordinating Center of the WHI. In March 1993, 16 university medical programs were awarded contracts as "vanguard clinical centers." Their charge was to test, refine, and implement the final study design and procedures to enroll women nationwide for the first stage of the WHI clinical trials by September 1993. Another 29 clinical centers were to be added in mid-1994. Altogether 45 centers would carry out the Women's Health Initiative, with each of the centers recruiting 3,490 women over a three-year period. A target of 20 percent was set for the enrollment of minority women. Harlan stated, "We will be vigilant in our efforts to ensure that the results of the WHI have meaning to all women from [all] socioeconomic and racial backgrounds."[21]

In November 1993, an Institute of Medicine committee expressed skepticism about the study, saying that smaller and better-focused projects could probably attain just as much at substantial savings. It recommended altering it. Healy argued that the study was needed to remedy the neglect of women's health in the many studies financed by the government. She said, "Billions of dollars have been spent to do research in men, and now a relatively modest study comes along to do studies in women, and it is subject to this kind of scrutiny."[22] Mary Haan, M.D., who is helping to direct the study at the University of California at Davis, said, "It sounds to me as if a lot of these recommendations are based on an interest in cost-cutting, not an interest in science."[23] Haan was disappointed at attempts to water down the proposal, which she feels is valid and deserved. She says the response from women, who have felt like second-hand citizens for so long, was positive. "I heard over and over again that [women participants] are so pleased that something finally is being done for women."

We've come a long way through the efforts of many women as well as men. In 1992, at the request of then vice president Dan Quayle (whose mother had died of breast cancer and whose wife was an outspoken breast cancer activist), the NCI director appointed the President's Cancer Panel Special Commission on Breast Cancer to examine and assess all aspects of breast cancer, including the state of research, prevention, detection, and treatment. The special 19-member commission held 11 meetings over a little more than a year and heard testimony from more than 190 scientists, clinicians, patient advocates, and experts in all aspects of breast cancer. Its report was issued in October 1993[24] (see Chapter 31).

The first woman secretary of Health and Human Services, Donna Shalala, addressed the impact women have made when she spoke at her Conference to Establish a National Action Plan on Breast Cancer in December 1993, saying, "The truth is that the changes we see in our federal budget for breast cancer research, the changes we see in the national media attention focused on breast cancer, and the changes this administration has made to increase resources for breast cancer have been motivated in large part by the power and anger of women all across this country."[25]

Breast cancer, the devastating disease women fear more than any other, which will take the lives of close to half a million women in this last decade of the twentieth century, the disease for which there is no sure cure or prevention, has finally pushed women into action. As the incidence of breast cancer rises, and more and more women speak out about it, the angrier we have become — and the more powerful. We are going into the twenty-first century wide awake with our eyes open, refusing to be an afterthought to the mostly male medical and political establishment. We have gotten more federal money for breast cancer research. We are determined that in the first decade of the new century, the number of women dying from breast cancer will dramatically decline.

2

Dollars and Sense

The money for breast cancer research is voted by a male-dominated and male-oriented Congress.

Rose Kushner, *breast cancer advocate*[1]

At present, only 13 percent of federal research dollars is directed at diseases which strike women. Women make up more than half of our population and contribute taxes to fund research. They are entitled to parity.

Congresswoman Louise M. Slater (D-New York)[2]

The federal government's involvement in cancer research, in general, started off slowly. In 1922 two Public Health Service laboratories started conducting cancer research. In the years that followed, a number of bills were introduced in Congress, including a law in 1927 that proposed offering a $5 million reward for the discovery of a successful cure for cancer. That law was not passed, but as of 1995, 68 years later, no one could have claimed the reward.

In 1937, the 78th Congress succeeded in passing the National Cancer Institute Act. President Franklin D. Roosevelt signed it into law. It was to "provide for, foster, and aid in coordinating research relating to cancer; to establish the National Cancer Institute; and for other purposes."[3] Congress authorized an annual appropriation of $700,000.

Congress also passed a law mandating the establishment of a National Cancer Advisory Board (NCAB). The board was to have 18 members appointed by the president for six-year terms. At most, 12 members could be from the health and scientific disciplines. The board would advise the director of NCI on programs and policies. The NCAB was to be an independent body, funded by the federal government and staffed by the NCI. It would have the authority to conduct activities such as promoting and lobbying that government agencies such as the NCI or NIH were not permitted to do. The board was to meet quarterly.

In 1971, the National Cancer Act was passed to launch the National "War on Cancer." The President's Cancer Panel was established by Congress to direct it. The panel consists of three presidentially appointed members, each of whom serves for three years. The NCAB and President's Cancer Panel are the most prestigious and influential of the NIH's more than 160 advisory committees.

Cancer is big business. The disease is commonly treated with surgery, chemotherapy (anticancer drugs), hormonal therapy, radiation, and biological therapy, the newest treatment. Any word of a possible breakthrough in a chemotherapy agent sends pharmaceutical company stock prices soaring. When the drug gets FDA approval, the drug company can see an increase of profits in the millions because of, at least in part, the high prices charged for drugs in the United States. In 1994, the U.S. General Accounting Office (GAO) found that 47 prescription drugs cost twice as much in the United States as in Great Britain.[4] Most of the differences in prescription drug prices cannot be attributed to a difference in manufacturers' costs. That was confirmed more than 25 years ago by George Squibb, former vice president of Squibb Pharmaceuticals, who admitted that the cost of manufacturing a drug had little relation to the price charged by the company.[5] The drug price differences are mainly due to lack of regulatory constraints in the United States. While drug manufacturers frequently blame their high prices on the costs of research and development of new products, it appears that these expenses may not be passed on to foreign markets. For example, the cost of tamoxifen is 242 percent higher in the

United States than in the United Kingdom.[6] "Chemotherapy costs more in this country than in any other country," says Devra Lee Davis, Ph.D., a senior science adviser with the office of the assistant secretary of health.[7] Davis's findings support those of the GAO. Yet, despite the fact that we spend more on chemotherapy per cancer patient, we do not cure more people of cancer.

Mary Katzke, a survivor of breast cancer, says that diagnostic procedures as well are far more expensive here. "I went in yesterday and had my sonogram and mammogram. It would have been $15 in Belgium. Here it can cost $500 to $600."[8] In general a sonogram and mammogram in the United States would not cost quite that much. However, the price would be far closer to that amount than to the $15 in Belgium, where health care is subsidized by the government.

Many drug companies do have special indigent programs for patients who cannot afford to pay for drugs. Jeff Soper, a spokesman for Zeneca, the company that manufactures tamoxifen, says the company has a multimillion-dollar program and that since its inception, in 1978, $40 million has gone into the program. (In 1991 alone there was $260 million in tamoxifen sales internationally.) He would divulge little other information, such as the amount spent on the development of tamoxifen, which he called proprietary information.[9] Much of the money for the research and development of the drug was provided by the federal government and private foundations. At a breast cancer conference I attended, two doctors from the Midwest were talking about a patient who could not afford to pay for tamoxifen, which can cost close to a hundred dollars a month. I told the doctors about the indigent program the drug company has. The doctor said that he knew about the program and had helped the elderly woman, on a fixed income, fill out the extensive paperwork needed to apply for the drug. The woman was turned down. She was not sufficiently destitute. As a result, she was *not* getting a treatment that could potentially make a difference in whether she lived or died.

Breast cancer costs more to treat than any other cancer in the United States. According to Lou Fintor, M.A., M.P.H., at the Centers for Disease Control, the total minimum cost of treating breast cancer in 1989, using 1990 dollars, was $6,599,000,000. That is $150 billion more than was spent on colorectal cancer, one and a half billion more than on lung cancer, and two billion more than on prostate cancer, the three next most costly cancers.[10] In 1995, 182,000 women were diagnosed with breast cancer, 169,900 people were diagnosed with lung cancer, and 244,000 men were diagnosed with prostate cancer.[11]

The cost of cancer is made up of direct and indirect costs, not to mention psychosocial costs. Direct costs are the use of resources such as medical care, diagnosis, treatment, continuing care of the patient, rehabilitation, terminal care, nursing home care, doctors' bills, medications, prostheses, transportation to health providers, getting someone in to cook, clean, care for the patient, items for rehabilitation and comfort such as humidifiers, installing an elevator in the home, and so on.

Indirect costs include the time and output lost by the patient, family, friends, and others from employment, housekeeping, volunteer activities, and leisure. A family member may have to turn down a promotion or make an unwanted job change or miss out on other opportunities.

Psychosocial costs include a general deterioration of quality of life for the patient as well as for family members, friends, and coworkers. The illness can result in anxiety, reduced self-esteem and feelings of well-being, resentment, family conflicts, antisocial behavior, and suicide, all of which ultimately have an economic impact.

The cost to the U.S. economy in 1993 for women diagnosed with breast cancer was approximately $23.1 billion, with business's share being over $10.2 billion according to an analysis based on data from the National Cancer Institute. Those costs include medical treatment and the loss of productivity and earning because of a premature death. They do not include nonmedical expenses. According to Medstat, a health-care consultant to 80 American businesses and government, nearly a third of the breast cancer claims were from women under the age of 50, and the annual cost for breast cancer treatment was seven times the cost of health care for women without the disease. Over a 27-month period, the average cost was found to be $34,000, but in some cases the bill could be over $345,000.[12]

"Dramatically underfunded," is how Amy Langer, executive director of the National Alliance of Breast Cancer Organizations (NABCO), describes past funding for breast cancer research.[13] In 1981, the NCI budget for breast cancer research was $33.9 million, but by 1995 that number was almost ten times as large, an estimated $323.7 million.[14] Surgeon Susan Love, M.D., director of the UCLA Breast Center, pointed out that in 1990 the United States spent roughly ten times more on AIDS research ($1.1 billion) than it did on breast cancer, even though breast cancer had claimed roughly six times as many lives.[15] Testifying before a House subcommittee in December 1991, when spending was $92.7 million, then NIH director Berna-dine Healy, M.D., commented on the increased money for breast cancer research, saying, "These funding levels attest to the high priority accorded breast cancer both by NCI and Congress."[16]

Angry, assertive, and vocal women can take much of the credit for the increase in funding as well as the increase in awareness of breast cancer.

Part II

Risk Factors, Cause, and Prevention

3

Startling Statistics

I've been told nothing is known about the biology of the normal breast. Without that information, it's impossible to know why some women are at high risk and others not at all. Unless more is known about "healthy" breasts, they can't understand why cells go berserk and become malignant.

Rose Kushner, *breast cancer advocate*[1]

I knew I was a person at risk, but none of my doctors seemed to want to do anything about that or even took it seriously. When is the message going to get out to general practitioners?

Loretta Steen, *diagnosed with breast cancer at 31, whose mother was diagnosed with breast cancer at forty-three*[2]

The biggest risk factor for getting breast cancer is being a woman. The biggest risk factor for not surviving breast cancer is being poor.

Ninety-nine percent of the breast cancer cases diagnosed in the United States occur in women, a risk factor over which we have no control. Although it is not known what causes breast cancer, various risk factors have been established. Russell Harris, M.D., of the Cancer

Prevention Program at the University of North Carolina School of Medicine, Chapel Hill, says that the only well-established risk factor is age, another risk factor over which we have no control.[3] According to the National Cancer Institute, for 85 percent of women the major risk factor is age. As you can see in the following NCI statistics, the older a woman gets, the greater risk she faces.

RISK OF GETTING BREAST CANCER BY AGE	
Age	Odds
25	1 in 19,608
30	1 in 2,525
35	1 in 622
40	1 in 217
45	1 in 93
50	1 in 50
55	1 in 33
60	1 in 24
65	1 in 17
70	1 in 14
75	1 in 11
80	1 in 10
85	1 in 9
95	1 in 8

Another major risk factor, which again is not preventable, is having a first-degree family member who has had premenopausal breast cancer. The more relatives diagnosed with breast cancer before menopause — for example, both a mother and sister or two sisters — the greater the risk. The risk decreases when the family member is postmenopausal. As many as 10 percent of breast cancer cases are a result of heredity. There is even some evidence that the risk of breast cancer can be increased if a father or brother has prostate cancer.[4] Other known risk factors include obesity, age at childbearing and nursing, and age at time of sexual maturation (start of menarche). These risk factors are, for the most part, well accepted and not controversial. However, they account for about 40 percent of the women diagnosed with breast cancer in the United States. Therefore, as many as 60 percent of women *who get breast cancer do not have any of the known risk factors,* other than, of course, being a woman and getting older. That raises an obvious question. If the established risk factors account for so small a number of breast cancer cases, what other factor or factors put so many additional women at risk? And are there risk factors that we can avoid so as to prevent or at least decrease our risk of getting breast cancer? Are there man-made risk factors, such as carcinogens in our environment, that cause or promote breast cancer?

Other possible, and controversial, risk factors that are not as well established include fat in the diet, pesticides, chemicals, oral contraception, estrogen replacement therapy, abortion, radiation, being African American, being a lesbian, use of alcohol, age at first pregnancy or no pregnancy, and smoking. Although studies have been done in most of these areas, in general there is little definitive data. There are researchers who would disagree with that, saying, for example, that there is plenty of evidence that environmental factors are responsible for many cases of breast cancer.

The risk factors or importance of various risk factors may be different for women who are premenopausal as opposed to postmenopausal. There may be differences in the actual biologic makeup of breast cancer tumors in younger and older women. While 60 percent of tumors in premenopausal women are estrogen receptor negative, only 20 percent of tumors in postmenopausal women are estrogen receptor negative.[5] (Tumors that are estrogen receptor negative are not believed to be affected by estrogen, whereas tumors that are estrogen receptor positive are stimulated by estrogen.)

There are also geographical risk factors. Women who have breast cancer in the United States have the greatest risk of dying from it if they live in Washington, D.C., where the mortality rate is 35.9 percent.[6] The lowest breast cancer mortality rate, 17.6 percent, is in Hawaii.[7] Rates are highest in the northeast part of the U.S.[8] For white women, death rates range from 20.4 percent in Hawaii to 32.9 percent in New Jersey. For women of races other than white, the mortality rates range from 14.5 percent in the state of Washington to 39.6 percent in Washington, D.C.[9]

Another risk factor can be spotted on a mammogram. I. Craig Henderson, M.D., director of the Clinical Cancer Center at the University of California in San Francisco, says that a woman's risk of developing breast cancer is increased if her mammogram shows an abnormal increase of cells that are atypical.[10] The condition is difficult to diagnose correctly and necessitates a biopsy. A woman who has the condition, called atypical hyperplasia, is at even greater risk if her mother had breast cancer before menopause. However, many women with atypical hyperplasia *do not* develop breast cancer.

Whatever risk factors are finally found, one dire statistic is all too well known. The rate of breast cancer has been increasing virtually every year in the United States since formal tracking of cases started in the 1930s. In Connecticut, which has the oldest cancer registry in the United States keeping track of breast cancer, the age-standardized incidence rose by an average 1.2 percent per year. Between 1982 and 1986, the incidence in the United States rose even more sharply at 4 percent a year. Since 1935, the incidence has risen in all age groups. In 1940, one in 20 women in the United States was diagnosed during her lifetime with breast cancer. In 1992, the figure was one woman in eight. Between 1950 and 1990, the annual incidence of breast cancer increased approximately 52 percent, while the death rate increased 4 percent during the same period of time. During the 1980s, the death rate from breast cancer among African American women increased about 21 percent, from about 26 deaths per 100,000 to nearly 32 per 100,000 women. In 1991, the death rate for African American women was 31.9, which was 19 percent higher than for white women. In white women, during the same period of time, the death rate was relatively constant, going up less than 1 percent.[11] In 1996, it was estimated that 44,300 women would die from breast cancer.[12] Although there are various theories as to why this is happening, such as earlier detection because of improved mammography and women living to older ages when they are more likely to develop breast cancer, there are no definitive answers.

Over the years the mortality rate of breast cancer has remained relatively stable, with virtually no progress being made in reducing the death rate. In 1995, the first hopeful sign in a long time was seen when NCI announced a drop in the breast cancer mortality rate from 1989 to 1992. White women were the major beneficiaries of the reduction, with their mortality rate dropping 5.5 percent. However, according to then NCI director Samuel Broder, M.D., the mortality rate among African American women during the same three years increased 2.6 percent.[13] In the 1990s, more than 1.5 million women will be diagnosed with breast cancer; nearly 30 percent will ultimately die of the disease.[14]

Devra Lee Davis says the surge in cancer deaths in women in the industrial world has yet to be explained and that more research must be done on the following risk factors:

- high-fat diet, including types of fats eaten
- low-fiber, low-anti-oxidant (green-yellow vegetables) diet, and low-calcium/vitamin D diets
- prolonged use of high doses of estrogen replacement therapy
- prolonged use of oral contraceptives before first pregnancy
- history of benign breast disease
- alcohol
- stress and exercise patterns
- exposures to pesticides and other fat-seeking synthetic organic chemicals that can bioconcentrate in fat[15]

The rising rate of breast cancer is distressing and unacceptable. There is no question that research must address this. Little is known about the causes of breast cancer. And while some of the risk factors for breast cancer cannot be avoided, such as inherited genes, there are risk factors that can be avoided. Identification of those factors is crucial.

4

Poverty

[Middle-class women are] more likely to have insurance that can handle their treatment and they're not restricted to where they can go for care. Poor women don't have that available to them. They don't have the resources.

Joyce Ford, *director, Breast Examination Center of Harlem*[1]

If you screen [for breast cancer] in a poor population, you're going to get more advanced cancer than in an affluent population because the affluent population has been constantly going in.

Harold Freeman, M.D., *head of the President's Cancer Panel*[2]

We have to address the disproportionate impact in poor women, African American women, Hispanic women.

Joycelyn Elders, *former U.S. Surgeon General*[3]

"Risk factors" usually refers to those things that can make someone more prone to getting a disease. There is another set of risk factors that makes it less likely you'll survive the cancer. Though poverty may or may not put you at greater risk of developing breast cancer, it indisputably puts you at a higher risk of dying of it. Women who are poor have a higher death rate from breast cancer. According to Harold Freeman, M.D., the poor, in general, have a 10 to 15 percent lower cancer survival rate regardless of race. "I feel the issue of poverty is a major risk, for women in particular," says Freeman. "It is also one risk factor that can be eliminated. Access to competent health care would go a long way toward reducing that risk. That doesn't require research or brilliant scientists. It does require money."[4]

In 1994, researchers at the State University of New York at Buffalo, who examined ten previous studies, six national and four regional or state, reported that the higher rate of cancer in the African American population in the United States was due more to socioeconomic factors than to racial differences.[5]

Arlene Draper, a Hispanic woman from Costa Rica who now lives in San Diego, California, is a survivor of breast cancer. Speaking at a breast cancer rally in Washington, D.C., in 1993, she said she was there to represent her daughter and all the women in San Diego who were experiencing delayed diagnoses and inaccessibility to treatment.

Many in our county are unable to seek and get medical care. Their personal limitations are many. The system of care available to them, when available, is substandard, Third World medical care. Their care is further limited by shortage of bicultural health professionals who could identify with this segment of the population. Forty-one percent of the population in San Diego speaks a foreign language. Most of us here [at the rally] are fortunate. We have medical insurance and access to good medical care is at our fingertips. Others are not so lucky. They can't have these medical services that we take so much for granted. Our standard of living is the highest in the world but not all citizens enjoy it. Our country is the most advanced. Our medical research is tops, yet this knowledge and benefit is not there for all. Ones experiencing these limitations are called the underserved. This word is not specific to a particular group. It represents all who encounter barriers to minimal care, including citizens who are indigent, the working poor, those without medical insurance, the elderly, the homeless, those with limited educations, or language barriers. It doesn't recognize race, color, or creed. Very often the underserved are shuffled, ignored, misdiagnosed, and treated without human compassion. They can't be swept under the rug as if they didn't exist.[6]

A survey done by Louis Harris and Associates in 1993 found that one in seven women failed to get treatment for an illness when needed, largely because of insurance gaps and high costs. One in three women did not get basic preventive health service during the previous year.[7] The mortality rate in women with breast cancer is 30 percent higher in poor women than in those who are not. Since a greater percentage of African American women fall into the poverty class than white women, 31 percent compared to 10.8 percent, there is a substantial difference in the mortality rate by race.[8] For example, in 1990 the five-year relative survival rate for white women was 80.5 percent compared with 64.1 percent for African American women.[9]

A study reported in September 1994 found that African American women were more than twice as likely as white women to die of breast cancer. J. William Eley, M.D., of Emory University, the chief author of the study, suggested that 40 percent of the higher death rate could be attributed to the cancer's being at a later stage when diagnosed. He said, "The importance of this study is to [show] how advanced the disease is when black women are diagnosed." An additional 15 percent difference in the higher death rate was attributed to the cancer's being more aggressive in African American women. Eley cited diet differences and environmental factors as possibly being related to the greater aggressiveness of the tumors.[10]

In October 1993, the President's Cancer Panel Special Commission on Breast Cancer reported that "access [to detection and treatment] is a particular problem for women who are low-income, minority, young or old, and living in rural areas." It pointed out that those women represented a large and expanding segment of the population and noted that they are unable to pay for early detection, diagnosis, and treatment and have inadequate or, more likely, no health insurance.[11]

In 1973, a study done at Howard University Medical School in Washington, D.C., showed a significant difference in the cancer incidence and mortality rate in African Americans compared to white Americans. It noted an "alarming increase" over the previous 25 years.[12] In 1989, Harold Freeman, head of the President's Cancer Panel, said that in breast cancer, in which early detection gives the best chance of survival, the five-year survival rate is 75 percent in white women compared to 63 percent for African American women.[13]

A review of over 500 women treated for breast cancer at Harlem

Hospital in New York City, an area in Manhattan with a predominantly African American population, showed a five-year survival rate of 39 percent. Joyce Ford, director of the Breast Examination Center of Harlem, which provides free breast screening for women who cannot afford it, says that 50 percent of the women in a 1976 study had late-stage breast cancer when it was detected. The later breast cancer — or virtually any cancer for that matter — is detected, the less likely it is that treatment will be successful. There are over 50,000 women in Harlem who fall within the recommended breast cancer screening guidelines. While the number of women coming in for breast screening has been increasing, Ford says that the center is severely restricted in the number of women who can be seen because there is not enough money available. The center could not possibly handle all the women in Harlem who should be getting a mammogram.[14]

Many studies have found differences in the stage of the cancer at diagnosis and survival between African American women and white women with breast cancer. A study published in 1993 confirmed the findings in previous studies that showed more advanced breast cancer in African American women than white women when diagnosed.[15] According to the study, whites from lower socioeconomic income strata also tended to have more advanced disease when diagnosed. The authors of the study say that the findings suggest that "the advanced stage of breast cancer at diagnosis is related, in part, to the poorer access to health care common to socioeconomically disadvantaged populations." The study also found that only 50 percent of the excess risk faced by African American women with Stages III and IV breast cancer, compared with white women, could be accounted for, which suggests that breast cancer may act differently in different races. Freeman raises the question as to whether race in itself can be a determining factor.

More and more evidence suggests that African American women may have a more virulent form of the disease. A study done at the University of Texas Health Science Center in San Antonio found that tumors from African American women had more actively dividing cancer cells than tumors from white women and that their tumors often lacked hormone receptors, which is another factor in a poorer prognosis.[16]

A study in which close to 1,000 newly diagnosed tumors were

examined found that breast cancer tumors from African American women were more likely to have histologic features associated with poor prognosis than white women. The study, done at the Louisiana State Medical Center, supported some of the findings in the Texas Health Science Center study.[17]

A third study, done at George Washington University, came up with similar findings. After examining tumors from women treated there, it was found that the tumors from African American women were more actively growing, were less likely to have hormone receptors, and appeared more abnormal.[18]

In the 1980s, the American Cancer Society (ACS) did a wide-ranging study to determine the extent of the role that the combination of poverty and ignorance plays in who survives and who doesn't survive cancer. Its survey examined the influence of socioeconomic status on the risk of developing cancer, time of diagnosis, access to medical care, quality of medical care, and other factors that could influence cancer incidence, survival rates, and mortality.

The landmark ACS report, published in 1986,[19] showed nearly 34 million Americans living below the poverty level. Of that number, 23 million were white Americans, 9.5 million were African Americans, and 1.2 million were others. That means one-third of the poor in America are found within the slightly more than 10 percent proportion of African Americans in the United State's population. A study in 1991[20] arrived at the same conclusions as the ACS study — that the disproportionate distribution of poor African Americans accounts for much of the higher cancer incidence and mortality rates. According to the 1990 census almost 60 percent of female-headed households are living below the poverty level.[21] Dr. Harold Freeman says that the ways poverty can impact on early detection, treatment, and survival of cancer include "unemployment, inadequate education, substandard housing, chronic malnutrition, and diminished access to medical care." Living in a continuing state of poverty can result in "a fatalism born of powerlessness and placing priority on sheer day-to-day survival."[22] Freeman says there is enough evidence to suggest that low socioeconomic status, regardless of race, is a major determinant of poor cancer survival. These problems are all compounded in women.

Women who are working are more likely than men to have low-paying jobs with no medical coverage or a very meager policy. Women who are covered by their husband's insurance are likely to lose it if their husband dies or they get a divorce. A study done by the Older Women's League (OWL) in 1992 reported that only 55 percent of women aged 40 to 46 have health insurance on their jobs, while 72 percent of men in the same age group have coverage at their jobs.[23]

Poor women are plagued by other problems as well. The education they've received is frequently limited, resulting in less access to information on breast cancer screening, prevention, and warning signs. Even when there is low-cost or free screening and treatment available, access to it is often affected by the woman's lack of funds for transportation and child care and the scarcity of doctors who are willing to practice in poor urban areas.

Freeman says that some progress is being made but that it is very slow and there is still a long way to go. For example, in 1993 the Centers for Disease Control and Prevention (CDC) provided $60 million for breast screening programs for underserved women in the United States. Sixty million dollars to set up screening programs for all the women in the United States who don't have access is far from adequate, but Freeman says it's a start. What concerns him is what kind of impact the programs that are developed will have on the survival rate of the women who take part and are diagnosed with breast cancer. Freeman says, "It's not so clear whether follow-up after mammography is available. I think they've left it to the local area to see that that's done. . . . If you don't have treatment, a system to follow them all the way through, you're really whistling Dixie. It doesn't help to say that everyone can have a mammogram."[24]

What kind of impact will the breast cancer advocacy movement have on this long-standing, pervasive, and complex problem confronting so many women? Ford says that the women speaking out are generally middle-class, white American women. She feels that poor women may benefit to some extent, but that the needs of this socioeconomic group are not the same as the needs of the middle class and says, "It's not fair to expect that those in the middle class will be able to address all the needs that the poor would have. Obviously the poor would not even think about some of the issues that might be of concern to the middle class because they're still dealing with problems on their level, some very basic problems." Ford describes the problems poor women face as a lack of resources to pay for screening or treatment and about how even to get into the system for any assistance that might be available. She says that a group is needed specifically to address the particular problems poor women with breast cancer face. Her hope is that that there will be advocacy groups for poor women and that the two groups, poor and not poor, would then "meet in the middle."[25]

It can be difficult finding statistics on minority populations because so few studies have included them or been done on them. For years women in general have faced discrimination, being denied access to top jobs, getting less pay for equal work, not being included in medical studies, being patronized by male doctors. But no one has been as severely affected as poor women.

Older women are also more likely to be diagnosed with breast cancer at a later stage, which puts them at a bigger risk of dying. A study published in 1993 confirmed other reports of an age-stage relationship in breast cancer. It found an increased risk of advanced stages of breast cancer among older women, particularly blacks.[26] "We are battling a medical ageism, a sort of nihilism about detection of breast cancer in older women," says Dr. Bernadine Healy, former director of the National Institutes of Health. She cites the need for "culturally sensitive approaches to education, community outreach, and physician information . . . for greater access to native, black, Hispanic, native Hawaiian, older women, and low-literacy groups."[27]

5

Heredity

When I lost [my mother], all of a sudden I started thinking, "Oh my gosh, this is going to happen to me. I'm doomed."

Joan D'Argo, *breast cancer survivor*[1]

I'm from a very high-risk family. [My] great-grandmother, my mother, and my three sisters have all had breast cancer. That was a long time ago, which is why it really angers me sometimes that we're now just giving the information that made practical sense so many years ago. We're just now telling women that genetics may just play a role.

Zora Brown, *president,*
Breast Cancer Resource Committee, Washington, D.C.[2]

There is no question that having a first-degree relative with breast cancer puts a woman at an increased risk of developing the disease. But how great a risk is it, really? At most, only about 10 percent of breast cancer cases are hereditary, or caused by an inherited gene.[3] According to Dr. Susan Love, director of the UCLA Breast Center, women whose mothers have breast cancer frequently think they're doomed and that they're automatically going to get it.[4] A survey of 150 women referred to Northwest Memorial Hospital's High Risk

Breast Center found they believed their risk to be five to ten times higher than the 6 percent that it actually was. All women have a one-in-eight risk of developing breast cancer during their lifetime. Women with a first-degree relative with breast cancer have a one-in-seven or one-in-six risk.

Love says, "It's not that you have a one hundred percent or even fifty percent risk of getting breast cancer. A lot of these risk factors are statistical. They increase your risk a little bit, but it's not that much, and the majority of women who have risk factors do not get breast cancer. The greater the number of first-degree relatives who have had breast cancer, the greater the risk. If the mother was diagnosed before menopause, the risk is greater than if she were diagnosed postmenopausally."[5]

It had been thought that breast cancer could not be inherited paternally, that only cancer on the mother's side could have an impact. Alison Estabrook, M.D., chief of breast surgery at Columbia Presbyterian Hospital in New York, says that is not true, that if the mother or sister of the woman's father had breast cancer before menopause, that can also be inherited. As Estabrook points out, "These things take a long time to tease out. It's genetics."[6] In addition, a study published in 1992 suggested that male breast cancer in a father (though it represents just 1 percent of all the breast cancer diagnosed in the United States) has the same effect on breast cancer risk in a woman as having a mother with breast cancer.[7]

A family history of prostate cancer may also be a risk factor for breast cancer. David E. Anderson, Ph.D., at M. D. Anderson Cancer Center in Houston, says that "studies indicate a genetic association between prostate cancer and breast cancer that is independent of other hereditary cancers."[8] And it apparently works the other way around. A study of 947 Icelandic women, published in 1992 in the *Journal of Medical Genetics*,[9] found that male relatives of women with breast cancer had a 40 to 50 percent increase in the risk of prostate cancer compared to a control population; researchers expect family history of prostate cancer to eventually be incorporated into assessments of an individual's risk of breast cancer.

In 1990, Mary-Claire King, Ph.D., a geneticist at the University of Washington, showed for the first time that familial breast cancer could be linked to a single gene. Heredity is governed by the DNA housed in the nucleus of each cell. Human cells contain three billion units [base pairs] of DNA arranged in linear sequence along 23 pairs of chromosomes. These long chains are known to contain the 50,000 to 100,000 functional segments, or genes, required to construct and operate the body. The gene, which researchers called BRCA1, is on chromosome 17q12-21. Mutations of this gene have been found to predispose women to breast and ovarian cancer. Researchers at the University of Michigan School of Medicine have screened families with a high rate of breast cancer for BRCA1 mutations. Their findings support data that some women with the gene are estimated to have an 85 percent risk of breast cancer.[10] It's estimated that one in 200 to 400 women may carry the mutated gene. In August 1992, researchers in Michigan tested a woman for the mutated BRCA1 gene.[11] The woman, who was 36 years old, had seen her mother diagnosed with breast cancer at age 46, her oldest sister die of breast cancer at age 38, and another sister diagnosed with breast cancer at the age of 41. The woman wanted to have a prophylactic mastectomy of both breasts to reduce her risk of developing breast cancer as much as possible. She tested negative for the mutated gene and did not undergo mastectomy.

In September 1994, researchers announced the culmination of a four-year international race to isolate the BRCA1 gene first identified by King. The team of researchers who beat out others trying to locate the gene were from Utah, the National Institutes of Environmental Health Sciences in Research Triangle Park, North Carolina, Myriad Genetics Inc., and several other institutions. They pinpointed the gene's exact location and made copies of it in a laboratory.

It is believed that between 5 and 10 percent of breast cancer is inherited and that the BRCA1 gene is responsible for half of the inherited cases, leaving 90 or 95 percent of breast cancer cases caused by other factors such as environment, lifestyle, and diet.[12] A test for the BRCA1 gene could be available by 1995 or 1996. But development of a test for the gene raises other issues, as pointed out by Kenneth Offit, chief of Clinical Genetics Services at Memorial Sloan-Kettering Cancer Center in New York City.[13] The information, which could help women make a more informed decision about preventive options, could mean a loss of medical coverage (since it would constitute evidence of a pre-existing condition), life and disability insurance, and employment. Offit says, "There are no guidelines to protect the privacy of individuals who decide to get a genetic test to determine their cancer risk." He cites a 1993 survey of insurance commissioners in 32 states. Forty-four percent felt that a family history of breast cancer would be sufficient cause to deny medical insurance. As of September 1994, only Montana had legislation banning such discrimination.

6

The Fat Factor

If the American diet were as low in fat as the Japanese was until recently, 10 to 20 percent . . . , we might expect our breast cancer death rate to be much lower, possibly as low as 11,000 [a year].

Peter Greenwald, M.D., *director of NCI's Division of Cancer Prevention and Control*[1]

We found no evidence to support the hypothesis that fat intake is a major cause of breast cancer.

Walter Willett, M.D., *director, Harvard Nurses' Health Study*[2]

The idea that diet, in particular fat in the diet, plays a role in breast cancer is not new. In the mid-1950s, studies were done to examine the role of fat in the diet. International comparisons have shown a strong positive relationship between breast cancer mortality and fat consumption. The United States, Great Britain, and the Netherlands, countries in which the consumption of fat is high, have among the highest breast cancer rates, whereas in Japan, Singapore, and Rumania, where a very lean diet is eaten, the incidence of breast cancer is one-sixth to one-half the rate in the United States.[3]

In 1963, a study found that Japanese women with breast cancer had a better survival rate than their counterparts in the United States. Studies that followed confirmed that finding.[4]

The National Cancer Institute finally approved the Women's Health Trial (WHT) for American women in 1983. It was to follow some 6,000 women for ten years. Half the women in the study would be on a diet containing a maximum of 20 percent fat. The rest would eat the way they usually did. It was the first trial in the United States that had breast cancer prevention as its ultimate goal. The feasibility trial, which started the following year, found that fat intake in the intervention group could be lowered from 39 percent to 21 percent of calories over a 12-month period. In 1987, tentative approval was given for the full trial by the Board of Scientific Counselors at NCI. But in January 1988, NCI announced that its advisory board had voted not to run the trial. Although it was decided that the full outcome study was feasible, it was canceled because it was concluded that for the trial to be effective in the ten years, 32,000 women would have to participate instead of the originally planned 6,000 women. That would quadruple the cost from $25 million to $100 million. Some opponents also focused on the issue of compliance, saying that women could not be trusted either to stay on the low-fat diet or to report accurately what they had consumed, despite the fact that the feasibility study had shown it was indeed possible.[5]

Samuel Broder, M.D., who at that time was director of NCI, received a letter from David Korn, M.D., the head of the National Cancer Advisory Board and Stanford University's medical school, urging dismissal of the study. The letter said, in part, "In the face of serious constraints on resources and the many important scientific opportunities in cancer research, it is not appropriate to fund a trial of this magnitude."[6] In her article "Breast Cancer Prevention: Diet vs. Drugs" in *Ms*, journalist Susan Rennie called the cancelation of the trial a "classic case of sticker shock." She claimed that scientists, who wanted funds for research into detection and treatment of breast cancer, were used to getting their way and did not want to see $10 million a year going to a prevention study. She claimed that, in making their decision, the scientists ignored the fact that if the WHT found as little as a 10 percent reduction in the number of breast cancer cases as a result of reducing fat in the diet, some $177 million a year could be saved.[7]

An attempt was then made to revise the study. Other diseases besides breast cancer would be included. That proposal was turned down by the NCAB in December 1990. Again, the question of the ability of the women in the study to comply with the diet and accurately to report it was raised. Korn said that there was "no way to measure fat intake." He suggested that as women in the trial aged, their memories could suffer. If they couldn't remember what they should eat and what they did eat, a costly and time-consuming study could prove to be invalid. The NCAB also said that the study would have to include poor women, especially poor women of color, and that it was not known if those women could comply with a diet containing a maximum of 20 percent fat. Korn was quoted in the *SF Weekly*, a newspaper in San Francisco, as saying, "It's one thing to develop behavioral changes in college-graduate, well-to-do white women, and quite another to talk to a bunch of high school dropout African-American women who worry whether they can get a bottle of milk for their kids, let alone whether they're eating high-fat food." Not surprisingly, his comments generated angry cries of racism and ageism from women.[8]

Women were up in arms about the cancelation of the trial. In the magazine *Science*, Congresswoman Pat Schroeder charged NCI with reneging on a commitment. She said that several months earlier, she and two other congresswomen had spent half a day talking to directors at the National Institutes of Health. "They said this study would be undertaken; they were emphatic about that." To Schroeder, the NCI decision to ignore the commitment they'd made was "unbelievable . . . outrageous."[9]

Breast surgeon Susan Love had her own questions and ideas about why the medical profession for the most part has been less than enthusiastic on this issue. Love says, "The dairy and meat lobbies are very strong: medicine is usually reluctant to go up against powerful lobbies. . . . It's unfortunate that big business can have such a great effect on the medical profession, but it does, all too often."[10]

Breast cancer survivor Ellen Hobbs, who founded the advocacy group Save Ourselves (SOS), agreed. She said, "There are plenty of studies that show the fact that breast cancer is much more prevalent in populations which consume more amounts of animal fat and dairy products. No matter what the research shows, we could probably go a long way toward reducing the incidence of breast cancer by getting rid of the American diet that's killing everybody. The dairy industry and chemical industry that produced the pesticides that end up in our foods should be targeted. That's where the American public is very ignorant if they're going to allow themselves to be manipulated by the American Cancer Society, the meat and dairy industry, the pharmaceutical industry. I don't know how you wake up a whole country. You still get women who get very upset on hearing these things."[11]

As to the claim that women would not be able to change their eating habits and would not be able to keep track of what they had eaten, various studies dispute that. In an ongoing study in Canada, in which close to 600 high-risk women were enrolled, at the end of two years 60 percent of the women were eating diets containing less than 20 percent fat and 80 percent were eating diets containing under 25 percent fat. Their compliance was assessed by frequent questionnaires and chemical analysis.[12]

In a feasibility study for the Women's Intervention and Nutrition Study (WINS), involving some 300 postmenopausal women with Stage I or II breast cancer, the American Health Foundation reported that the women in the intervention group were able to comply with a low-fat (20 to 25 percent of calories) diet for the two-year period of the study.[13]

The strong positive relationship that has appeared to exist between breast cancer and fat consumption has resulted in the assumption by many people that fat must play some role in breast cancer. Larry Norton, M.D., chief of breast and gynecological medical service at Memorial Sloan-Kettering Cancer Center in New York, says that the epidemiologic evidence is clear-cut, that countries with high-fat diets and high-calorie diets have more breast cancer.[14]

The role of fat in the diet has been shown in laboratories where rodents fed a diet high in fat develop more mammary tumors. Researchers have known for forty years that high-fat diets promote the growth of mammary tumors in laboratory animals.[15] Norton says, however, that "most of the intervention studies have not yet shown that diet is that related."[16] It remains an unresolved, controversial issue, with some studies supporting and other studies not supporting the hypothesis.

In 1989, a study was published in which a high-fat diet and a high-calorie diet were shown to increase the risk of breast cancer.[17]

The study involved some 750 Italian women in a northwestern province of Italy, 250 of whom had breast cancer. The study concluded that "a diet rich in fat, saturated fat or animal proteins may be associated with a twofold to threefold increase in a woman's risk of breast cancer." Results indicated that a diet with less than 28 percent fat would achieve a substantial reduction in the risk of getting breast cancer. The study, although using a relatively small number of women, was considered to be particularly well done.

In 1991, researchers at the University of Toronto said that a study involving some 56,000 women found that the risk of developing breast cancer rose in relation to the amount of fat in the diet; that every 77 grams, or 693 calories, of fat consumed a day increased a woman's risk of breast cancer 35 percent.[18] The study also found evidence that a woman whose fat intake represented 47 percent of her daily calories was 50 percent more likely to develop cancer than one who limited her fat intake to 31 percent of calories a day.

The Women's Health Initiative, announced by then NIH head Bernadine Healy in 1991, included an expanded version of the Women's Health Trial. As many as 57,000 women would be followed for an average of 14 years. The women in the study would be between 50 and 79 years of age. There was immediate criticism of the trial. Because the intervention group would be on a 20 percent fat diet, critics said it would probably prove nothing because fat intake has been decreasing in the United States. Since the control group was likely to reduce their fat intake even more, it would be difficult to find an effect even if one exists. In addition, even under the most optimistic circumstances, the reduction in risk that could be achieved in the post-menopausal years is likely to be small and difficult to detect. Critics of the study concluded that it was highly unlikely that even this large trial could resolve the debate.

In October 1992, Walter Willett, M.D., at Harvard Medical School, reported on an eight-year follow-up in the Nurses' Health Study in which over 89,000 nurses were taking part. The study concluded that fat intake had no "adverse influence" on breast cancer in middle-aged women. It noted that a fat intake of 30 percent of calories, as advised by numerous groups, would not substantially reduce the incidence of breast cancer, although a weak association could not be ruled out. Another conclusion was that eating fiber had no protective effect. As for why there was a much lower rate of breast cancer in Japan, where much smaller amounts of fats are consumed, that was attributed to other lifestyle differences, including reproductive practices. Researchers involved with the study said that the evidence was strong enough to settle the debate about diet and breast cancer. The researchers also acknowledged that the data, based on eight years of follow-up, could not exclude a very weak association, an effect of fat intake earlier in life, or an influence of substantially lower levels of fat consumption, such as below 20 percent. Willett said that overall calories may play a more important role than fat and pointed out that breast cancer rates tend to be highest in prosperous countries where people are well nourished. In those countries girls start menstruating at an earlier age and have children later in life.[19]

The reaction from the medical world to the study was mixed. Some agreed that the study had resolved the question of diet and breast cancer. Others contended that there were a number of factors not taken into account in the study — that the fat intake may have not been low enough or that perhaps an intervention has to come at a younger age.

Marc Lippman, M.D., director of the Vincent T. Lombardi Cancer Research Center at Georgetown University, called the study "excellent." A *New York Times* article quoted him as saying, "A lot of people who look at it will wind up saying, 'If your goal is to do something really substantial with breast cancer risk, you're wasting your time with fat reduction.' "[20]

NCI issued an immediate statement. Peter Greenwald, M.D., director of NCI's Division of Cancer Prevention and Control (DCPC), said that since the Nurses' Study looked at women with a dietary fat intake ranging from 27 to about 50 percent, the conclusions of the study would be restricted to women who eat within that percentage range. To have an impact on breast cancer, women might have to limit their fat intake to 20 to 25 percent. He added that the planned Women's Health Initiative, in which the low-fat eating pattern [of 20 percent of total calories from fat] will be examined, will play a great role in resolving the conflict.[21] Ross Prentice, M.D., of Fred Hutchinson Cancer Research Center in Seattle, who is coordinating the study, says the fat/breast cancer link is still "a good hypothesis that needs to be fully tested."[22]

Also disputing the findings was Joel Fuhrman, M.D., a member of the Physicians' Committee for Responsible Medicine. He argues, "Everybody in this study was eating a high-fat diet. That's like, in a study on smoking, measuring the effects of two packs a day versus three packs a day." Fuhrman says studies suggest that fat must be limited to 15 to 20 percent of total calories, starting in childhood.[23]

Like Fuhrman, many researchers continue to believe that a diet lower in fat will show the fat/breast cancer link. David Rose, M.D., chief of the Division of Nutrition and Endocrinology at the American Health Foundation, says, "We believe the percentage for risk is a maximum 20 percent of fat. . . . We have to reduce fat to that level to get benefit." He adds that there may be a threshold at which the percentage of fat in the diet makes no difference and that the "optimal" level of fat in the diet may be 20 percent or less to have a protective effect on the development of breast cancer and its spread.[24] Early in 1994 the American Health Foundation started a seven-year outcome trial of the Women's Intervention and Nutrition Study (WINS) to see if a low-fat diet would prevent the recurrence of breast cancer in a patient. Rose says there is a strong scientific rationale for thinking that such a study may well be beneficial. It took over a decade to persuade NCI that such a study should be done. In the study, patients with Stage I or II breast cancer will be randomized to go onto either a low-fat diet with 15 to 20 percent of calories from fat or the currently recommended diet containing 30 percent fat. Rose says, "Almost certainly, another benefit would be to reduce the risk of developing a new primary breast cancer in the other breast."[25]

Besides the amount of fat eaten, the type of fat eaten appears to be an important factor. For example, in Mediterranean diets, although the fat intake is not low, most of the fat is not from an animal source. In Spain, Portugal, Greece, and southern Italy (where the diet traditionally is very different from that in northern Italy), people consume a lot of monounsaturated fats, like olive oil, which may put them at a lower risk of breast cancer. There are data that suggest monounsaturated fat may have an inhibitory effect on breast cancer promotion and progression. A survey in Greece of women with and without breast cancer, published early in 1995, found that the cancer-free women consumed more fruits, vegetables, and olive oil than the women with breast cancer. [26]

Samuel S. Epstein, M.D., professor of occuptional and environmental medicine at the University of Illinois Medical Center, says that there is a great deal of evidence that shows it's not the amount of fat that you eat, but what is in that fat. Contaminants that can be present include organic chlorine pesticides, chlordane, aldrin, and dieldrin, which for decades have been known to induce breast cancer in rodents. Epstein points out that the pesticides mimic the effect of estrogens, producing "estrogenic effects in the body and [acting] biologically and biochemically in the same way estrogens do."[27]

The other question raised about diet is fiber. Studies have shown that decreasing fat intake and increasing fiber intake substantially lowers the risk of developing colon/rectal cancer. Could that work the same way in breast cancer? In Finland, the fat intake is similar to that of women in the United States — the rate of breast cancer is not. Finland has a lower rate of breast cancer; however, their fiber consumption is much higher than the fiber intake of women in the United States.[28] That suggests that fiber may play a role in reducing the risk of breast cancer.

7

Hormonal Hazards

If a woman wanted to conduct her entire life so as to reduce her risk for breast cancer, she could have ten to fifteen kids and breastfeed continuously from age seventeen on. But that's clearly not a good solution.

Lynn Rosenberg, Sc.D., *Boston University School of Medicine*[1]

Since there is an undefined risk for women taking oral contraceptives, why hasn't more been done to develop a male contraceptive?

Devra Lee Davis, Ph.D. *founder of the International Organization for Breast Cancer Prevention*[2]

The female hormone estrogen has long been implicated in breast cancer. In the late eighteenth century, the English physician Sir George Thomas Beatson was the first to control the spread of breast cancer by removing the woman's ovaries, her primary source of estrogen.[3] Estrogen is the name for a group of steroid hormones that control female sexual development. In the woman's body, estrogen is produced primarily by the ovaries. A small amount is secreted by the adrenal glands. Estrogen can be bad or good. It breaks down into either a stronger, long-lasting form that is bad, or a weaker, short-acting type that is good. Although there is substantial evidence that estrogen can increase the risk of breast cancer, the exact role it plays has not been defined and is still being investigated. There are a number of different theories.

Richard Theriault, M.D., at M. D. Anderson Cancer Center in Houston, says that there are no data to suggest that estrogen is an initiator of breast cancer or that it is itself a carcinogen. It is likely that estrogen promotes the cancer once it has developed.[4]

In the 1970s, Harvard epidemiologist Brian MacMahon, M.D., did a study[5] in which he concluded that the following factors put a woman at risk:

- the younger a woman is when she starts menstruating (in the last 200 years, the average age of menarche has declined dramatically; in 1860 it was 17 and in the early 1990s it was 12)
- the older a woman is when she has her first child
- the older a woman is at menopause (women who start menopause at 55 or older have twice the risk of breast cancer as those with menopause before 45)

Other risk factors are believed to be the length of time between menarche and first pregnancy and not having any children. All the risk factors mentioned above result in a prolonged, uninterrupted presence of high estrogen levels in the body.

The way estrogen is metabolized in the body may be a factor in predicting the risk of breast cancer. Michael Osborne, M.D., at the Strang-Cornell Breast Center in New York, examined breast tissue from women with breast cancer. He found an elevation of the level of a natural estrogen called 17-beta-estradiol.[6] According to Daniel Nebert, M.D., at the University of Cincinnati, a product of that estrogen is known to cause DNA damage. Therefore, 17-beta-estradiol may be tumor promoting.[7]

Pregnancy

Many studies have established that early full-term pregnancy decreases the risk of breast cancer. However, it appears that the benefit may appear when the woman is older. Studies in Italy and England have indicated a temporary increase in the risk of breast cancer after pregnancy. A large Swedish study reported in the *New England Journal of Medicine* in July 1994[8] came up with similar findings: that having a child may increase the risk of breast cancer in younger women (when the incidence of breast cancer is rare), while reducing the risk as the woman gets older, when breast cancer is more common. For the first 15 years after giving birth, the mother's risk of breast cancer was found to be greater than for women who have not had a child. The older a woman is when she has her first child, the higher the risk of breast cancer right after giving birth. For example, a woman who had her first child at age 35 faces a 41 percent higher risk of breast cancer than does a childless woman. But by age 59, the mother's risk is 29 percent lower than that faced by the childless woman. The risk is lowest in those who give birth at age 20. By the time they're 30, their risk is just 2 percent higher than that of a childless woman, and at age 59 it is 32 percent lower. The researchers suggest that a woman's risk of breast cancer may rise for a period of time after giving birth because of stimulation of cells that were already in the early stages of cancer. The findings indicate that the relationship between pregnancy and breast cancer may be more complex than had been thought.[9]

Researchers at M. D. Anderson Cancer Center in Houston came up with similiar findings. Their study, published in the British journal *Lancet* in June 1994, found that a mother's risk of getting breast cancer decreased the longer she remained cancer-free, until her risk was lower than that of a woman who had not had a child. The researchers also found that if a woman in her twenties is diagnosed with breast cancer while she is pregnant, she is three times as likely to die of the cancer than a woman who is not pregnant when diagnosed.[10] Lest women in their twenties panic, Eugenia Calle, M.D., of the American Cancer Society, points out that women in their twenties represent less than 1 percent of all cases of breast cancer.[11]

As for why pregnancy eventually lowers the risk of breast cancer, the theory has been that an early pregnancy would result in a change in hormone levels, most likely in the levels of estrogen. However, according to Dimitrios Trichopoulos, M.D., chair of the Department of Epidemiology at the Harvard School of Public Health, that is not the case. He says a consensus is gradually emerging that the protective effect of early pregnancy is mediated through terminal differentiation of mammary gland cells. Terminal differentiation (fully matured cells) has been demonstrated in experimental settings. The effect of terminal differentiation is really reduction of the number of cells in the breast that are susceptible to cancer. Decreasing the number of cells in the cellular population at risk decreases the number of possible cells that can become cancerous.[12] If Trichopoulos's theory proves to be correct, it is an obvious explanation of why an early pregnancy could decrease the risk of breast cancer. Leon Bradlow, Ph.D., director of the Laboratory of Biochemical Endocrinology at Strang-Cornell Breast Center in New York, agrees, saying that many scientists believe that the cell differentiation that takes place during a pregnancy offers a protective benefit. This phenomenon shows the importance of the number of cells present that are at risk for becoming cancer cells. The fewer the number of cells at risk, the less likely it is that cancer will develop. The most important factor in determining the number of cells may be the number of calories one ingests early in life, probably because well-nourished females generate a greater number of ductal stem cells than less-well-nourished women do.

Another theory, espoused by Malcolm Pike, M.D., at the University of Southern California, is that full-term pregnancy stimulates cells in the lining of the milk ducts to differentiate into mature forms, which are less likely to turn cancerous. Pike theorizes that early pregnancy transforms breast cells so that fewer are susceptible to harmful effects of estrogen. Therefore, the earlier you go through pregnancy, the earlier this protection kicks in. It works that way in animals as well. Pike is testing a birth control/breast cancer prevention pill in women that enables the woman's body to simulate pregnancy while at the same time postponing the real thing. He uses GnRH (gonadotropin-releasing hormone) to suppress ovulation and small doses of progestin and estrogen to replace hormones the body isn't making. Mammograms performed on women taking his pill showed less-dense breast tissue, which Pike says is a good sign.[13]

And yet another theory is that breast cancer is promoted by the monthly bombardment of breast tissue by hormones, which has its greatest effect on immature, or undifferentiated, breast cells. Pregnancy pushes breast cells to mature (differentiate) and gives breast tissue a nine-month break from the hormonal bombardment. According to Mary Costanza, M.D., at the University of Massachusetts Medical Center in Worcester, the estrogen present during pregnancy is in the estriol form, which may be more protective than the estradiol that is pumped out by the ovaries every month.[14]

Breastfeeding

A large study done at the University of Wisconsin, in which over 13,000 women responded to a phone survey, found that the risk of breast cancer before menopause decreases the longer a mother breastfeeds her baby and the younger she is when she begins.[15] According to the study, published in 1994, no reduction of risk was seen in postmenopausal women with a history of breastfeeding. The number of women who may benefit is relatively small since postmenopausal women develop 80 percent of all breast cancer. Some earlier studies have come up with similar results, while others have found no connection. A review in 1985 of previous studies suggested that breastfeeding might reduce the risk of breast cancer in premenopausal women. Other studies since then have had contradictory results. Studies in China, where more than half the women breastfeed for at least three years, suggest that long-term breastfeeding reduces breast cancer risk in both premenopausal and postmenopausal women.[16] Researchers speculate that the reduced risk may be a result of changing hormone secretions, interrupted ovulation, or an actual physical change in the breast.

Menopause

Early menopause or oophorectomy (removal of the ovaries) at an early age, which results in a virtual absence of estrogen, has a marked protective effect. A woman who stops ovulating at age 35 has about a 70 percent reduction in her lifetime risk of breast cancer. Dr. Larry Norton says that women who are born without ovaries and don't produce estrogen have essentially no breast cancer, or such a low incidence of breast cancer that it's in the range of less than 1 percent of the incidence of normal women with intact ovaries. And he says that when breast cancer cells are studied in the laboratory, their stimulation by estrogen can be seen.[17]

Women who have been obese before going into menopause are at a decreased risk of developing breast cancer. The reason may be that young obese women tend to ovulate less frequently and therefore have lower estrogen levels and less exposure to the hormone. On the other hand, postmenopausal women who are obese are at an increased risk of breast cancer. Their risk rises because body fat itself produces estrogen. So when hormonal levels are declining in women because of ovulatory cycle decline during and after menopause, excess body fat may become more important. Dr. Walter Willett says these innate biological processes may account for the different risk levels and not fat intake per se.[18]

Abortion and Breast Cancer

There is some evidence that having an abortion may put a woman at a greater risk of breast cancer. Joel Brind, professor of biology at the City University of New York, says recent studies suggest a heightened risk for women who have abortions before their first full-term pregnancy and charges that the information has been suppressed.[19] That charge is refuted by many, including Dr. Marc Lippman, who says the information has not been at all suppressed, adding that the research on the subject is not conclusive.[20]

The reasoning behind the theory that abortion may be a risk factor goes like this. During the first part of pregnancy, increased concentrations of estrogen stimulate breasts to grow, whereas during the second half of pregnancy, the breast cells differentiate to allow milk production. If, as some believe, cell differentiation is protective, when pregnancy is spontaneously or intentionally aborted, the woman has high levels of estrogen but misses out on cell differentiation. Hence, she is at an increased risk.

There have been charges made by religious and civil libertarian watchdog organizations that the issue is being pushed by prolife groups which have managed to publicize the studies that support their view and ignore those that show no relationship. Ann Thompson Cook, executive director of the Religious Coalition for Abortion Rights, says it is one of many "unscrupulous attempts to misrepresent medical science and religious tradition in order to sway women's decisions concerning abortion."[21] Following are a few of the studies, most of which show no connection.

In 1981, Malcolm Pike, M.D., at the University of Southern California, reported finding a very small 2.4-fold increase in the risk of breast cancer in women under 33 years of age who had had an abortion before having a full-term pregnancy.[22] Over a decade later, Pike acknowledged that he hasn't examined recent data so couldn't comment on whether abortion does increase risk.[23]

Holly Howe, Ph.D., with the New York State Department of Health, looked at 1,451 women under the age of 40 diagnosed with breast cancer between 1976 and 1980. In 1989, she reported that she'd found a slightly higher relative risk — between 1.5 and 1.9 — of breast cancer in women who had had abortions.[24]

While Janet Daling, Ph.D., professor of epidemiology at Fred Hutchinson Cancer Research Center, says that a study shows an increase in risk for women under 18 who have an abortion, she is quick to point out that "we can't make generalizations for all women."[25]

Lynn Rosenberg, Sc.D., at the Sloan Epidemiology Unit at Boston University, did a study examining 3,200 women with breast cancer and 4,844 women without breast cancer in 1988. She found that the breast cancer of the women in her study was not related to abortions. "At the moment there is no convincing evidence that abortion affects risks."[26]

And if risk is increased by having an abortion, Kevin J. Cullen, M.D., at Georgetown University Medical Center, says, "It's not something that we think is globally important for breast cancer." He says other factors like a family history or exposure to carcinogens are far more significant.[27] Dr. Walter Willett, at Harvard Medical School, says if there is an increased risk, it is not because of abortion. "Of course the risk is higher among women having an abortion, not because abortions are a risk factor, but because a full-term pregnancy is protective."[28]

An evaluation of the relationship between abortion and breast cancer published in the *1993 Epidemiological Review* concludes that it is difficult to reach any kind of definitive resolution because of the inconsistency of the results as well as inaccuracies in reporting spontaneous and induced abortion.[29]

At the end of October, a headline in the *New York Times* read, "New Study Links Abortions and Increase in Breast Cancer."[30] The study suggested that "induced abortion in the last month of the first trimester [of pregnancy] is associated with nearly a doubling [50 percent] of breast cancer risk." At the same time it noted that "prior studies of breast cancer in relation to spontaneous abortion have not yielded consistent results." The authors of the study said more research was needed.[31] Noel Weiss, M.D., one of the authors, said that the findings were "provocative," but that women "should not give this study any weight in making a decision now."[32]

In an editorial responding to the study, Lynn Rosenberg said, "A difference in risk of 50 percent [relative risk of 1.5] is small in epidemiologic terms and severely challenges our ability to distinguish whether it reflects cause and effect or whether it simply reflects bias." She acknowledged that the findings did add to the "limited evidence" currently available linking abortion and breast cancer, which she described as "neither a coherent body of knowledge nor [establishment of] a convincing biologic mechanism."[33]

An epidemiologist at the Harvard School of Public Health, Karin Michels, said that her review of 40 published studies on abortion and breast cancer found no evidence of an increased risk.[34]

The majority of studies show no link between abortion and breast cancer.

Estrogen Replacement Therapy (ERT)

The question of estrogen replacement therapy in postmenopausal women and whether it can put a woman at greater risk of breast cancer remains controversial and of great concern to many women. During and after menopause, a woman's estrogen level drops dramatically, resulting in some unpleasant, and in some cases debilitating, symptoms such as hot flashes. In addition, a decrease in estrogen puts a woman at a greater risk of developing osteoporosis and heart disease.

In 1990, 375,000 women died of heart attacks.[35] Studies have suggested a minimum mortality drop of 50 percent when the woman has been on ERT. Some studies have shown the decrease to be as high as 85 percent. A reduction of coronary heart disease by 50 percent would have a major impact on women.

Osteoporosis in the general population results in 1.3 million fractures a year at a cost of $1.3 million.[36] Estrogen replacement therapy has been shown to have an impact on the development of osteoporosis.

The probability of ERT causing breast cancer in otherwise healthy postmenopausal women is hardly resolved. Studies have been done and there is some data, but it is far from definitive.

After reviewing some 24 studies and 3 meta-analyses in 1992, Janet Henrich, M.D., of Yale, reached the conclusion that "in women who use estrogen for short periods of time, most of the evidence indicates that there is not an increased risk of breast cancer." She and several other experts say women can take estrogen for five years and perhaps longer without putting themselves at higher risk for breast cancer.[37]

A study of close to 900 women between the ages of 45 and 65, published in early 1995, confirmed the benefits of ERT in reducing cardiovascular risk factors. There was no hint of an increase of breast cancer in the women who were on ERT. However, the study was conducted for just three years, which researchers acknowleged is not long enough to assess such a risk.[38]

It appears that the length of time a woman is on ERT may be the key. Various studies have shown a 25 to 50 percent increase in risk of breast cancer in women who are on ERT for 15 or 25 years. It appears that, overall, per year of ERT there's a 3 percent increase in breast cancer risk, whereas normally there is a 2 percent increase per year in women during the postmenopausal period. The women at greatest risk are those with a family history of breast cancer. However, as Barbara Hulka, M.D., head of epidemiology at the School of Public Health at the University of North Carolina, and others point out, the possible increased risk of breast cancer in healthy women must be weighed against the well-documented health benefits of estrogen, including lowering the risk of heart disease, osteoporosis, and increasing HDLs, the "good" cholesterol.[39]

Another unanswered question is whether women who have had breast cancer can ever take estrogen. Since estrogen appears to be a factor in the development of breast cancer, estrogen is generally not prescribed for women who have had breast cancer, regardless of whether the tumor is estrogen-receptor positive or negative, out of concern that the estrogen will lead to a recurrence of the disease. However, it's not known which would be most beneficial to women with breast cancer — withholding estrogen therapy and putting them at a greater risk of heart disease and osteoporosis or giving them estrogen therapy and increasing their risk of breast cancer. A woman who is a long-term survivor of breast cancer has competing risks of mortality — breast cancer recurrence, heart disease, and osteoporosis.

In the 1990s, nearly two million women will develop breast cancer and as many as half a million of those women will be premenopausal. Chemotherapy causes early menopause in 54 percent of women under 35 and 84 percent of women ages 35 to 44.[40] Therefore, as more and more women are diagnosed with breast cancer, more will face prolonged estrogen deficiency as a result of an early chemotherapy-induced menopause. Those women experience the symptoms associated with menopause and many ask that ERT be available under medical supervision. Dr. Richard Theriault says a clinical trial of ERT in breast cancer patients needs to be done.[41]

Rena Sellin, M.D., associate professor of medicine at M. D. Anderson Cancer Center in Houston, says a five-year study comparing ERT with no estrogen therapy in a specific population of estrogen-deficient women with breast cancer started enrolling patients in July 1992. Before starting the study, Sellin and colleagues collected 220 anonymous surveys from women with breast cancer who attended outpatient clinics at the hospital. Most women were concerned that ERT could lead to a cancer recurrence; most women were also concerned about osteoporosis and heart disease. About half of the women who responded said they'd be willing to consider ERT under medical supervision at some time. Of physicians who responded to a survey about ERT, 32 percent were aware of women on ERT who had had breast cancer. Fifty doctors said they would prescribe ERT to specific patients who had had breast cancer. Most of the doctors who responded did not personally believe that ERT increases the risk of breast cancer recurrence.[42]

Although it has been customary not to prescribe ERT for any woman who has had breast cancer, a group of doctors questioned the assumption that ERT would put a woman at risk of recurrence, saying there was little data either way. In 1994, members of the breast cancer committee of the Eastern Cooperative Oncology Group (a consortium of several thousand cancer specialists) expressed concern about the increasing number of women who are going into early menopause as a result of cancer treatment and the menopausal side effects they experience as well as the increased risk of osteoporosis and heart disease.[43] Melody Cobleigh, M.D., said that NCI should sponsor a pilot study of ERT along with tamoxifen on several hundred breast cancer survivors.[44]

There is no question that many women with breast cancer are concerned about their long-term increased risk of heart disease and osteoporosis as well as the immediate side effects of menopause. Studies have shown that the anti-estrogen drug tamoxifen, which many postmenopausal women with breast cancer take as adjuvant therapy, can also reduce the risk of heart disease and osteoporosis.[45] It is believed that this is a result of the weak estrogen-like effects that tamoxifen has. Tamoxifen's use in the possible prevention of breast cancer is discussed later in this chapter.

Oral Contraceptives — "the Pill"

Oral contraceptives, better known as "the Pill," were first marketed in the United States in 1960. As of 1994, some 11 million women in the United States were taking them.[46] Are these women putting themselves at a greater risk of developing breast cancer? Cynthia Pearson of the National Women's Health Network thinks it is a very real possibility. At an NCI conference in 1993, she said, "Four years ago my group and others asked the Food and Drug Administration [FDA] to inform women that long-term use of the oral contraceptives might increase the risk of breast cancer." At that time they requested that a warning be put on the package inserts. The FDA declined. Pearson said that since the original request was made, other studies have come out which suggest a possible risk.[47] Should there now be a warning? Responding to the question, Dr. Janet R. Daling, a researcher at Fred Hutchinson Cancer Research Center in Seattle, said that if the data, some of which were not yet published, and additional new data supported the findings, then it should and would appear on the package inserts.[48]

The study to which Daling referred was published in April 1994.[49] It found an increased risk for breast cancer among women under the age of 35 who took the Pill for more than ten years and supported other evidence that long-term use of oral contraceptives may increase the risk for the early onset of breast cancer. The researchers at Hutchinson found that women under 35 who used oral contraceptives for more than ten years had a 70 percent increased risk of breast cancer compared to women who had never taken them or had taken them for less than one year. In addition, they found that women who took the Pill within five years after they started menstruating faced a 30 percent increased risk. Two meta-analyses (combining findings from many studies, analyzing the findings, and summarizing the overall results) of data from different oral contraceptive use studies found a similar 11 percent increased risk for breast cancer for women under 45 who had ever used the Pill and a 40 percent increased risk for women in this age group who were long-term users.[50, 51]

During the 1980s, evidence started to emerge that suggested a link between early onset of breast cancer and both long-term use of the Pill and use at a young age. Some studies have also suggested that women of all ages with a family history of breast cancer or a history of benign breast disease may be at a particularly increased risk for breast cancer if they've used the Pill.[52]

An analysis of data from the U.S. Cancer and Steroid Hormone Study found that women aged 20 to 34 who had ever used the Pill had a 40 percent increased risk of breast cancer.[53] No increased risk was found for women aged 35 to 44.

A study in Boston found an overall twofold increased risk for breast cancer among women under age 45 who used the Pill.[54] Risk was increased for short-term and long-term use, and risk increased as duration of use increased.

In England, a study found that women under the age of 36 who had taken the Pill for four to eight years had a 40 percent increased risk for breast cancer, while women who took the Pill for more than eight years had a 70 percent increased risk.[55]

Researchers in Sweden found that women who started to use the Pill before the age of 25 increased their risk for breast cancer nearly sixfold.[56] However, the amount of time the woman used the Pill did not appear to increase risk.

Dr. Janet Daling said a review of some studies found two possible risk factors for breast cancer associated with taking the Pill — the use of oral contraceptives in women under 20 years of age, and use for 5 to 10 years or more. Daling qualified the statement by saying that the data is not conclusive, but there is the suggestion that early and prolonged use may put women at greater risk, although there is no consensus on this. For the most part the risk was confined to premenopausal women who developed breast cancer before the age of 35. At the same time Daling noted that oral contraceptives offered other benefits beside preventing pregnancy. The use of oral contraceptives can decrease the risk of endometrial cancer and ovarian cancer.[57]

A study in 1991 at Memorial Sloan-Kettering Cancer Center in New York found a strong consensus among reported studies that the Pill had not increased the risk of breast cancer in women over age 45, even when the Pill was used for long periods of time.[58] The report stated that the controversy was confined to studies of younger women and that there was little data to show that the use of oral contraceptives put women at risk. It concluded that the "lack of consistency [in the various studies] and the potential for bias and confounding argue strongly against concluding, at this time, that there is causal relationship between oral contraception and breast cancer."

Two years later a meta-analysis of reports that compared categories of women who had ever used oral contraceptives, long-term oral contraceptive users, and oral contraceptive use before a first full-term pregnancy found no association in the first two categories. A significant correlation was found between use of the Pill and breast cancer among the women who took the Pill before their first full-term pregnancy. The analysis also questioned the methodology used in some of the studies. The conclusion was that there is a possible increased risk for breast cancer in women who use oral contraceptives before a first full-term pregnancy. Another conclusion, and possibly a more significant one, was that the findings in the studies used in the analysis were confounded by studies that were generally of low quality. The report also recommended that further studies be done addressing the risk of breast cancer in women who use the birth control pill, and that the studies be done with the proper methodology so as to limit any biases in the findings.[59]

Most studies have found no overall increased risk for breast cancer associated with the Pill. One of the reasons it is difficult to do a meaningful comparison of studies is that there have been so many different combinations of the Pill used by women. So once again, the jury is out.

In explaining why the use of oral birth controls may appear to put a woman at greater risk, breast surgeon Susan Love says the oral contraceptives allow a woman to delay the first pregnancy and a later first pregnancy is a risk factor for breast cancer. She adds, "Birth control pills have never been shown to increase breast cancer risk."[60]

Darcy Spicer, M.D., at the University of Southern California, says that the doses of estrogen and progestin administered in the oral contraceptive have decreased substantially. "I think one can fairly conclusively say that oral contraceptives formulated as they are do not increase the risk of breast cancer, presumably because they replace ovarian estrogen and progesterone in amounts which would have been produced by a normal ovary." She said that preliminary findings in an ongoing clinical trial suggested that reducing estrogen and progesterone in the Pill may be helpful in reducing the risk of breast cancer.[61]

8

Environmental Enemies

Extensive evidence exists to indicate that cancer is an environmental disease.

Rita Arditti, *breast cancer survivor*[1]

I wonder about everything . . . radio waves in faxes, how often do you do transcontinental trips, radiation exposure in airplanes . . . the water's polluted, the air is polluted.

Alison Estabrook, *chief of breast surgery,*
Columbia Presbyterian Hospital[2]

What if we find out that electricity causes cancer, are we willing to give up electricity?

Sharon Green, *executive director, Y-ME*[3]

Radioactive releases from nuclear power plants appear to be an important and hitherto neglected factor in the otherwise unexplained recent rise of cancer in most industrial nations.

Ernest Sternglass, *professor emeritus of*
radiology, University of Pittsburgh[4]

The female breast is one of the most radiosensitive human organs.

Roy E. Shore, Dr. P.H., Ph.D.[5]

Chemicals

The chemical environment we inhabit today is both grossly and qualitatively different from that of the 1700s as well as that of our grandparents and even our parents. Before the Second World War, our exposure was limited, as we didn't have the ability to make massive quantities of chemicals. David Ozonoff, M.D., at the Boston University School of Public Health, says environmental chemicals are "not a legacy from the industrial revolution of the nineteenth century, but [a result of] the rise of the chemical industry in the twentieth century." He calls the chemicals "recent and unwelcome newcomers."[6] Today, more than 70,000 chemicals are being used in the United States.

In its National Toxicology Program, the United States government has identified some 30 known carcinogens, including benzene, arsenic, DES, and mustard gas. The list of suspected carcinogens runs much higher. According to Joan D'Argo, of Greenpeace, most of the tens of thousands of chemicals in use have not been effectively tested and regulated.[7] Besides man-made contaminating chemicals, we now also have in our environment man-made radiation and electromagnetic fields.

Many in the scientific community continue to dismiss the idea that environmental factors play any significant role in the development of breast cancer. At the same time, an increasing number believe that environmental factors could be the reason, at least in part, the rate of breast cancer is steadily increasing while most women who are diagnosed with breast cancer do not have any of the known risk factors.

Dr. Samuel Epstein, professor of occupational and environmental medicine at the University of Illinois Medical Center, says we are being exposed to tremendous environmental hazards. He cites an extensive body of evidence including

- Production and manufacture of synthetic organic chemicals, particularly industrial carcinogens, went from one billion pounds in 1940 to over 400 billion pounds annually by the 1980s.
- Just 10 percent of the new chemicals have been adequately tested for carcinogenicity.
- Of some 120 substances identified as carcinogens in experiments in animals over the last 20 years, less than 10 percent have been subjected to epidemiologic study by NCI or industry.

Epstein charges that for two or three decades the federal government has ignored threats to our well-being that include contaminants in the food we eat, radionuclides from civilian reactors that end up in our water and food, estrogenic food additives, and occupational exposures to petrochemicals and other chemicals.[8]

Amy Langer, head of the National Alliance of Breast Cancer Organizations (NABCO), charges the Environmental Protection Agency (EPA) with not doing its job. "That," she says, "has been shown by a number of recent studies. Dogs whose owners use pesticides die of increased rates of certain cancers. In some homes where children have been exposed to pesticides indoors, there's an increase in leukemia and brain cancer. We know from twenty studies in eight different countries that farmers and gardeners are at an increased risk of some cancers, which we think is related to their exposure to pesticides."[9]

Some pesticides have the ability to remain in body fat. In a woman's body, those pesticides can mimic estrogen and produce estrogenic effects. There is a lot of evidence that the greater the amount of contaminants contained in the fat in your body, the more harmful they are.[10] The major contaminants of fat fall into these categories: organochloride pesticides such as DDT (and its metabolite DDE) and other estrogenic pesticides such as methoxychlor, toxaphene, dieldrin, endosulfan, chlordane, and aldrin. Some were shown to induce breast cancer in rodents as many as 30 years ago. If the theory is true that as estrogen in the body increases so does a woman's risk of breast cancer, then exposure to pesticides (which end up as estrogen in fatty breast tissue) may very well be a significant risk factor in the development of breast cancer.[11]

According to Ana Soto, M.D., at Tufts University School of Medicine, the most common hormonal property among environmental chemicals is their ability to mimic estrogen.[12] And she says that there are many of those chemicals out there. Besides being found in pesticides, Soto says, estrogenic chemicals are found in many commonly used products. For example, the chemical nonyl phenol, used in plastics, may contaminate food during processing or packaging. (Soto and her colleague, Dr. Carlos Sonnenschein, M.D., made the discovery inadvertently when they found that plastic they were using in their lab shed estrogen-like chemicals.) Chemicals that may eventually become estrogenic are found in detergents, cosmetics, condom lubricants, spermicidal foams, and other products. Soto and colleagues have developed a test called the E-SCREEN that can measure the estrogenic activity of chemicals. She says that chemicals should be tested for their estrogenic activity before being released into the environment because of the possible hazards of their cumulative effect. And she proposes a study to see if increased incidence of breast cancer correlates with the cumulative dose of all estrogenic chemicals in our body.

Studies have found higher levels of pesticide residues in the breast fat of women with breast cancer compared to residues in women with benign conditions, according to Ruby Senie, Ph.D., associate attending epidemiologist at Memorial Sloan-Kettering Cancer Center. She says that other studies indicate that exposure to pesticides influences hormonal levels in lab animals.[13]

A 1992 pilot study by Frank Falck, Jr., Ph.D., at the University of Michigan, found that the breast tissue in women with breast cancer had 50 to 60 percent greater concentrations of contaminants such as PCBs and pesticides like DDTs (organochlorines) than the breast fat tissue of women without breast cancer.[14]

In Finland, the breast tissue of 44 women with breast cancer and 33 women without breast cancer was checked for residues of the organochlorine beta-HCH, a pesticide. Women with significant levels of the residue had a tenfold higher risk of breast cancer than the women with lower levels.[15]

Breast surgeon Alison Estabrook compared levels of DDT in the blood and in cysts of women with gross cystic disease at Columbia Presbyterian Hospital in New York. Estabrook found higher levels of DDT in the fluid of breast cysts than in the blood, as well as higher levels of estradiol (a potent form of estrogen) and other substances. She says that women with gross cystic disease are at a slightly higher risk of breast cancer. Estabrook notes that Long Island, New York, which has elevated levels of breast cancer, had many farming communities that used DDT to spray crops; and that even if it hasn't been used in 20 years the residue might still affect the drinking water.[16]

Research into the biologically active chemicals that accumulate in a woman's body over her lifetime is being done by Mary S. Wolff, Ph.D., at the Mt. Sinai School of Medicine in New York. She and her colleagues have compared the breast tissue of women with breast cancer with the breast tissue of women who do not have breast cancer.

Wolff says, "These lines of research are fairly unusual, although they seem quite simple and straightforward in terms of the kind of stuff that's out there to be done."[17]

Studies like the ones done by Wolff have not been well supported for a variety of reasons, one being skepticism on the part of the male medical establishment; another being major efforts by companies that produce various suspect products to denigrate the idea of there being any problems. In 1987, Wolff found levels of DDE (a by-product of DDT) and PCBs elevated about 40 percent in breast cancer tissue.[18] A study published in 1993, comparing the levels of DDE in the blood of women with breast cancer and women without breast cancer, found women with the highest levels of DDE in their blood were four times as likely to have breast cancer as those women with the lowest levels.[19] The level of DDE in the blood of women with breast cancer was 35 percent higher than in women without breast cancer. When food contaminated with the pesticide DDT is eaten, the residue accumulates in the fatty tissue of the breast and stays forever. If DDT is a factor in the development of some breast cancers, the women at the greatest risk are those women who had the greatest exposure to DDT when it was being used in the United States from 1945 until it was banned in 1972. The study suggests that DDT may be one of the factors accounting for the sharp rise in breast cancer in women over 50, since they would fit right into that category. Although the study showed a significant statistical link between breast cancer and DDT, Wolff acknowledges that more work is needed before a clear cause-and-effect link can be established.

Wolff's study came under criticism from Lawrence J. Fischer, Ph.D., at the Institute for Environmental Toxicology, Michigan State University, who charged that the study had "serious scientific deficiencies" because women were not asked about their diet, lifestyle, age of menarche, family history, and reproductive history. He contends that without that information it is impossible to know if the two groups were comparable in regard to other known risk factors.[20] Wolff says her original work was in a small pilot study and acknowledges "we didn't collect enough data on background." But the results of the pilot study enabled her to get funding for a bigger study, which is now under way.[21]

Another pesticide under investigation is endosulfan. Endosulfan enters the food supply as a pesticide on carrots, lettuce, spinach, to-matoes, and other crops. A study by the Environmental Working Group, a private organization, found that two million pounds of en-dosulfan is applied to crops each year.[22] According to Dr. Ana Soto, endosulfan has as potent an estrogen-like effect as DDT. Soto found that estrogenic pesticides accelerated the reproduction of breast can-cer cells and that different estrogenic pesticides, like endosulfan, di-cofol, and methoxychlor, accumulate together as if they are the same chemical.[23] If that's true, estrogenic pesticides that are not banned are potentially adding to the banned pesticides like DDT that are still in a woman's body. When the EPA gauges the safety of pesticides, it uses tests that assume different chemicals do not interact with each other or have an additive effect. Endosulfan, dicofol, and methoxychlor en-dosulfan are all still on the market. According to Dr. Samuel Epstein, various chemicals and carcinogens do interact, becoming more haz-ardous. He says, "There is excellent evidence that DDT will promote the formation of breast cancers after somebody has been exposed to low doses of other carcinogens."[24]

In the mid-1970s, consumers in Israel put pressure on the Israeli government to take action against pesticides. The government com-plied, phasing out the use of organic chlorine pesticides at dairy farms. One study found that breast cancer mortality rates dropped overall 8 percent between 1976 and 1986.[25] The authors of the study contend that the true rate of decrease was probably near 20 percent if trends seen before the ban were factored in.

Some researchers have argued for years that industrial chemicals with estrogen-like effects in the body contribute to an increased risk of breast cancer. Scientists believe that estrogenic pesticides may affect a woman either through repeated exposure or through exposure during some crucial phase early in her sexual development.

A study published in the fall of 1993 looked at previous studies on the possible link between chemicals that could act like estrogens, such as DDT, and other organochlorides. Most of the breast cancer risk factors, such as the early onset of menstruation, late age of meno-pause, late or no pregnancy, and caloric intake relative to body weight, can be linked to the total exposure to estrogen over a lifetime. If exposure to chemicals can increase the total amount of exposure to estrogen a woman faces, decreasing that exposure, as was done in

Israel, may serve as a way to reduce risk and prevent some breast cancers. The authors of the study called for the development of major epidemiologic studies to evaluate whether the incidence of breast cancer is increasing because of increased exposure to these chemicals.[26]

A study done by the Kaiser Foundation Research Institute in Oakland, California, found no overall link between breast cancer risk and levels of DDE in the blood as had been found in previous studies.[27] The April 1994 investigation found a slight positive association in African American women. Nancy Krieger, director of the study, said the findings do not "by any means definitively disprove the hypothesis" that DDT exposure is associated with an increased risk of breast cancer. She says that further serious investigation is needed. Krieger added that the breast cancer itself can mobilize organochlorines in breast tissue, causing elevated levels, which may have been the reason Dr. Mary Wolff found elevated levels in her study.[28] Dr. Brian Mac-Mahon at the Harvard School of Public Health, said that while further research was needed, "for the moment, we must conclude that the available epidemiological evidence overall is not supportive of an association between exposure to DDT and increased risk."[29] Robert Hoover, M.D., chief of the epidemiology branch at NCI, said that he didn't disagree with the analysis of the study, but with the interpretation of the findings. "I wouldn't have written it so strongly negative," said Hoover.[30] PCBs and other organochlorines were also measured in the study. As in some earlier studies, no link was found between breast cancer risk and PCB levels.

On Long Island, where the breast cancer rate is significantly higher than the national rate, a study by the New York State Health Department reported that women who once lived near large chemical plants had a greater risk of developing breast cancer after menopause.[31] Women who lived less than a mile from plants producing chemicals, rubber, and plastics between 1965 and 1975 had a greater than 62 percent increased risk of getting breast cancer, with the risk increasing as the number of chemical plants grew. Itzhak Goldberg, M.D., chairman of the radiation oncology department at Long Island Jewish Medical Center, cited the study as a "wake-up call for all of us." He noted the dearth of studies in the past to discover why a particular patient had breast cancer. "This study," said Goldberg, "puts the issue on the front burner."[32] Wolff called the study the "first credible report of its kind," a comment echoed by other researchers. She said that even though a link between the chemicals and breast cancer was not established, it nevertheless "casts suspicion in that direction, and that has to be followed up with more research."[33] According to Mark Chassin, the New York State health commissioner, if the association proves to be real, "it will be the first time that an environmental risk factor that is avoidable has been identified." Chassin also said that the findings could account for up to 5 percent of the breast cancer cases on Long Island. He qualified that by saying that he still believed the traditionally accepted risk factors, such as early menstruation, late birth of first child, late menopause, etc., could account for the higher rate of breast cancer there if a greater proportion of women living on Long Island had those risk factors than women in other locations.[34] Previous studies on Long Island, including one by the CDC, had failed to find any environmental cause.

In 1995, scientists from NCI and the National Institute of Environmental Health Sciences (NIEHS) started a five-year intensive environmental study on Long Island. The Long Island Breast Cancer Study Project (LIBCSP), created by congressional mandate in response to the loudly voiced concerns of Long Island residents, calls for a case-control study to assess "biological markers for environmental and other risk factors contributing to the incidence of breast cancer on Long Island."[35] Schoharie County in New York and Tolland County in Connecticut are also part of the study. Iris Obrams, M.D., director of the study, says it presents "an opportunity for groundbreaking epidemiologic research that may serve, ultimately, as a research model for the nation."[36] The study will look at past and current exposures of women, with and without breast cancer, to contaminated drinking water, indoor and ambient air pollution, including aircraft emissions, and pesticide levels in the dust in household carpeting, electromagnetic fields, and hazardous and municipal wastes.

In April 1993, NCI announced a number of current or new studies looking at breast cancer and environmental factors.[37] In conjunction with researchers from NIEHS, NCI researchers would look at how recognized risks and specific environmental exposures may be contributing to the increasing number of breast cancer deaths. In much of the Northeast, many mid-Atlantic states, and some Midwestern states, breast cancer rates are above the national average. The environmental factors under examination in six epidemiologic studies include electromagnetic fields, pesticides, and contaminants in the food and water supply.

In Michigan, where contamination of animal feed with PCBs in the mid-1970s led to widespread contamination of farm animals, milk, and residents in the area, researchers will compare the levels of PCB residues from the breast fat of women with breast cancer with that of women without cancer.[38]

In a rural area of Alabama, residents were exposed to high levels of DDT from about 1947 to 1971, when a chemical company discharged tons of DDT into a nearby river. People in the area regularly ate fish caught in the river. When CDC investigated blood levels of DDE, they were about ten times higher in this group than the average level elsewhere in the country. NCI is planning to develop a case-control study to compare DDE residues in breast fat and blood of women with and without breast cancer.[39]

The Agricultural Health Study in Iowa and North Carolina, both of which have a large population of farmers using pesticides, will assess exposures to agents such as pesticides, chemical solvents, engine exhausts, animal viruses, and sunlight in 100,000 farmers, their spouses, and their children. As cancer cases are diagnosed, breast cancer cases will be incorporated into special studies to collect even more detailed information on possible exposures and risk factors.[40]

Radiation

The link between breast cancer and radiation has been known for some time. The first documentation to show an excess of breast cancer associated with radiation appeared in 1965.[41] Women who had large doses of radiation during multiple fluoroscopic examination (a diagnostic procedure using continuous X-ray rather than individual films) were found to have a greater risk of developing breast cancer. A Canadian study found that women in whom tuberculosis had been diagnosed with fluoroscopy in the 1930s and 1940s had a higher rate of breast cancer.[42]

It was originally believed that radiation would not have any effect on younger, prepubescent girls. That theory proved false when Japanese women who were exposed to fallout from the atomic bombs as children during World War II showed an increase of breast cancer.[43] A study at the University of Rochester School of Medicine and Dentistry confirmed findings that showed exposing girls to X-rays before puberty increased their risk of developing breast cancer.[44] The study showed that women who received X-ray treatments for enlarged thymus glands as infants were nearly four times as likely to get breast cancer once they reached their thirties as their sisters who did not have X-ray treatments.[45] In Sweden, researchers compared women treated with radiation for benign breast disease with women not treated with radiation for the same condition. They found that the total dose, age at first treatment, and time since first exposure were all factors in the risk of developing breast cancer.[46]

A study of radiation in the treatment of breast cancer concluded that the radiation contributed marginally to developing a cancer in the other breast. The risk was greatest among women who had the radiation at a relatively young age, under 45.[47]

Dr. Samuel Epstein, professor of occupational and environmental medicine at the University of Illinois Medical Center, holds the cancer establishment responsible for a significant proportion of the increase in breast cancer incidence in the 1980s and 1990s.[48] In the early 1970s, the ACS and NCI went on a large-scale mammography program. Epstein charges that radiation doses known clearly and unequivocally at that time to be carcinogenic were used on women who were being told that mammography was safe and effective. He says the breast in premenopausal women is 40 times more sensitive to radiation than the breast in the postmenopausal woman.

The Swedish study referred to earlier said its findings should be considered when weighing the relative risks versus benefits of generalized screening of young women by mammography. However, Ellen Mendelson, M.D., chief of mammography and women's imaging in the Department of Radiology in West Pennsylvania Hospital, counters that the radiation risk of mammography to any woman getting a mammogram now is negligible because the amount of radiation used is so low.[49] That, of course, assumes that the mammography machine used is state-of-the art, dedicated (used only for mammography), and calibrated regularly. (See Part III, Mammography: Miracle or Myth?)

Ernest Sternglass, M.D., professor emeritus of radiology at the University of Pittsburgh, has been studying the effects of radiation extensively and is certain it has led to an increase in cancer incidence. He has focused his research on radiation emissions. He says there are two dozen studies that show a link between airborne releases from nuclear power sites and mortality rates on Long Island, N.Y., and Connecticut, areas which were exposed to those releases. He contends that there is a large risk associated with small doses and charges that information has been virtually ignored. The effect appears to be greatest where nuclear plants are close to metropolitan areas, especially when they're close to nearby surface drinking water supplies or farming areas that supply cities with fresh milk. In Sternglass's opinion, the effect has been devastating. "It now appears that chronic exposure to nuclear fission products in the diet and drinking water may be the single largest factor in the rise of most forms of malignancies in the general population since World War II."[50]

Although it's been known for decades that radiation produces cancer, it wasn't understood that very small amounts of radiation, such as from fallout from bomb testing in the 1950s and 1960s and small releases from nuclear reactors (military and commercial), could result in what look like very large changes in cancer rates in different countries and different parts of this country.[51] Epidemiologic studies show a relationship with cancer occurrence when emissions from nuclear reactors in different regions are compared with incidence of cancer in those regions, which confirms the idea that effects of very small amounts of radiation added into the drinking water have been underestimated.

Some of the evidence that Sternglass cites includes the following:

- Two years after Three Mile Island was shut down, infant mortality in Pennsylvania dropped 30 to 40 percent.
- Some 5 to 8 years after New York City started getting 80 to 90 percent of its drinking water from sources far upwind from the Indian Point power plant, cancer rates in New York City decreased. However, just north of New York City, in Westchester County, where most of the water supply is from a source within a few miles directly downwind from the Indian Point plant, there has been a continuing increase of over 35 percent since the early 1960s.
- A tumor registry in Connecticut started in 1935 shows the incidence of breast cancer from 1935 to 1944 (before the nuclear age

began in 1945) declining. The increase in breast cancer began
with the nuclear age.

- Between 1970 and 1975, the Millstone reactor, in Waterford,
  Connecticut, 12 miles from eastern Long Island, released quanti-
  ties of radioactive iodine that were double the amount released by
  Three Mile Island in 1979. The releases were never publicized.
  After the Millstone reactor was opened, there was another large
  increase in breast cancer.
- Peak releases from the Brookhaven National Laboratory on Long
  Island occurred between 1958 and 1964. Some 20 years later, an
  increased incidence of breast cancer started to appear, with the
  highest incidence within 12 miles of Brookhaven.

Sternglass contends that radioactive contamination of the air,
drinking water, and food is the single most important factor that was
not considered in the investigation into higher breast cancer rates on
Long Island. He believes that radioactive contaminants of the diet
probably act synergistically with ordinary chemical carcinogens in the
body to both initiate and promote the development of breast cancer.[52]

Electromagnetic Fields (EMF)

The combination of electric fields and magnetic fields that radiate
from electric cables, power lines, wires, fixtures, and appliances was for
years thought by scientists to be harmless. However, in 1989, as a
result of a number of studies, the Congressional Office of Technology
Assessment concluded that it could not be assumed there are no risks
from EMF. James Melius, M.D., director of the Division of Occupational Health and Environment in New York State, says that EMF is
an issue of serious concern because of how common exposures are and
because of the growing scientific literature about problems associated
with cancer and other diseases. He says that some studies have looked
at male breast cancer and associated it with men in occupations with
high EMF exposure.[53] NCI is currently funding a large study in the
Northwest looking at EMF exposure in the home.

A Swedish study published in 1993, in which about half a million
participants were followed over a long period of time, reported a
doubling of the childhood leukemia rate in children exposed to
EMF.[54] In Sweden it is now proposed that the standard be set that a

400-kilovolt line would require 150 feet on each side of a bumper zone within which people could not live and schools could not be located.

Researchers at the University of North Carolina at Chapel Hill found that women in electrical occupations had 38 percent excess mortality from breast cancer relative to other employees.[55] The study, published in June 1994, was done to test the hypothesis that breast cancer risk is increased by electromagnetic fields. The investigators acknowledged possible study limitations. Although they believed the findings were broadly consistent with other evidence supporting the association, they still urged further investigation.

Studies on EMF are continuing. The University of Washington is conducting a study on EMF and breast cancer, as is Patricia Coogan, M.P.H., at the Boston University School of Public Health, who is looking at breast cancer risk in women exposed to EMF at work. Coogan says that the association is plausible because it is hypothesized that EMF disrupt the functioning of the pineal gland, which produces melatonin. Melatonin inhibits the synthesis of estrogen and prolactin in the body, so a lowered level may mean an increased level of exposure to estrogen.[56]

"None of the 30 or 40 studies done in the last ten years has provided any convincing evidence that EMFs cause birth defects, childhood cancers, breast cancer in women, and other problems," says Patricia Buffler, dean of the School of Public Health, University of California at Berkeley. Since 1987, Buffler has chaired an independent committee of scientists that commissions and reviews studies on the health effects of EMF for the Electric Power Research Institute, an organization sponsored by major utility companies in the United States. She says there is no sound basis for the scientific community to be cautioning consumers against low-level emissions from appliances or power lines.[57] In April 1995, the American Physical Society, the world's largest group of physicists, took a similar stand, saying it could find no evidence that EMF from power lines cause cancer. The society called the public's fears groundless and said that billions of dollars were being spent for mitigation work when "more serious environmental problems are neglected for lack of funding." It concluded, "The conjectures relating cancer to power line fields have not been scientifically substantiated."[58]

Not everyone agrees. In June 1994, Washington State's Department of Labor and Industries granted worker's compensation to a 50-year-old man who claimed his cancer was caused by EMF exposure. James Brewer had worked as a smelter at Kaiser Aluminum in Tacoma, Washington, where he was exposed to high levels of EMF. Lawyers on the case said it was the first time that a government body had acknowleged such a link.[59] The company is appealing the ruling.

It's been known for several centuries that cancer can be caused by exposure to environmental factors. For example, in the eighteenth century in England, when many chimney sweeps developed scrotal cancer, an association was made with exposure to the chemicals in soot. In 1962, in her book *Silent Spring*, biologist Rachel Carson wrote: "For the first time in the history of the world, every human being is now subject to contact with dangerous chemicals, from the moment of conception until death." However, during the twentieth century, when industrialization wreaked havoc on our environment, little attention was paid and few studies were done. That is no longer acceptable. Today, more and more groups are holding conferences on the environmental factors that contribute to the development of breast cancer and breast cancer advocates are demanding more research into environmental issues such as pesticides, radiation fallout from nuclear power plants, and the hazards of power lines and electromagnetic fields. In 1992 the National Breast Cancer Coalition made research into environmental exposures one of its priorities, as did other organizations. If, as it appears, environmental factors do play a role in the development of breast cancer, studies must be done to find out how those factors can be eliminated or at least neutralized.

9

Other Risks

Current smokers may be at an increased risk of fatal breast cancer.

Eugenia Calle, Ph.D.,
American Cancer Society epidemiologist[1]

There have been weak to moderate associations between alcohol and breast cancer risk and between hormone levels and breast cancer risk. Our study . . . suggests a linkage between the two factors.

Marsha E. Reichman, Ph.D.,
formerly with the National Cancer Institute[2]

It has been known for years that cigarette smoking can increase the risk for many diseases—most notably heart disease and lung cancer. However, smoking had not been linked to breast cancer. Now it is. Other factors are also being questioned as possible factors in the development or promotion of breast cancer, such as alcohol, sexual orientation, silicone implants, to name just some. Although it is generally not believed that these factors, in and of themselves, cause breast cancer, it is thought that they may combine with other factors in promoting the disease. Following are some of the possible risk factors being considered. No doubt, other factors will eventually join the list.

Smoking

Women with breast cancer who smoke increase their risk of dying of breast cancer by at least 25 percent. According to an ACS study reported in June 1994, the risk grows with the number of cigarettes a woman smokes. Women smoking two or more packs a day have an escalated risk of dying from breast cancer compared to nonsmokers and former smokers. Eugenia Calle, Ph.D., the epidemiologist who directed the study, said the findings did not suggest that smoking causes breast cancer. She said there were several possibilities for the increased mortality risk, which include the facts that "smokers may have impaired immune systems; they may not obtain routine [mammograms]; or smoking may cause a direct deleterious effect on survival."[3] Oncologist and epidemiologist Mary Daly, M.D., at the Fox Chase Center in Philadelphia, said, "The study should be taken as provocative and should be looked at further."[4]

Frederica Perera, D.P.H., at the School of Public Health at the Columbia Presbyterian Cancer Center in New York, reported in 1995 that carcinogens from cigarette smoking have been found in the breast tissue of smokers.[5]

Researchers in Japan found that wives of men who smoke more than a pack of cigarettes a day have a significant excess relative risk for developing breast cancer solely from passive smoke. They believe smoking could be an initiator of breast cancer.[6] In the United States, there are data to suggest that adolescent smoking is something to be concerned about in relation to breast cancer. Young women between the ages of 15 and 24 are showing the greatest increase in smoking. (In 1986, lung cancer replaced breast cancer as the biggest cancer killer of women.)

Alcohol

Although there are data to suggest that the consumption of alcohol can put a woman at a greater risk of breast cancer, questions still remain. A study published in 1987 reported that women who consumed a moderate amount of alcohol increased their risk of breast cancer by approximately 50 percent.[7] What that means is that if a woman's lifetime risk of developing breast cancer were 3.3 percent, her lifetime risk would increase to 5 percent.

Another study published in the same issue was conducted by NCI. That study showed an increased risk of breast cancer of 1.5 percent in women who were regular drinkers.[8] Another NCI study, also published in 1987, found that the women whose risk went up as a result of drinking alcohol were those who had started drinking regularly before the age of 30.[9]

In 1992, early results from a five-year study at Harvard University and the University of Wisconsin involving some 16,000 women found that women who had two drinks a day had a 50 percent increase in breast cancer risk compared to women who did not drink alcohol.[10] Harvard epidemiologist Brian MacMahon, one of the authors of the study, said, "This is the biggest study so far to confirm it."[11]

Another study by the Harvard School of Public Health was conducted in Spain.[12] Results, reported in 1993, showed a 50 percent increase in risk in women who had just one 8-ounce glass of wine a day, and a 70 percent increase in women who had two or more glasses of wine a day. At that time, Dr. Walter Willett, who is also conducting the Nurses' Health Study at the Harvard School of Public Health, said that there were some 30 studies linking the rise in breast cancer with a moderate consumption of alcohol. "Although the cause-and-effect relationship is only suggested," Willett said, "no other plausible explanation has been put forward."[13]

Why would moderate drinking increase a woman's risk of breast cancer? A possible answer is suggested in a small study done at NCI by Marsha E. Reichman, Ph.D.[14] She found that two drinks a day raised the level of estrogen in premenopausal women. Reichman says, "This is the first study to suggest that the mechanism by which alcohol affects breast cancer rise may be the increase in hormones caused by alcohol."

Homosexuality

Being a lesbian puts a woman at greater risk of developing breast cancer, according to epidemiologist Suzanne G. Haynes, Ph.D., at NCI. She collected surveys done on lesbians that asked about factors known to put women at a greater risk of developing breast cancer. Haynes concluded that lesbians have a two to three times greater risk of breast cancer than heterosexual women.[15]

A statement from NCI, following the release of Haynes's statement, said that Haynes's conclusions were based on an analysis of factors known to increase the risk of breast cancer, including not having children, or having them after 30, and heavy drinking.[16] Ed Sondik, M.D., deputy director of NCI's Department of Cancer Prevention and Control (DCPC), says, "There is no evidence that being a lesbian intrinsically increases the risk."[17] The reason there is no evidence is that at that time, February 1993, no study had been done measuring the actual incidence and mortality from breast cancer in lesbians.

Katherine A. O'Hanlan, M.D., associate director of the gynecologic cancer service at Stanford University School of Medicine, agrees that demographic information about the population is "entirely lacking." But that is just one part of a much more global problem, much of which involves the rights and treatment of gay women. O'Hanlan says studies document homophobic attitudes among many doctors and nurses. The homophobic attitude of a caretaker is often perceived by the patient and, as a consequence, the woman may stop going for a yearly exam or for screenings out of concern that she will not receive the best treatment or simply out of discomfort.[18] In one survey, 94 percent of the lesbians who responded agreed with the statement "You'd get poorer care if they knew you were [gay]." Forty percent agreed with the statement "It's like putting your life in someone's hands who really hates you."[19] Any woman, regardless of sexual orientation, who does not go for breast screening regularly (clinical exams and mammography) is at a greater risk of having breast cancer diagnosed when it is more advanced and therefore less likely to be treated successfully.

There is evidence that many lesbians internalize the oppression they experience, according to O'Hanlan. As a result they are more likely to overeat (be overweight), use cigarettes, and drink more than heterosexual women. In addition, they are also less likely to have children.[20] These are all risk factors for breast cancer. If some of these factors, such as overeating, drinking in excess, smoking, and limited doctor visits are linked to the oppression lesbians experience, they are risk factors that can be turned around.

A position paper on health care was approved by the American Medical Women's Association in 1993. Among other things, it called for research into health issues and recognition by all health care providers that homophobia is a health hazard and that "sensitivity to lifestyle and sexuality issues should be present in the interview, examination, diagnosis, and treatment of lesbian, gay, and bisexual patients."[21]

Milk

Early in February 1994, the drug bovine somatotropin (BST) went on sale. The milk-production stimulant, a growth hormone, is the first economically important product of genetic engineering to be used in farming in the United States. Besides raising a cow's output of milk 5 to 20 percent, BST has raised considerable controversy.

John Shumway, a dairy producer in upstate New York, told the Wisconsin Farmers Union that he stopped using BST after 34 of his 200 cows developed mastitis, a potentially severe udder infection. A dairy farmer in Michigan reported that two of his cows had died after he used BST.[22]

Monsanto, the drug's manufacturer, said that in the first 6 months of sales it received 95 complaints about BST from dairy farmers, including the deaths of 36 cows. John O'Hara, an FDA spokesman, said that the rate of deaths reported in BST-treated cows was lower than would be expected among the cow population in general.[23]

According to Dr. Samuel Epstein, professor of occupational and environmental medicine at University of Illinois Medical Center, BST could potentially put a woman at greater risk of breast cancer. He says there is evidence linking milk from treated cows with an increased risk of breast cancer. He charges that the FDA has ignored that evidence. The hormone induces an increase in an insulin-like growth factor, IGF-1, in cow's milk. Epstein says that IGF-1 promotes the transformation of normal breast epithelium to breast cancer. Epstein says he has notified both the FDA and NCI of his concerns.[24]

According to the FDA, "The suggestion that IGF-1 in milk can induce or promote breast cancer in humans is scientifically unfounded and misguided." The FDA says that the milk from treated cows has not been found to be different from the milk of nontreated cows.[25]

Occupation

According to some epidemiologic studies, the type of work a woman does may increase her risk of breast cancer. The Centers for Disease

Control and Prevention reviewed some 2.9 million women's death certificates from 1979 through 1987. The study found that professional women, such as executives, teachers, librarians, and religious workers, had the highest incidence of breast cancer, while homemakers, women in the service, farming, and transportation had the lowest rate.[26] Epidemiologist Carol Burnett says the most likely explanation is "delayed childbirth by professional women."[27] Paul Seligman, M.D., of the National Institute of Occupational Safety and Health also says that the occupational risk has more to do with the delayed pregnancies of so many professional women than the work they do.[28]

Silicone Implants

Studies have confirmed that silicone breast implants with polyurethane plastic coatings do break down and send potentially carcinogenic chemicals into women's bodies in small amounts. The research was done by Bristol-Myers Squibb, whose subsidiary Medical Engineering Corporation made the implants until 1991. Sibyl Goldrich, founder of the Command Trust Network, a consumer information group, wasn't surprised by the finding. "We have known for some time that doctors were not taking seriously enough the issue of polyurethane in our bodies. But the question is, now what? I can't imagine any woman with this cancer-causing stuff coursing through her body just leaving them in place."[29] The FDA says that 2-toluene diamine, or TDA, was found in the blood and urine of women who have the implants. TDA has caused cancer in rats when fed to them.[30] In 1991, the FDA suggested that the risk was so small that removing the implants might pose a bigger risk than leaving them in place.

That same year, implants without the coating were scrutinized as well because of concern that the silicone in the implants might also cause health problems such as immune system breakdowns. The FDA requested the removal of all silicone gel implants from the market. (See also Part V, Psychosocial Impact.)

It is an outrage and tragedy that so little is known about the risk factors for a disease that kills 46,000 women a year. Seventy to 80 percent of the women diagnosed with breast cancer have none of the "known" risk factors. And of those known risk factors, most are ones over which women have no control. There was tremendous publicity and lots of back-patting when a breast cancer gene was finally identified. However, the gene accounts for only 5 percent of breast cancer cases. Undoubtedly, over time, more risk factors will be identified and more fully explained. But for thousands of women each year, time is running out.

10

Prevention

We have to stop business as usual. We have to change the direction and really put our emphasis on basic science and prevention, and not such a large emphasis on treatment.

Susan Love, M.D., *director, UCLA Breast Center*[1]

We think it [tamoxifen] has the potential to prevent as many as 40 percent of new cancer cases each year.

Peter Greenwald, M.D., *National Cancer Institute*[2]

I'm quite concerned that this is the best idea researchers have got, giving a drug [tamoxifen] intended to prevent recurrence of breast cancer to young, well women when there's no clear evidence that it will behave the same way in that population.

Maryann Napoli, *associate director of the Center for Medical Consumers in New York City*[3]

Prophylactic mastectomy may possibly be the most effective intervention we have at the present time to prevent breast cancer.

Kelman Cohen, M.D., *Medical College of Virginia at Richmond, January 1993*[4]

Discovering the causes of breast cancer will be a major and significant accomplishment. However, that does not necessarily guarantee the elimination of breast cancer. Knowing what causes a disease and how to keep it from developing are, unfortunately, not always one and the same. The ultimate goal of breast cancer research is to find a way to prevent its development.

There are three types of prevention: primary prevention to keep breast cancer from ever occurring (which is obviously the best prevention); secondary prevention, which seeks to detect the cancer as early as possible so as to ensure the best chance of survival (an example is mammography); and tertiary prevention, which is reducing the rate of recurrence and disability in the women who have breast cancer.

The best way not to die of breast cancer is not to get it in the first place. The question, then, is why prevention research into breast cancer is so sparse compared to repeated studies on treatment, which has had a relatively small impact on the lifetime survival of women with breast cancer.

Before going into possible answers to that question, it is important to note that not everyone believes there is insufficient research into breast cancer and its prevention. According to Elaine Blume, with the National Cancer Institute Office of Cancer Communications, "It is ridiculous to think that all NCI is doing is making new combinations of chemotherapy. We've done incredible things with basic science — biochemical mechanisms, genetics, treatment." Blume says, "People like Dr. Susan Love who say that NCI doesn't promote study into prevention and cure simply are ignorant of what's being done."[5] Dr. Love has been critical of the way money is spent on research, contending that far too much money is spent investigating different variations of the same treatment. She continues to call for more research into possible promoters of breast cancer like diet, oral contraception, hormone replacement therapy, as well as genetic research, to identify women who are predisposed to develop the disease. Love says, "We have to identify the genetic markers for breast cancer and the molecular changes that lead cells to uncontrolled growth. We need to identify the environmental factors that cause these mutations." She contends that too frequently the responsibility for the disease is placed on the woman, for having a late pregnancy or eating too much fat.

"But," Love asks, "what of the societal causes? What about the carcinogens and hormones in fat?"[6]

One possible reason for the small number of studies on prevention of breast cancer is the belief of some researchers that, without understanding the mechanism of breast cancer, finding a way to prevent it is not possible. To many that sounds like a cop-out. For example, for years scientists theorized that smoking was a cause of lung cancer. The common response was that it could not be causing lung cancer because no mechanism had been found that linked smoking and cancer. At that time, the rising incidence of lung cancer was often attributed to better detection methods. It is now well established and acknowledged by all, with the exception of cigarette manufacturers, that smoking does cause lung cancer. As breast cancer advocate the late Rose Kushner so aptly put it, "We must always remember that yesterday's quackery may be tomorrow's breakthrough."[7]

Scientists and breast cancer advocates all have their own theories as to why research into the prevention of breast cancer has been minimal. In 1992, some 68 cancer and public health experts called a news conference to say that the war on cancer is not being won, and that in past years only one in 20 dollars of the NCI budget has gone into research on preventing cancer.

One more excellent reason for prevention research in breast cancer is that a large portion of the population does not have access to the best treatment. Knowing how to prevent breast cancer would make that almost a nonissue. While conducting primary prevention research will be slow and expensive in the short run, Davis says its promise is great and can't be overestimated. In the end, prevention will save money and lives.[8]

The Tamoxifen Prevention Trial

A major study in the prevention of breast cancer began in the early 1990s. The Breast Cancer Prevention Trial (BCPT) has gotten lots of hype, both good and bad. It was on the drawing board as early as 1984 but didn't actually start recruiting women until eight years later. The five-year $70 million study was designed to evaluate whether tamoxifen, an artificial anti-estrogen drug used to treat some women with breast cancer, can also prevent the development of new breast cancers. The trial is being conducted at 270 cancer centers throughout the United States and Canada.

When BCPT started enrolling women in April 1992, the immediate response from women wanting to participate exceeded expectations. During the first four months, about 60 women each day applied to enter the study. The goal is eventual enrollment of some 16,000 women in the trial. As of June 1993, some 50,000 women had volunteered. During the screening of those women for eligibility to take part in the study, 100 cases of existing breast cancer were found.

At times it looked as though the trial would never get underway. A month before it was scheduled to start, two researchers at the University of Texas Medical Branch in Galveston reported that female rats given tamoxifen had indications that bits of DNA were damaged in their liver cells. The greater the number of injections, the greater the number of damaged DNA bits. The nature of the damage and the mechanisms of the damage, they said, "aren't yet known and require additional studies." They speculated that the damage might lead to mutations and other cell changes, "which must be examined as part of a safety evaluation of this drug."[9] The response from NCI was that the rat data was somewhat misleading because the rats were given doses far greater than those planned for women in the trial and rat livers also have many more cells capable of processing estrogen than do human livers, which could account for the damaged bits of DNA that were found in the rats.[10]

Another question raised was the cost factor. Could the United States afford to give healthy women an expensive drug to prevent a disease that many would never get anyway? Indeed, tamoxifen is expensive, costing as much as $90 in 1996 for a month's supply. As Devra Lee Davis points out, "Chemotherapy costs more in this country than in any other country."[11]

The following October, after the start of the trial, a congressional hearing was held. Congressman Donald Payne (D-New Jersey), chair of the House subcommittee that started looking into the trial before it began, said there was reason for further caution because "in the last year, new research has been published about the dangers of tamoxifen and new concerns about the study have been raised."[12]

Testifying at the hearing, Dr. Bernadine Healy, then head of NIH, called the study "precedent setting." She said that the study would assess the tumor-suppressive effects of tamoxifen and was a means of evaluating a lot of risk factors for breast cancer in women in the study, including family history in at least one first-degree relative, reproductive factors such as early first period, late menopause, late first birth, no children, biopsy of benign breast disease with excessive growth and/or atypical cells. Healy cited estimates that tamoxifen could reduce the incidence of breast cancer in women at risk by 30 to 50 percent.

Another enthusiastic supporter was Victor Vogel, M.D., director of the Breast Special Risk Clinic at M. D. Anderson Cancer Center, University of Texas in Houston. He pointed out that prior to the approval, the study had undergone extensive evaluation and a long approval time. "No trial that I know of has ever had better preliminary data and substantiation to begin studying humans than this [prevention] trial has," Vogel said. He also urged that tamoxifen be prescribed as a preventive measure only for women participating in the clinical trial.[13]

When women began taking tamoxifen for the treatment of breast cancer, there had been concern that they would be at a greater risk of heart disease and osteoporosis, since the absence of estrogen in the body can result in a greater occurrence of those diseases. However, studies done by Richard Love, M.D., professor of oncology at the University of Wisconsin, show that tamoxifen treatment for breast cancer does not appear to put the woman at a greater risk of osteoporosis and heart disease because of the weak estrogen-like effect that tamoxifen has. He reported in March 1992 that tamoxifen increased bone density in 140 women by three percent.[14] Although that is less than the 5 to 10 percent increase seen in studies using estrogen, it is the same as the anti-osteoporosis drug etidronate. Other studies have also shown that tamoxifen slows osteoporosis, as well as decreasing cholesterol and, therefore, the risk of heart disease. Noting those studies, I. Craig Henderson, M.D., director of the Clinical Cancer Center at the University of California at San Francisco, called the tamoxifen trial "exciting." He said, "We're developing a therapy that may have the potential to deal with the three most common causes of death for women over 60: heart disease, osteoporosis, and breast cancer." He predicted that at some point women may consider taking tamoxifen instead of estrogen for postmenopausal symptoms.[15]

Many women who had persistently called for research into the prevention of breast cancer were just as adamantly opposed to this trial. Adrian Fugh-Berman, M.D., medical adviser to the Women's Health Network, who had already voiced opposition to the study, testified before the House subcommittee hearing, saying that "the women eligible for enrollment are not truly at high risk for breast cancer and tamoxifen is too toxic for use in healthy women. . . . While the benefits of tamoxifen for primary prevention are highly questionable, the risks are well-documented."[16] Arthur Caplan, Ph.D., director of the Center for Bioethics, University of Pennsylvania, said it would be the first major government study in which a substance known to have significant harmful side effects would be given to healthy people to get information about its preventive properties. He also expressed doubt about the premise that tamoxifen could reduce new cases of breast cancer by as much as 40 percent. He said that would depend on a 30 to 40 percent reduction in cancer of the second breast among women with breast cancer treated with tamoxifen, which may have no relevance for women who do not have cancer. The second breast of a woman with breast cancer has been exposed to exactly the same genetic, hormonal, dietary, and toxic influences that the cancerous breast received. "While our society commonly views women as collections of body parts," said Caplan, "surely using one half of a woman's body as a healthy control for the other half is taking things a bit too far." Caplan contends that while the benefits of tamoxifen for healthy women are debatable, its risks are undeniable, with the most serious being a fivefold increase in the risk of endometrial cancer.[17]

Dr. Samuel Epstein says that there is not "the slightest scrap of evidence that tamoxifen will prevent breast cancer. It is a powerful liver carcinogen and also produces cancer of the uterus." Epstein charges that women entering the trial are not really told the full risks involved. He says that the consent form is misleading, minimizing the risk and maximizing possible benefits. He warns that "participating oncologists and institutions clearly risk future malpractice claims."[18] Epstein charges that tamoxifen may actually be a more potent human carcinogen than is currently recognized for the following reasons:

- It is structurally related to DNA.
- It induced liver tumors in 15 percent of rats at doses equivalent to

the daily 20 mg low dose in human adjuvant therapy, and 71 percent at the higher 40 mg dose; the tumors were highly malignant.

- In Sweden, two of 931 women in Stockholm receiving adjuvant therapy of 40 mg dose daily were diagnosed with liver cancer; the Stockholm trial documented 6.4 relative risk of endometrial cancer.
- Very few women have taken tamoxifen for more than five years, so that long-term effects are unknown.

Epstein also claims that there is "no valid evidence that [tamoxifen] will reduce osteoporosis. . . . There's little or no evidence this will reduce the incidence of heart attack."[19]

Ellen Hobbs, a breast cancer survivor and advocate, had not been won over by the tamoxifen study when I spoke with her late in 1993. She noted that there were likely to be big gains for drug companies and few, if any, gains for women. Hobbs says, "There's a good example of where a pharmaceutical company saw an opportunity to create a whole new market for a drug that they didn't previously have. 'Let's try it out on healthy women and maybe we can sell it to them.' Do you realize how much money that would make for them? [Women are] ignorant if they're happy about the tamoxifen study, because they could limit risk by changing their diet. That would give them just as big a chance as tamoxifen and wouldn't be giving them a risk of liver or uterine cancer. The trouble is, people want a quick fix."[20]

In March 1994, new data emerged suggesting that tamoxifen may be riskier than previously thought. It appeared to have the potential of causing fatal uterine cancer. Experts assured women that the drug's proven benefit in preventing new breast cancers in women who have had breast cancer outweighs its risks and that the debate is only about healthy women taking the drug.

Trudy Bush, Ph.D., an epidemiologist at Johns Hopkins University, called the discovery of the uterine deaths "very frightening." It had been thought that any uterine cancer caused by tamoxifen would be easily treated. The finding that the uterine cancer can be fatal, said Dr. Bush, "was a surprise and is of great concern." She reviewed the risk estimates for the tamoxifen study because of her increasing concern that the study might have promised too much and glossed over the drug's dangers. Bush believes the heart disease benefit was exaggerated and that designers of the study underestimated the risk of clotting disorders and failed to account for another side effect, swelling of the macula at the center of the retina. In her analysis, the bad effects outweighed the good.[21] Dr. Richard Love said his analysis also concluded that the risks outweighed the benefits and said, "I think the study should be stopped."[22]

For the most part, those who had supported the trial were not swayed by the new data. Dr. Craig Henderson said the study should go forward since so many women who were afraid of developing breast cancer were already taking tamoxifen. He said it is important to see whether the drug is beneficial overall. "My concern is, if we don't do the trial, we're going to continue to use the drug." If the trial is not completed, and tamoxifen continues to be used, its role, if any, in preventing breast cancer and the full extent of its possible hazards will not be known.[23]

At the end of March 1994, recruitment into the trial was stopped, but not because of concerns over its safety. The discovery of falsified and fabricated data in some of the breast cancer trials being conducted in the United States and Canada by the National Surgical Adjuvant Breast and Bowel Project (NSABP) resulted in the NCI's calling for a temporary halt in recruitment into 14 cancer studies, including the tamoxifen prevention trial. (See also Part IV, Treatment: Slash, Burn, and Poison.)

At a congressional hearing in mid-April, chaired by John Dingell (D-Michigan), Harold Varmus, M.D., director of NIH, and Samuel Broder, M.D., who was then director of NCI, testified on the new data on uterine cancer deaths related to tamoxifen. When asked if women in the BCPT had been notified of the data on possible new risks, they insisted that the responsibility for informing patients belonged to the institutions carrying out the NCI-sponsored trials. They acknowledged that they didn't know for sure whether the patients had been informed but said they surely hoped so. Congressman Dingell said notification of the patients was a "simple moral question." Dr. Varmus replied that "all sites [had] been notified to inform the patients," but, under close questioning, admitted the possibility that they might not have been notified.[24]

Opponents of the trial again called for its end. Dr. Fugh-Berman was one of those angry about continuation of the study. "Both old and new information make it unconscionable to continue this trial. . . .

At what point do the risks become high enough to stop this trial?"[25] Cynthia Pearson, of the National Women's Health Network, was angry as well. "To let this trial proceed is to watch women die of trust."[26]

In early April, Zeneca Pharmaceuticals, the manufacturer of tamoxifen, and the FDA warned physicians about the increased risk of endometrial cancer. A letter sent to doctors notified them that the package insert for tamoxifen had been revised to update it on the drug's toxicity. Among things changed on the insert was the information that while most of the uterine cancers were diagnosed at an early, curable stage, there had been some deaths reported, and that, outside of clinical trials, tamoxifen should be prescribed only for breast cancer patients. Two weeks later, letters about the risk of uterine cancer were sent to women taking part in the study.

In the second week of May, the Board of Scientific Counselors recommended to NCI that the breast cancer prevention trial start accruing new participants as soon as possible on condition that measures be put in place to increase monitoring for endometrial cancer and to individualize informed consent of women in the trial. The Independent Data Safety and Monitoring Committee recommended that all participants receive annual endometrial aspiration biopsy in addition to the previously required pelvic exam, and that women interested in joining up or already enrolled be given individualized information about potential risks and benefits. The Endpoint Review, Safety Monitoring and Advisory Committee (ERSMAC), an independent committee of the Breast Cancer Prevention Trial (BCPT), recommended that additional endometrial monitoring be instituted.

In June, the FDA's advisory committee said the study should be resumed immediately. Charles Schiffer, M.D., of the University of Maryland and chair of the committee, said, "Losing the opportunity to evaluate this drug would hurt the group that probably needs it the most." The ruling meant that the FDA would not block resumption of the trial. The FDA panel also rejected NCI's proposal for annual biopsies, saying there's no proof that biopsies effectively detect the hard-to-find uterine cancer.[27]

NCI contended that tamoxifen's benefits still outweighed its risks and that it could conceivably prevent 133 cases of breast cancer while causing 83 cases of uterine cancer. Critics continued to say that tamoxifen could do far more harm, linking it to blood clots, and possibly liver and gastrointestinal cancers. They also say that uterine cancer in tamoxifen patients appears to be deadlier than in other women.

On June 8, federal health officials said it intended to continue the BCPT but held back on giving full authorization to enroll new women into the study. Officials at the University of Pittsburgh said they had received approval to resume interviewing potential volunteers for the study and to assess their risks for breast cancer. But approval had not been given to resume the selection of new participants. Resumption depended on completion of a revision of the forms that women must sign before entering the study, saying that they have been informed of possible risks.

The BCPT was officially reopened September 23, 1994. According to NCI, since then 40 to 50 women a month have been accepted into the trial, a great reduction from the number of women admitted before the trial was closed, which was about 300 women a month. Results of the study are expected in the year 2000 or 2001.

Prophylactic Mastectomy

A drastic way a woman can prevent, or greatly reduce her risk of developing, breast cancer is to have her breasts removed. Some women at particularly high risk of breast cancer decide to have prophylactic mastectomies before there are any signs of cancer. But even having both breasts removed is not a guarantee that a woman will not, at some time, be diagnosed with breast cancer. Prophylactic mastectomies do reduce the risk nearly 100 percent; it would be highly unlikely that a woman undergoing the operation would get breast cancer. But even when the breasts are removed, there is always the possibility of some minuscule amount of breast tissue remaining and that is what makes it impossible to offer any guarantee. Kelman Cohen, M.D., chief of plastic surgery at the Medical College of Virginia in Richmond, says that one of his patients who underwent a prophylactic mastectomy developed breast cancer afterward, and that he knows of several other women to whom this has happened as well.[28]

There was a period of time when it was not unusual for a woman to undergo prophylactic mastectomy. According to Dr. Cohen, in the late 1970s and early 1980s, many mastectomies that were not needed were performed because symptoms were misread. Women were incorrectly diagnosed with breast cancer or told they had fibrocystic disease, "which," says Cohen, "is really a wastebasket diagnosis now in disfavor because it refers to a plethora of conditions, most of which are benign."[29]

Someone who has been an eyewitness to, and even participant in, the overenthusiasm for prophylactic mastectomy is John R. Jarrett, M.D., a plastic and reconstructive surgeon in Eugene, Oregon. During the 1970s and 1980s, Jarrett performed some 500 prophylactic mastectomies on healthy women. He says, "There are a lot of things that we know now that we didn't know in the late '70s," and that going by the standards of 1993, he probably would have performed only half that number. He notes improved mammographic techniques and greater knowledge and understanding of benign conditions.[30]

Dr. Marc Lippman, director of the Vincent T. Lombardi Cancer Research Center at Georgetown University, says about a dozen prophylactic mastectomies are done each year at the center. He says women should be made aware of all their options before undergoing the procedure, but believes there are situations in which prophylactic mastectomy may be the best solution.[31]

Mary Jo Kahn was diagnosed with breast cancer at the age of 39. She saw her mother die of breast cancer at the age of 47 after being diagnosed at the age of 39. She says that she was 14 when her mother was diagnosed and that her mother told her that they'd gotten the cancer early and she wouldn't die. She had a radical and disabling mastectomy and underwent chemotherapy. Kahn says,

> It was a time of silence. After two years she had a recurrence. Then she had another recurrence and died at forty-seven. I was twenty-one, my older sister was twenty-three. It was traumatic for all of us. We felt emotionally orphaned when she died. Our father really wasn't there for us. We all knew we were at risk. While I was in the hospital, my older sister was diagnosed with breast cancer. While we were on chemo, my younger sister and her husband came up. They were adamant that this not happen to her. She checked with many doctors. In the end she had five doctors she conferred with. None said to do it. They said it was a viable option. In the end, when she decided to do the prophylactic mastectomy, she went to a surgeon who said, "I would have never told you to do it, but I'm delighted you're doing it."

The mammograms for my other younger sister were impossible to read. After she had her second biopsy she started looking into prophylactic mastectomy. She had it when she was thirty-three. She was tired of biopsies. Both sisters are happy with it.[32]

There are some doctors who advocate prophylactic mastectomy for any woman with two immediate family members diagnosed with breast cancer before menopause, but both critics and supporters agree that prophylactic mastectomy is a very radical option to prevent the development of breast cancer. Most physicians are reluctant to recommend it and do not like to perform it. Susan Love, who is one of those physicians, acknowledges that she has performed a few prophylactic mastectomies in her practice, but only after much time is spent with the woman going over her breast cancer risk and the other options open to her, such as very close observation. Love is concerned that that is not always the case and that there may be women undergoing this procedure unnecessarily. She says, "I think a lot of times women are being sold a bill of goods, and that worries me." Love adds that there have been no studies and consequently no data to show that the procedure really does reduce risk. She acknowledges that intuitively it makes sense, but "a lot of things in medicine that are later proven wrong or harmful, like DES [diethylstilbestrol, the drug given to prevent miscarriage and later found to cause cancer], made sense at the time."[33]

Vitamin A

Many laboratory studies on rats have shown and continue to show that retinoids (vitamin A or synthetics of vitamin A) at high doses reduce breast cancer. Adrianne Rogers, M.D., Department of Pathology, Boston University School of Medicine, explains that the dose of vitamin A given the rats was extremely high, as much as 300 times the requirement, and that given to humans at that level, it would be very toxic. But she says there are many studies being done with different synthetic retinoids in hopes of finding ones that will reduce the risk of breast cancer without toxic effects.[34] The chief obstacle in terms of long-term use of retinoids for the prevention of breast cancer is toxicity, as most accumulate in the liver and can cause liver failure. A relatively nontoxic retinoid called fenretinide has been developed and is being investigated in a long-term clinical trial for its effectiveness in preventing second primary breast tumors.

Clifford Welsch, Ph.D., at the Department of Pharmacology and Toxicology, Michigan State University, says that studies using lower levels of vitamin A had no effect, that near-toxic levels are required to get an antitumor effect in animals. Welsch calls retinoids a "double-edged sword" because of the studies that show retinoids inhibiting tumor growth and other studies showing retinoids exciting and enhancing the tumor process. In 1992 a study was conducted in which large doses of retinoids were given to human subjects. There were no apparent serious side effects, other than occasional night blindness that was relatively easily reversed.[35]

Diet

Diet has remained controversial in its possible role in affecting the inhibition and development of breast cancer. ICZ, a chemical by-product of a compound found in broccoli, cabbage, brussels sprouts, and cauliflower, can inhibit breast cancer tumor growth by acting as an anti-estrogen. However, it can also promote tumor growth by mimicking the effects of estrogen, according to Hong Liu, Ph.D., at Texas A&M University. In a laboratory study, he measured the estrogenic and anti-estrogenic effects of ICZ on human breast cancer cells and found both effects. The authors of the study believe that environmental estrogens may contribute to some breast cancer but say that much more information is needed on dietary levels, potencies, and the interactive effects of estrogenic and anti-estrogenic chemicals.[36] Barry R. Goldin, Ph.D., at Tufts University School of Medicine, says that what needs to be studied is which compounds have a higher anti-estrogenic effect than estrogenic effect in order to prevent or treat estrogen-related cancers such as breast cancer.[37]

A study of women in Greece found that women of all ages who ate the most vegetables had a 48 percent lower cancer risk than those who ate the fewest vegetables. And women who ate the most fruits reduced their breast cancer risk 32 percent compared with women who ate the least amount of fruits. The study, published early in 1995, supported similar findings in some previously conducted half-dozen studies in several countries. Harvard epidemiologist Dimitrios Trichopoulos, who coauthored the Greek study, said, "Even though diet doesn't go to the root of the breast cancer problem, the findings of the various studies indicate that a prudent diet containing plenty of vegetables with olive oil may lower the risk of this disease." The same study found that consumption of olive oil reduced the risk of breast cancer. Trichopoulos pointed out that the Greek women who consumed the smaller amounts of olive oil still had much more in their diets than their counterparts in the United States and predicted that American women could conceivably lower their risk of breast cancer by as much as 50 percent if they consumed more olive oil and decreased their intake of other fats.[38]

Some studies have indicated that the low incidence of breast cancer in Asian women who do not leave their homeland may be a result of a diet consisting of large-scale consumption of soybeans and soybean products. In the United States, most soybeans are consumed by domesticated animals. Soybeans make up a very small part, if any, of the average American's diet. A study published in 1990 found that soybeans in the diets of rats resulted in the chemoprevention of mammary tumors, suggesting that the active substances in soybeans are the phytoestrogens potentially acting as inhibitors of estrogenic action.[39] (Phytoestrogens are compounds in plants that act like estrogens.) A study of Chinese women in Singapore concluded that soy products may protect against breast cancer in premenopausal women. Besides soy products, high intakes of polyunsaturated fatty acids and beta-carotene were also associated with a decreased risk of breast cancer.[40]

At a September 1994 symposium of international scientists, the possibilities of a diet rich in soybean products and other plant-based foods that contain phytoestrogens were discussed. The agent getting the most attention was genistein, a soybean component, that is an isoflavonoid (a compound that has about 0.5 percent of the activity of natural estrogens). Coral A. Lamartiniere, Ph.D., a researcher at the University of Alabama's Department of Pharmacology and Toxicology, claimed to have evidence that genistein retarded the development of breast tumors in female rats. Steven Barnes, Ph.D., at the University of Alabama, said the impact of phytoestrogens on estrogen-sensitive diseases such as breast cancer has not been studied in detail, but several researchers said the effects of phytoestrogens on the treatment of breast cancer should be of high research priority. One enthusiast was Mark Messina, Ph.D., of the North Central Soybean Projects in Port Townshend, Washington. He said, "We know soy is safe. We could replace tamoxifen with soy." Daniel Sheehan, Ph.D., at the National Center for Toxicology Research in Arkansas, disagreed, saying that soy has not been proved safe. He said it could take decades to fully understand the compound's activities. Researchers identified the areas which should get top priority for research funding in order for the field to evolve:

- the actions of phytoestrogens that are weakly anti-estrogenic
- the actions of anti-estrogens that are weakly estrogenic
- factors that influence dietary absorption of phytoestrogens
- how endogenous hormones (manufactured within the body) and exogenous hormones (from sources outside the body) work

The researchers were in agreement about the need for much more research into the possible cancer-prevention qualities of soybean and other phytoestrogenic plants.[41]

Exercise

Women who exercise an average of four hours a week during their childbearing years will reduce their risk of breast cancer by almost 60 percent. That was the finding in September 1994 in a study on the benefits of exercise. The women who profited most were those who had had children and those who were physically active in their teenage years and early twenties.[42] Lynn Rosenberg, an epidemiologist at Boston University School of Medicine, said the findings could be "extremely important. . . . There's not any method at the moment that women could practically use to reduce their risk of breast cancer." And if the results are not confirmed, Rosenberg asserts, "there are a thousand other reasons why women should exercise."[43]

Some studies have shown that exercise may reduce the risk of cancer by lowering the level of hormones in the body. Other studies have shown that high levels of exercise in young women can delay the start of menstruation, cause longer cycles, or halt ovulation altogether, thereby lessening exposure to crucial hormones believed to play a role in breast cancer. A study reported by Harvard researchers in 1981 found that college-age women athletes were less likely to develop breast cancer.[44] Louise Brinton, chief of the environmental studies section at NCI, said it was a "well-conducted study that confirms what probably most of us would have believed."[45] The study results are only for women 40 years of age and younger. Leslie Bernstein, Ph.D., at the University of Southern California, the leader of the study, says that additional research on women aged 55 to 64 is now being done.[46]

As a result of pressure from breast cancer advocates and others, more research is being done on ways to prevent breast cancer. The tamoxifen study is the biggest commitment that has been made by the federal government to find a way to prevent breast cancer. If the study does prove the usefulness of tamoxifen in preventing breast cancer in some women at high risk, the fact remains that the drug is not without side effects. What is promising is studies of possible nontoxic ways of preventing breast cancer such as exercise and diet.

Part III

Mammography: Miracle or Myth?

11

The Revealing Photo

[Mammography] was indeed invented by a man, and I think there's a
good [tool] we could invent for them with a little of our money.

Susan Love, M.D., *director, UCLA Breast Center*[1]

I went to get a mammogram. At 20 years old I was rejected. They told
me, "Oh, you don't need to worry about it."

Dusharme Carter, Miss Oklahoma, *diagnosed at age 20*[2]

Mammography is a relatively new technique that was first used experimentally in 1913 by a German pathologist, A. Soloman. He X-rayed
some 3,000 amputated breasts and defined different problems he
found — tumors, microcalcifications, and irregularities in breast tissue. Based on his findings, he suggested that cancer in the breast
might be found before it could be felt by X-raying the breast. From
that time on, X-rays were used for that purpose *on a very limited basis*
in the United States and abroad.[3]

In 1930, Stafford Warren, M.D., reported in the *American Journal
of Radiology* on the potential use of mammography in the diagnosis of
women with symptoms. Seven years later other researchers reported
on the possibility of its use to detect breast cancer in women without

symptoms. It was many years before mammography was viewed as a real possibility for the screening of women for breast cancer.[4]

In 1959, a woman was referred to a surgeon by I. S. Ravdin, M.D., president of the American College of Surgeons, for a biopsy despite the fact that her breast was clinically normal. No lump, thickening, or abnormality could be felt during a physical examination. The reason for the biopsy was a suspicious mammogram. The mammography had been performed by Dr. Ravdin. The biopsy was positive. Ravdin became an advocate of mammography.[5]

Mammography in the early 1960s, which required long exposure times, resulted in an unacceptable amount of radiation and produced a less than optimal picture quality, in large part because all-purpose X-ray machines were used. Dedicated mammography machines (used only for mammograms) were introduced in the mid-1960s.

Other forms of screening were also explored, such as Xeromammography, developed by the Xerox Corporation. Introduced in 1972, the Xerogram was printed on paper. At that time, it provided a clearer picture than a mammogram. However, the development of film-screen mammography resulted in a more precise picture of the breast with less radiation. Xerography is now rarely used and the machines are no longer being manufactured. Thermography, another method that was tried, does not use radiation. An infrared camera is used to measure and display heat patterns. The method has a smaller detection rate of breast cancer than either a clinical breast exam or mammogram. Transillumination, like thermography, uses no radiation. It is based on the idea that light will shine through a breast but will be blocked by a lump. It has not proved to be a successful screening device. Ultrasound, which is also called sonography, is frequently used after a mammogram, when necessary, to get additional information. A sonogram of a lump that was seen on a mammogram can often show whether it is a cyst filled with fluid or a solid tumor.

In the 1970s, the technological standards for mammography varied widely, as did acceptance of mammography by women as well as doctors. And it wasn't always easy to find a facility that offered mammograms. Consequently, before 1980 few women in the United States were getting mammograms. As the amount of radiation exposure during mammography declined and reports of studies showing benefits of screening were published, mammography usage increased and it was no longer difficult to find a facility.

During the late 1970s and early 1980s, the supply of mammography machines increased rapidly. One study estimates that from 1981 to the end of 1990, nearly 10,000 mammography units had been installed.[6] In 1990, it was estimated that the limited demand for mammography would require only about 2,600 machines.[7] The underutilization of mammography machines is one factor that led to the frequently high cost of mammography.

According to the American College of Radiologists (ACR), in 1994 there were approximately 11,000 mammography facilities in the United States. At that time the ACR deduced that even if every woman who should be getting a mammogram under the current guidelines did so, there would still be underutilization of these machines.[8] In other words, there are still significantly more mammography machines available than are needed.

That raises another issue. A lot of money has been invested in those facilities, many of which are not operating at capacity. The *New York Times* has had, on a fairly regular basis, a full-page advertisement with a large picture of Whoopi Goldberg sitting with her hands under her chin, smiling broadly. Underneath in large letters the ad reads, "Don't mess with your life. Have a mammogram." Another line in the ad says that it is "a public health message from the following accredited mammography centers." The names, addresses, and telephone numbers of accredited facilities are listed. There are no guidelines given as to who should get a mammogram, but the text explains that a mammogram can often detect cancer before it has spread to other parts of the body and that early detection could save your life. The ad also talks of the importance of getting a mammogram at a facility accredited by the American College of Radiologists (ACR), which assures you of "the safest possible radiation dose . . . dedicated equipment . . . a highly trained, experienced medical staff." The ad goes on to warn the reader, "Don't take chances. Not all mammography facilities have been accredited by ACR. Make sure you have your mammogram at an ACR accredited facility." Nowhere does it say that the ACR program is a voluntary program, that the application fee for accreditation for the first unit is $700 and for any others at that facility $600 a unit, and that not having ACR accreditation does not mean the facility does not meet the criteria for performing high-caliber mammography. The ad also does not mention that there are many other accredited facilities in the area and that they can be located by calling a toll-free number. And it fails to inform women that as of October 1994, every mammography facility was required to have FDA certification. Without providing information about which women are the best candidates for mammography and where women could get more information about it, the ad is pehaps of more use to those who paid for it than to the women who see it. Unfortunately, the motives of some radiologists in promoting mammograms may be questionable and not always in the best interest of women. Annette Brown, M.D., assistant professor of radiology at the State University of New York, who is ACR accredited, says she got mail and a phone call asking if she wanted to be part of the ad. Participating in the ad four times would cost $6,000. "It's just 'business,' " says Brown,[9] who did not buy a share of the ad.

Up to 15 percent of abnormal lumps that can be felt in a breast exam won't show up on a mammogram. So a normal mammogram is no guarantee that everything is fine. Mary Katzke was 37 when she found a lump in her breast. The fact that her mother had died of breast cancer about ten years earlier just added to her concern. She went to a gynecologist, showed the doctor the lump, and related her family history. After examining her, the gynecologist told Mary that she didn't think it was anything but that she'd send Mary to a breast specialist because of her history.

> This man felt the lump. I was crying. I couldn't stop crying. I was a wreck. He patted me on the head and told me I was being paranoid because my mother had had breast cancer and that he was sure this was just fibrocystic disease and that if it would make me feel better I could go and get a mammogram so that I would stop worrying. Nothing showed up [on the mammogram] and he never said anything to me about coming back. So I waited a year till the next exam. For the entire year, I was feeling it and touching it all the time, getting more and more anxious. Then I went to a different doctor. I said to him, "Would you just look at this? I've had two doctors tell me it was nothing." He felt it and immediately flushed red. He said, "You're not going anywhere until our breast person looks at this. It feels very suspicious to

me." So I went to this woman, who gave me a sonogram instead of mammogram, and there it was. It also showed up on a chest X-ray, and I'm thinking why didn't the other doctor do those two things? . . . The tumor was one point one centimeters [it was malignant]. It was removed but had margins that extended out. I think if it had been removed when I first found the lump, I would have been able to keep my breast.[10]

Susan Honig, director of the Comprehensive Breast Center at the Vincent T. Lombardi Cancer Research Center in Washington, D.C., advises women to think about switching doctors if the doctor takes no further action on a suspicious lump that can be felt but doesn't show up on the mammogram.[11]

To some, mammography is viewed as a lifesaver, close to miraculous. It is frequently promoted that way. It has occasionally been touted as the best way to "prevent" breast cancer. That, of course, is ridiculous. Mammography does not and cannot prevent breast cancer. To many, mammography is mostly hype, misleading thousands of women. They point out that mammography can produce false positives as well as false negatives, resulting in unjustified reassurance and unnecessary anxiety. Each side has its zealous supporters. Virtually all doctors endorse mammograms for women aged 50 or over. And that is where any consensus ends.

There has been plenty of concern from women that mammography is oversold, and that women are being given a less than accurate message. In her 1991 article "The Politics of Breast Cancer," Alisa Solomon says that the public campaign for mammography can make it look like a "miracle" cure.[12] Judith Brady, an activist in California and the editor of the book *One in Three: Women with Cancer Confront an Epidemic*, says that there is a subtle message that if you're a "good girl" and get your mammogram, you won't be punished by getting breast cancer.[13] Noted breast surgeon Susan Love puts it this way: "The medical profession and the media have sort of colluded to make it sound like if you do your breast self-exam and you get your mammogram, your cancer will be found early and you'll be cured and life will be groovy."[14] Activist and breast cancer survivor Sheila Swanson is also critical of the message that's going out. She says, "The information that's disseminated by the National Institutes of Health

(NIH) and the American Cancer Society (ACS) makes women feel that all they have to do is have their mammogram and do their breast self-examination and they'll be saved. That is complete fiction."[15]

While it is true that mammography can detect a lump two years before it can be felt, by the time it's reached that stage, it's been growing in the breast for eight to ten years. During that time, the cancer has access to blood vessels that can carry the cancer cells to other parts of the body. It is therefore possible that when mammography detects something in the breast that turns out to be cancer, the cancer may already have spread.

Regardless of the controversy, early in 1995 mammography was still the best method available to women for breast cancer screening and early detection. Dr. Larry Norton, head of gynecologic services at Memorial Sloan-Kettering Cancer Center, says, "If everybody did what they're supposed to with mammograms, probably the breast cancer death rate would drop by about 30 percent — that's a lot. It still means that, *doing everything you can with modern breast cancer diagnosis, 70 percent of women who are doomed to die of breast cancer will still die of breast cancer.* I think that mammograms are extremely important but they're not the whole answer."[16]

Another means of breast cancer detection that requires no special equipment, is not in any way invasive, is done by a woman, and costs nothing, is breast self-examination (BSE). For years it has been touted as an invaluable tool in the fight against breast cancer. About a third of women in the United States practice it monthly and another half practice it occasionally.[17] Victoria Champion, D.N.S, R.N., F.A.A.N., at the Indiana University School of Nursing, calls BSE "the most controversial of the screening recommendations" because of the lack of data on its efficacy in reducing mortality. Nevertheless, she points out that the "overwhelming majority" of tumors are found by women themselves.[18] Cynthia Pearson, program director at the National Women's Health Network, says, "Maybe we don't have perfect knowledge about BSE because no one can make lots of money off of it, so no one wanted to invest the money to study it."[19]

There is increasing evidence that BSE done correctly can detect a tumor that is relatively small at diagnosis, according to Cornelia J. Baines, M.D., associate professor, Department of Preventive Medicine, University of Toronto. She says a study being conducted in

Toronto and Finland appears to show that cancer deaths were reduced by BSE.[20] The Finnish study followed 29,000 women who were taught BSE and regularly performed it over two years. The study found that the women's breast cancer mortality rates were 25 percent lower than in Finland as a whole.[21] A large, ongoing study by the World Health Organization indicates a significantly higher number of breast cancers detected among the women doing BSE than in women not examining their breasts. In the BSE group, the tumors discovered were smaller than in the control group. However, data on possible mortality reduction was not yet available.[22] Two major studies of BSE are also under way in Russia and China.

Polly Newcomb, associate professor at the University of Wisconsin Comprehensive Cancer Center, says, "If a woman is going to do BSE, she should learn to do an outstanding job."[23] Agreeing with that is Suzanne Fletcher, M.D., a professor at Harvard Medical School, who asserts that "women have to train and they have to practice — this isn't something that's easy to do correctly."[24] But Dr. Susan Love contends that too often women are not shown properly how to examine their breasts and what to look for, adding that "the importance of BSE in the containment of cancer has been greatly exaggerated." [25]

Since proficiency with current techniques is so low, Victoria Champion addresses the need for simplified methods of doing BSE.[26] A simple, inexpensive device was designed to do just that. The Sensor Pad, invented by Earl Wright and manufactured by Inventive Products, is made of two latex-like sheets that contain a small amount of silicone between them. When placed over the breast, it is supposed to aid detection of an abnormality. Its cost is under $20. It is available in many European and Asian countries but not in the United States, despite the fact that it originated here. In September 1994, the FDA once again failed to approve the Sensor Pad. In handing down its rejection of approval, the FDA said clinical trials had to be done to show that the Sensor Pad actually saves lives. But Wright argues, "There is no good way to do a human trial [because] there are so many variables [such as arm position and level of skill] in breast self-examination."[27] He says it would take a minimum of 82,000 women to produce statistically meaningful results and claims that in two trials he did conduct with simulated breasts, the Sensor Pad generated more accurate results than using just the hand.[28] He says the device is not meant to replace screening but to aid a woman in doing BSE.[29] At the end of the 1994 hearing an angry Wright said his company would work with the FDA "to see what we have to do."

In the nine years that Wright has tried to get the Sensor Pad approved, numerous women and doctors have praised it, saying it makes examination of the breast easier, less threatening, and more likely to detect a small tumor.[30] Mary Gorman of Chevy Chase, Maryland, says she found a lump using the Sensor Pad four months after a mammogram turned up nothing. She says, "I feel like it saved my life. . . . [Lumps are] easier to detect."[31] But not everyone agrees. Cynthia Pearson contends, "Inventive Products has persuaded a lot of women and influential reporters that the Sensor Pad saves lives when they don't have the proof to back up their claims."[32]

In December 1995, the FDA finally approved its use based on the results of a study done in Japan. The study found that women who were trained in using the pad detected their own lumps almost as frequently as did trained nurses who also used the pad.

12

Who Gets It

There's no question that mammograms for women over 50 work great, and yet only 30 percent of these women are getting them.

Susan Love, M.D., *director, UCLA Breast Center*[1]

Too few women are getting mammograms. The percentage of women who should be getting them, according to the breast screening guidelines that were in use in 1993, has been increasing. However, it remains appallingly small. Of the women who do get a mammogram, many get just one and don't bother to get another. A National Health Interview Survey (NHIS) in 1987 found only 17 percent of women over 40 reported having a mammogram in the previous year; only 36 percent of women 40 and older had ever received a clinical breast exam and mammography.[2] The statistics broke down as shown below.

Group of Women	Women >40 Who'd Ever Had a Clinical Breast Exam and Mammogram
White	38 percent
Black	28 percent
Hispanic	20 percent
Age 70 and over	25 percent
Less than high school education	23 percent
Family income <$10,000	22 percent

The NHIS done three years later, in 1990, found that the rate of women more than 40 years of age who had had a mammogram the previous year had doubled over the 1987 survey. Although the doubling is a substantial increase, it still means that two-thirds of the women questioned did not have a screening mammogram in the previous year. Another 38 percent of the women had never had a mammogram.[3] The Centers for Disease Control and Prevention reported that in 1990, 58 percent of women age 40 and older said that they had had a mammogram in the previous two years.

A survey done by NCI found that in 1990, fewer than 25 percent of women over 65 were having regular mammograms. The women least likely to get a mammogram were older Americans, women in rural areas, native Hawaiians, low-literacy groups, African Americans, and Hispanics.[4]

In an attempt to find out why so few who should be getting mammograms were doing so, the Jacobs Institute of Women's Health in Washington, D.C., conducted studies in 1990[5] and 1992[6] on attitudes toward mammography and its use. Martha Romans, director of the institute, says that in their survey, the number of women aged 40 and older who reported having had at least one mammogram went up from 62 percent in 1990 to 74 percent in 1992. But the major increases occurred among a very specific population — white women with at least a high school education, making over $25,000 a year. The study showed no change in the percentage of black women who had ever had a mammogram. Screening rates increased most in women aged 40 to 59. Screening rates for women age 60 and over declined.[7]

The reason given by most women (76 percent) for having had the mammogram was that their physician had recommended it. The other 24 percent had decided on their own to get a mammogram.[8]

Fran Visco, president of the National Breast Cancer Coalition (NBCC), was one whose physician recommended a mammogram. Her breast cancer was discovered in her first mammogram at the age of 39. "My doctor advised me to get a baseline [mammogram]. I was absolutely stunned. I was very uninformed about breast cancer. I thought because I didn't have a family history, I didn't have to worry about it, and then I found out that 80 percent of the women with breast cancer don't fall into a high-risk category — *why don't we know this?*"[9] Fran Visco is not unique.

The reasons women gave in the 1992 Jacobs Institute study for not getting a mammogram include:

- no family history of breast cancer
- no suggestion by the doctor
- the high cost of mammography (more women cited this as a barrier in 1992 than in 1990)

The study also found an increase in the number of women who followed the ACS screening guidelines. In 1990, 31 percent of the women said they followed the guidelines. In 1992, that number increased to 41 percent. However, just the opposite was found in women over 60, whose screening rates and compliance with the ACS guidelines declined.

Martha Romans told a House subcommittee hearing in 1992 that the women least likely to get screening mammograms were older women, minority women, and women of lower income and education. She said that special efforts had to be made to reach those women, and that a way must be found to circumvent the economic barriers that stand in the way of so many women.[10]

Those economic barriers can be insurmountable for some women. Isabelle Hammond, executive director of the American Italian Foundation for Cancer, reported that in Caracas, Venezuela, a woman can get a mammogram for about $10, while it can cost upward of $250 in the United States.[11]

A report done for ACS in 1992 came up with findings similar to those of the Jacobs Institute of Women's Health. It found that the women most likely to get a mammogram were middle- to upper-class, white, and educated. The women least likely to follow the ACS breast cancer screening guidelines were minority, low-income, and over the age of 65. Those women are also the least likely to be knowledgeable about mammography and its benefits. Of the women who did get mammograms, most said they went at the recommendation of their doctor.[12] An earlier ACS study in 1986 found that only 49 percent of primary care doctors had ordered mammograms for women without symptoms and that only 11 percent followed the ACS guidelines.[13]

Other studies have found the same thing. The Cancer Epidemiology Program at the Department of Health and Rehabilitative Services in Tallahassee interviewed over 700 women aged 40 and found that about half had had a mammogram during the previous two years. Of the 34 percent of women who had never had a mammogram, about a third said their doctor had never told them to do so.[14] Lawrence Bassett, M.D., of the Iris Cantor Center for Breast Imaging in Los Angeles, says one way to increase the use of mammography is to persuade doctors to recommend it![15]

Congresswoman Barbara F. Vucanovich (R-Nevada) is a survivor of breast cancer and a fortunate one at that. When she was first elected to Congress in 1983, at the age of 61, she'd never had a mammogram. She told me that no doctor she saw had ever suggested she go for one. The congressional physician Vucanovich went to when she first got to Washington after being elected urged her to get a mammogram. She got the mammogram, cancer was detected, and she was successfully treated. Vucanovich says, "My feeling is that I don't think a woman should have to be elected to Congress to find out about a routine mammogram! We need physicians to be better educated."[16]

At an ACS conference in August 1993 in Boston, it was reported that younger women, who benefit least from mammography, are more likely to get the breast X-ray than older women, who have the most to gain. Robert Smith, Ph.D., senior director of detection for ACS, said that older women, as well as their doctors, need to become more knowledgeable about the importance of getting regular mammograms. Half of the women diagnosed with breast cancer are over 65.[17]

Mary Costanza, M.D., professor of medicine at the University of Massachusetts Medical School, concurs, saying that the women getting the fewest screening mammograms are the ones who are at the greatest risk — while women who are at the lowest risk are getting mammography screening at a greater rate. One reason, says Costanza, is that women who are 65 and older have a low perception of their risk and are unaware that they're in the highest-risk group. They think younger women are more likely to get breast cancer. In addition, younger women have a much better appreciation of the fact that a mammogram could save their life.[18] (That's not too surprising, since public service ads on television and in magazines advocating mammography virtually all use young women models.) Ironically, as women get older, a mammogram is of greater and greater value for another reason as well. As women age, their breasts become less dense, making the mammogram easier to read.

Costanza says many doctors do not tell older women to get a mammogram because they are not aware that the average 75-year-old woman will live another 12 years. In addition, women who are post-menopausal are much less likely to go to a gynecologist as they get older, and the gynecologist is the physician most likely to recommend mammography. The older woman's primary doctor is likely to be an internist, family doctor, or cardiologist.[19] Robert Smith of ACS says those doctors are not well informed about the importance of older women having a mammogram. He says that in one survey of physicians, over half did not know that there were no upper limits for mammography.[20]

In late summer of 1991, the American Association of Retired Persons (AARP) sponsored a telephone survey to examine the rate at which women over 65 got mammograms.[21] Some of their findings were that

- Over two-thirds of the women called had had a mammogram at some time in their lives.
- Seventy-three percent of the women who had ever had a mammogram had the last one because their physician recommended it.
- Four out of ten women (40 percent) had had a mammogram within the last year.
- Women who had had a mammogram in the last year tended to be younger, wealthier, and better educated.
- Forty-seven percent of the women 65 to 69 had had a mammogram in the last year, as opposed to 33 percent of the women 80 and older.
- Forty-nine percent of the women with a household income of $25,000 or more had had a mammogram in the last year, as opposed to 37 percent of the women with incomes of less than $15,000.
- Fifty-seven percent of the college-educated women had had a mammogram in the last year, as opposed to 37 percent of the women with a high school education or less.

The survey also found that a little over a third (36 percent) of the women knew something about Medicare coverage of mammography. However, about half of those women did not know how much Medicare provided for mammography, how often they could get a mammogram, how much Medicare would cover, etc. (Medicare started partial reimbursement for mammography every other year in 1991. In 1994, the maximum amount it would pay for a mammogram was 80 percent of $59.63.) The study concluded that although the risk of getting and dying of breast cancer increases with age, the likelihood of a woman's having had a mammogram within the last year decreases with age. A study done at Columbia University in New York and reported in the *New England Journal of Medicine* in 1995 also suggested that cost was an issue for older women. It found that the older women on Medicare most likely to have a mammogram were those who had supplemental insurance that would pay for the part not covered by Medicare.[22]

Sandy Warshaw, a breast cancer survivor and a member of the national board of the Older Women's League (OWL), says the biggest issue regarding breast cancer for older women today is the potential limit on care because someone declares that an older woman doesn't have a long enough life expectancy to benefit from mammography and treatment. "I don't believe anyone should have care denied for any reason," she says. "I think, too, that older women in general, over sixty-five, are not treated well. We're either invisible or outcasts."[23]

Another group of women not likely to get a mammogram are those who are poor, medically underserved, and/or members of a minority group. Many studies have found differences between black women and white women with breast cancer in the stage of the cancer at diagnosis and survival.

As of September 1994, only nine states had laws mandating the establishment of breast cancer screening programs for underserved populations — Colorado, Kentucky, Michigan, Nebraska, New York, South Dakota, Utah, West Virginia, and Wisconsin.[24]

As cutbacks are made in federal spending on health care, the number of women who are denied access to mammography because of its cost will only increase. Those women who will be most affected are minority, poor, and elderly women.

13

But Does It Save Lives?

There's no evidence that the mammogram will help save a younger woman's life.

Cynthia Pearson,
National Women's Health Network[1]

It is well established that mammography can detect breast cancer in a woman before she or her physician can feel it by palpating her breast; hence, the cancer can be detected as early as possible, when it is most treatable. I don't think anyone would question that. What is questionable is whether the earlier detection actually saves lives. And that's what numerous studies have been trying to determine for years.

Philip Strax, M.D., and Sam Shapiro can be credited with starting the first major study of mammography in the United States in 1963. The Health Insurance Plan (HIP) of Greater New York Study included some 62,000 symptomless women aged 40 to 64.[2] The women were randomly divided into two groups. Thirty-one thousand were to receive mammograms and clinical exams. The other women were to receive only the clinical breast exam. Of the women chosen for mammography, 10,000 refused to have the mammography and did not take part in the study. After seven years of follow-up, the landmark study showed a 30 percent reduction in breast cancer deaths in the women over 50 who had had mammograms. No reduction of deaths was found in women in their forties, although the study did suggest that mammography detected tumors at an earlier stage than breast self-examination (BSE) in women in their forties. In the HIP study, mammography was able to detect 39 percent of the cancers in women 40 to 49 and 60 percent in women 50 to 59. The study is still widely quoted.

In 1973, ten years after the HIP study began, ACS initiated the Breast Cancer Detection Demonstration Project (BCDDP). NCI soon joined the project. The BCDDP involved more than 280,000 women, 35 years and older, in 28 centers. Women were told that the mammogram could detect breast cancer earlier than they could by examining their breasts and earlier than a doctor could. When breast cancer was found before it could actually be felt, it usually meant that the cancer was in its earliest stage, when chances for successful treatment, even a cure, were highest.

John C. Bailar III, M.D., who at that time was NCI's deputy associate director for cancer control, expressed some concern about including women under 50 in the project, for the following reasons:

- the known sensitivity that breast tissue has to radiation — and its cancer-causing effect. (*Other than a developing fetus, breast tissue is the most sensitive tissue to radiation in the body.*)
- the high dose of radiation women would be exposed to (in 1973)
- the cumulative effect of radiation damage
- the difficulty in getting accurate results from a mammogram on young women because of the density of their breasts

Bailar thought the screening in younger women might actually cause more breast cancers than it would find.[3] In addition, at that point the HIP study had shown no reduction in deaths among women in their 40s.

His warnings went unheeded, and the study, including women 35 and older, progressed as planned. Within three years, the highly lauded demonstration project ran into trouble. In 1976, the BCDDP stopped screening women under 50 after Bailer's report about the dangers that younger women faced from exposure to the radiation generated by mammography was published in the *Annals of Internal Medicine*.[4] The dangers were the ones he had warned of when the project was started.

Published in a respectable medical journal, the warnings generated a great deal of discussion and concern, especially among women. This time Bailar's voice was heard, clearly. Women under 50 were banned from the screening. Many older women dropped out of the study as well. Why was Bailar's first input and warning virtually ignored? Why did it take a journal article to get the ACS and NCI to eliminate women from the project who were under 50 — three years after the BCDDP was started?

Samuel Epstein, M.D., professor of occupational and environmental medicine at the School of Public Health at the University of Illinois Medical Center and chair of the Cancer Prevention Coalition, says that the radiation danger had been established even before 1973, the year that the demonstration project was started.[5] He says that significant studies had shown in the *late 1960s* the risks that radiation presented, especially in younger premenopausal women, whose breasts are highly sensitive to radiation. Epstein claims that there had been clear evidence since the 1970s that before menopause a woman's breasts are 40 times more sensitive than the breasts of postmenopausal women. In 1972, it was reported that for every one rad exposure to the breast, the risk of breast cancer would increase by 1 percent. The minimal dose given to the women getting the mammograms in the screening project was two rads, and could be as high as five rads. That meant that a premenopausal woman who had a yearly mammogram with five rads exposure for five years would increase her cancer risk by 25 percent.[6]

Epstein charges that the women recruited for the screening were never told the risks. At the time of the project, the amount of radiation received was considerably higher than in later years, when more technically advanced mammography machines used a lower dose, as you can see below:

MAMMOGRAPHY RADS	
Early 1960s	7–9
Mid 1960s	4–5
Early 1970s	3–4
Mid/late 1970s	1–2
1980s	0.3–0.4
1989	0.1

Epstein has a theory about why the project, which included women under 50, went forward in 1973 and why those women under 50 were not warned of the known risks. He says the project was viewed as offering advantages to both NCI and ACS. Epstein bases this on a confidential memo written by Nathaniel Berlin, M.D., a senior NCI physician, who was in charge of the project. The memo said, in part, "Both the [ACS] and NCI will gain a great deal of favorable publicity [from screening, and] . . . this will assist in obtaining more research funds for basic and clinical research which is sorely needed." Epstein contends, "Once again, suspect technology was applied to women on a large scale in spite of warning signals and with insufficient knowledge of the likely consequences."[7]

Cancer detection in the BCDDP project was high. In women aged 40 to 49, mammography detected 91 percent of the cancers, and in women aged 50 to 59, 92 percent of the cancers were detected. There was no indication, however, that the women in the younger group, 40 to 49, survived any longer as a result of the early detection of their breast cancer.[8]

The question of whether mammography increases survival in women under 50 was addressed in 1988 in a new analysis of the HIP data done by the NCI. The results suggested that mammography with clinical breast exam reduced mortality in women under the age of 50 as well as women over 50. The investigators said that longer follow-up (18 years) and more efficient statistical analysis were probably responsible for those new findings. Kenneth Chu, M.D., who was the lead author of the NCI analysis, said, "Perhaps the new data will encourage those people who do not currently advocate mammography for women under 50 to reassess their position."[9]

Bailar was doing no reassessment. He called the new analysis "seriously biased."[10] Swedish radiologist Laszlo Tabar, M.D., from the Falun Central Hospital in Sweden, said that the HIP trial had little relevance anyway because the way mammography was done during that trial and the way mammography was done in 1988 were so different.[11] There is no question that substantial improvements have been made in mammography over the years. Just how those improvements affect the findings in the study is a matter of opinion.

The United States was not the only country doing mammography studies. Studies of the efficacy of mammography were being done, and have been done, in Canada, Italy, the Netherlands, Sweden, and the United Kingdom. It is hard to compare the studies because virtually each has different criteria. Some compare mammography with no mammography. Some compare mammography with and without breast self-examination (BSE). Different intervals between screenings are used, and so on. As for the benefits of mammography on younger women, Kathy Albain, M.D., associate professor of medicine at Loyola University Medical Center in Illinois, points out that "younger is not consistently defined — it can be under 30 or under 40 or under 50, etc."[12] That aside, none of the studies definitively showed statistically significant benefits to women under 50. Annette Brown, M.D., says the samples were too small, although there seemed to be some benefit in five of eight trials.[13]

In 1993, the study that had the biggest impact, generating tremendous controversy, was the Canadian National Breast Screening Study (NBSS). It began in 1980, after years of debate and two years of pilot studies. The study was designed to include some 50,000 women aged 40 to 49 over a period of seven years. It was specifically designed to study mammography in that age group. A second part of the study looked at 50,000 women aged 50 to 59.

Preliminary findings of the study were released in May 1992.[14] The findings suggested that screening for breast cancer in women aged 40 to 49 showed no benefit. As a result of the preliminary findings, authors of the study advised against screening women aged 40 to 49.

The Canadian study was formally published in November 1992.[15] The findings were the same as the earlier preliminary findings — that although cancers were found at earlier stages, mammography showed no benefits in terms of reducing the mortality rate from breast cancer in women under the age of 50. There also appeared to be a slightly higher mortality rate among the women in that age group who were screened than the women who did not have mammography. Not surprisingly, there were staunch supporters of the study and just as staunch critics.

Even before the formal release of the study findings, the preliminary findings generated a good deal of varied and heated response. David Eddy, M.D., Ph.D., a professor of health policy and management at Duke University, said, "This study is important because it is the only one that is specifically designed to evaluate mammography in women under 50."[16] Maryann Napoli, associate director of the Center for Medical Consumers and editor of the newsletter *Health Facts*, talked about the "profitability" of mammography, saying, "Screening women has become a lucrative business. . . . Too many vested interests would not want to see the field of mammography candidates narrowed in any way."[17] There is no question that doctors and hospitals have invested millions of dollars in machines for mammography and in updating the machines and, as noted earlier, many mammography facilities are underutilized.

Napoli also contends that screening has become politically correct, that it is a good way for politicians to show their concern over women's issues. They can fund mammography programs for the underserved and minority women (which frequently are the same) and tell their constituents the good they are doing. But Napoli raises the question about follow-up. Once the women are diagnosed, what kind of follow-up is there? Will these women get timely and competent treatment? Will they get any treatment at all?[18] The fact is that many women in these mammography programs who are diagnosed with breast cancer do not receive any follow-up. And if they do get follow-up treatment, the treatment they receive rarely compares to the treatment received by women with full medical coverage. Brown's experience has been with the New York City public hospital, Kings County Hospital, which serves a predominantly minority population. She says that follow-up services are available in New York City public hospitals. But she adds, "Whether or not they [women with breast cancer] make use of it is another story."[19]

In 1993, several medical conferences were held in the United States, primarily to examine the findings of the NBSS and other studies, in order to reassess whether the current breast screening guidelines were correct or should be changed. The biggest question (and for practical purposes the only real question) was efficacy of mammography in detecting breast cancer and *prolonging survival in women under 50.*

In February, a *New York Times* headline read, "Early Mammogram Gets Endorsement."[20] Barely a month later, another *New York Times* headline read, "Studies Say Mammograms Fail to Help Many Women."[21] Both articles were written by reporter Gina Kolata. There were similar headlines in papers big and small throughout the United

States, reporting the different conclusions reached at the NCI conference and the ACS conference.

After its two-day meeting, "Workshop on Breast Cancer Detection in Younger Women . . . A Current Assessment," in early February 1993, ACS said it would not change its guidelines at that time because the studies and the testimony heard did not warrant a change. Walter Lawrence, M.D., a former ACS president, said, "We have found more than sufficient data to support the usefulness of mammography as a lifesaving procedure for women 40 to 50 years of age." He said the studies for which there were data were not conclusive enough to say without doubt that women would not benefit from early screening.[22] The people who neither liked nor agreed with the ACS assessment charged that the jury was stacked in favor of the current guidelines. The jury was stacked in another way. Of the seven doctors on the panel (five M.D.'s and two Ph.D.'s), who were assessing something of vital importance to women, all were male.

At the hearing, Gerald Dodd, M.D., head of diagnostic imaging at M. D. Anderson Cancer Center in Houston, said that the Canadian study did bring up the question of whether women under 50 should be screened with mammography but did not answer the question. He added that the American Cancer Society "does not exist in a vacuum and it's not in our best interest to further confuse women or their doctors [by changing the guidelines]."[23]

Dr. Laszlo Tabar quoted from preliminary findings of an analysis of five Swedish studies, which found a 13 percent mortality rate reduction among younger women getting mammograms. And while he conceded that 13 percent was not statistically significant, he noted other findings that he thought were. He said that there was no difference in survival between younger and older women based on the biology of the tumor — specifically the grade, node status, and tumor size. Tabar urged shortening the time between mammography screenings in younger women from every two years to 18 months at the maximum. He asserted that is the only way to reduce mortality in women aged 40 to 49. Tabar called the Canadian study "disastrous . . . with no statistical relevance."[24]

One of the panelists, Curtis J. Mettlin, Ph.D., at the Roswell Park Memorial Institute in Buffalo, New York, noted a number of methodological concerns in the Canadian study. He believed the results should be considered preliminary because there was not enough follow-up time. Previous studies had shown no evidence of reducing mortality in young women seven years after their cancer was discovered by mammography.

Cornelia Baines, M.D., coauthor of the Canadian study, came to the conference from Toronto. She had not been invited to be one of the speakers. She was given a short time to defend the study. She described it as "a study conducted at the major teaching hospitals across Canada." She said women in the trial would continue to be monitored for any delayed benefits, but that at this time there was still no hard evidence that mammography improves survival for young women. As to whether she would change the ACS guidelines, she said she could never recommend changing guidelines on the basis of one study. As a result of the evidence given by the panel members, the ACS reached the conclusion that, for the time being, the mammography screening guidelines should stay as they are.

There were many other critics of the Canadian study. Stephen Feig, M.D., who is the director of breast imaging at Thomas Jefferson University in Philadelphia, was an adviser to the study. He resigned from it in 1984, after serving just one year. He says that he pulled out when his recommendations for improving the study were not followed.[25] A review of the quality of the mammograms for the first five years of the Canadian study, performed by three independent researchers, reported that 25 to 50 percent of the mammograms were not of acceptable quality.

Dr. Victor Vogel, assistant professor of medicine and epidemiology at M. D. Anderson Cancer Center at the University of Texas in Houston, said the study is flawed for the following reasons:

- There was no special training for technologists or radiologists.
- A review of the mammograms taken during the first four years of the study found that half were of poor quality or completely unacceptable.
- An internal review of the mammograms by reference radiologists for the study suggests that interpretation of the mammograms may have been a problem, that some cancers were missed: 42 percent of 102 cancers were missed when the mammograms were initially reviewed but seen when the films were looked at retro-

spectively; 17 percent of cancers were found to have been present on mammograms two to five years before they were detected in the study.

- Biopsies were not performed in 25 percent of the women for whom they were recommended.
- Symptomatic women were included in the study.

Therefore, the Canadian study does not answer definitively the question of whether mammography under 50 is beneficial or possibly harmful. Vogel acknowledges that other studies show no apparent benefit in women under 50 but says, "I don't think it is possible, based on this data, to conclude that this settles the question of whether or not screening mammography will lower mortality in women under the age of 50."[26]

The NCI named its own panel of five to review data from eight randomized, controlled trials, including the Canadian study. Its report said that the trials show mammography screening under the age of 50 does not significantly reduce breast cancer mortality in the first seven years after the test and that there was an uncertain marginal reduction in mortality after 10 to 12 years.[27] The panel was not charged to come up with recommendations and it didn't.

In addition to those done in the United States and Canada, studies of the efficacy of mammography have been done in the Netherlands (two studies), Sweden (five studies), and the United Kingdom (two studies). In 1995, another meta-analysis was done of eight breast cancer screening trials, using the latest data available. The results suggested mammography screening could reduce the mortality rate of women aged 40 through 49. Combining all the data, there was a 14 percent benefit. When the analysis was done without the controversial data from the Canadian study, there was a 23 percent benefit to younger women.[28]

In 1993, Alvin Mushlin, M.D., at the University of Rochester, called the question of younger women getting mammograms "probably the most controversial issue in medicine today."[29] Dr. Daniel Kopans, associate professor of radiology at Harvard Medical School, says that controversy over mammography is primarily due to economics. Large numbers of healthy women have to be evaluated to find the relatively few cancers that will be detected. Kopans maintains that numerous studies show that mammography can detect smaller cancers at earlier stages and that an earlier stage is associated with a better prognosis.[30] And he estimates, "If you screened all the women in the United States aged 40 to 49, you would save 3,000 lives a year."[31]

The issue of cost was addressed by Dr. David Eddy as well. He evaluated breast cancer mortality rates for 1969 through 1971 in women aged 40 through 49. His conclusion was that any mortality benefit from mammography in women under the age of 50 was not cost effective in terms of the cost of mammography screening.[32]

By 1993, it was well documented that mammography could decrease the mortality rate in women 50 and over. Although mammography could detect cancer earlier in women under 50, there remained minimal evidence of benefits in terms of reducing the mortality rate. The debate and studies continued, with a major issue being what the guidelines should be: at what age should a woman start to get mammograms and how often? Also in question was whether there should be a cut-off age when older women should be advised not to get mammography. Virtually no studies have included women over 75, so its possible benefits in that population are unknown. With cost an ever more important factor, and Medicare a growing burden, it is unlikely that such a study will ever take place. Of course, the real issue is why we still don't have a more reliable, inexpensive, and quick method of breast cancer detection that will eliminate virtually all of the questions now being debated as well as the need for any future studies on mammography.

14

The Guidelines Guessing Game

Even now the ACS insists on proceeding with premenopausal mammography, when there's no evidence that it's effective.

Samuel Epstein, M.D., *School of Public Health, University of Illinois Medical Center*[1]

Is it reasonable to restrict access [to mammography] only to those age groups, ethnic groups, racial groups or socioeconomic groups that were specifically evaluated through clinical trials?

G. Marie Swanson, Ph.D., M.P.H., *professor of medicine, Michigan State University*[2]

The question of which women should be getting a mammogram and how often they should be getting it is still unresolved and controversial. The first informal guidelines were created in 1973, when women aged 35 and older in the Breast Cancer Detection Demonstration Project (BCDDP) were to be screened yearly with a clinical breast exam and mammography. That changed four years later, when women under 50 were banned from the BCDDP because of possible danger from radiation.[3] New guidelines were issued by ACR in 1980[4] and again in 1983.[5]

In 1988, ACR met with interested organizations in an effort to come up with more universal breast screening guidelines. Not surprisingly, a major area of disagreement was guidelines for women under 50. Twelve of the organizations agreed that the screening of women without symptoms should begin at age 40 and be done once a year or every other year. Two of those organizations, NCI and the American Medical Association (AMA), questioned the need for a baseline mammogram. The American College of Physicians and the United States Preventive Services Task Force disagreed with screening women under 50, saying the data didn't support it. The guidelines that came out of that meeting were as follows:

- Starting at age 40, women should have a yearly clinical breast exam and a screening mammogram every one or two years.
- At age 50, both a clinical exam and mammography should be done yearly.
- Women with symptoms or at high risk should consult with their doctor about the appropriate screening.[6]

The 12 organizations that supported those guidelines were the American Academy of Family Physicians, the American Association of Women Radiologists, ACS, ACR, AMA, American Osteopathic College of Radiology, American Society for Therapeutic Radiology and Oncology, American Society of Clinical Oncology, American Society of Internal Medicine, College of American Pathologists, NCI, and the National Medical Association.

In 1991, ACS reevaluated its guidelines and concluded that they were fine, with the exception of a baseline mammogram at 35, which it eliminated.

Dr. Susan Love questions just how both the original and subsequent guidelines were arrived at. She says, "When the American Cancer Society came out with their guidelines, they were just making them up because we didn't have any data and we wanted to give women some recommendations." And she says that everyone "jumped on the bandwagon." Love says the guidelines must be reassessed as new data comes in. Speaking at the time when the Clinton administration was working on a health plan, Love said that if she were setting up the plan, "I wouldn't pay for mammograms [for women] under 50 for screening."[7] Love's statement probably would not sit well with the many American women in their 40s who are fighting to get their insurance companies to pay for screening mammograms and who feel this is the only real defense they have against breast cancer.

As noted, in 1993 the issue of mammography screening of women under 50 was discussed at conferences held by the ACS and NCI. The ACS concluded that the guidelines should remain as is; there was not sufficient evidence to show that women aged 40 to 49 did not benefit from mammography. It appeared that the NCI would go the other way and eliminate women under 50 from its guidelines.

In an NCI survey conducted during January and February of 1993, 71 percent of the 1,100 women questioned said that they would be concerned if ACS and NCI had different guidelines for mammography.[8] If the guidelines were to be changed to recommend that only women over 50 should get regular mammograms, 85 percent of the women said that women under the age of 50 should continue to get mammograms just to be on the safe side; 63 percent said women should get mammograms more frequently as protection, regardless of the guidelines.

Meanwhile, there were constant discussions among women's groups, physicians, and politicians as to whether the guidelines should be changed. Ellen Mendelson, M.D., the chief of Mammography and Women's Imaging in West Pennsylvania Hospital, argued that mammography in young women is expensive and difficult to read because of the dense breasts younger women usually have. She pointed out that only 1 percent of breast cancer cases occur in women under 30, and 3 percent occur in women under 35. She said that the only younger women, under 30, who should get a mammogram are those who have symptoms and possibly women at a very high risk of getting cancer because of heredity. She concluded that "screening mammography probably, in general, is not indicated for the group between 20 and 34 because of the low cancer incidence, the breast density, and the greater radiosensitivity, which over a lifetime may lead to a cumulative dose of radiation that may be higher than optimal." However, Mendelson does recommend that any woman with a breast problem should get an imaging workup.[9]

Dr. Larry Norton not only thinks that mammograms should be done on women in their forties, he says they should probably be done more often. "Frankly, we're considering doing it yearly [at Memorial

Sloan-Kettering Cancer Center] instead of every other year because breast cancers in young women tend to grow faster." He is convinced that mammograms save lives. "The very week that the Canadian trial [showing no benefit to women under 50] hit the newspapers, we diagnosed two tiny breast cancers in women in their early 40s, both of whom had breast conservation and minimal therapy because the disease was diagnosed at such an early stage. Both would have had much more pronounced disease if they had not had mammograms. Everyone has anecdotes like that and the anecdotes are compelling."[10] Swedish radiologist Laszlo Tabar agrees. He had been doing mammography every other year on women 40 to 50 years of age, but now thinks the screening should be done more frequently since breast cancer in younger women is more aggressive.[11] Regardless of the guidelines, there are doctors and hospitals in the United States that recommend a yearly mammogram starting at age 40.

Many researchers are convinced that breast cancer is more aggressive in premenopausal women. At both the University of Cincinnati in Ohio and the University of Nijmegen in the Netherlands, researchers concluded that breast cancer in women in their 40s typically develops twice as fast as in women over 50 from a microscopic lesion, which can only be detected by mammography, to a tumor large enough to be felt in a breast palpation. Because of that, they argue for more frequent mammograms in women in their 40s.

William C. Wood, M.D., chief of surgery at the Emory University Medical Center in Atlanta, also thinks breast cancer in younger women is more aggressive. He says there is some evidence that tumors grow more rapidly in women under 50, and adds that infrequent mammograms in younger women may defeat the purpose. "If you only have a mammogram every other year," he says, "by the time you get the test the tumor might have grown large enough to be felt." His opinion is that it is more important for women in their 40s to be getting mammograms than women over 75, because younger women who die lose many more years of life than older women.[12] Other physicians agree, citing the frequency of other diseases in women over 65.

This argument is far from convincing to Dr. Mary Costanza, professor of medicine at the University of Massachusetts Medical School, who says that many doctors seem unaware that the average 75-year-old woman will live an additional 12 years. However, there is very little data on the effectiveness of mammography on women 75 and older. Costanza says older women must be included in studies to see if they do benefit from mammography.[13]

It is generally agreed that the purpose of screening is to lower the mortality rate from a disease. It's fine that mammography can detect breast cancer earlier. However, if that early detection means that the woman simply lives longer knowing she has cancer, and that she dies at the same time that she would have died had her cancer been diagnosed at a later stage, what is the benefit?

Mary Jo Kahn is a breast cancer survivor and advocate with the Virginia Breast Cancer Foundation. She does not believe that there is any evidence that getting a mammogram before the age of 50 prolongs life:

> I don't know that I'll live longer because I was diagnosed two years earlier than I would have been without a mammogram. If we have set up a false hope, that's a big mistake. We need to ease gently into any changes in guidelines. We need a transition period before we throw [the guidelines] out completely. We have to make sure we're doing the right thing. I am opposed to false hope. . . . I think the medical profession is confused and misinformed and patients are as well. The dangers of mammography to younger women must be considered. Once they determined that mammography done on my sister wasn't readable, why did they keep doing it?[14]

While the two major cancer agencies in the United States, NCI and ACS, were debating and finally sticking with their breast screening guidelines during the first half of 1993, 17 European breast cancer experts were meeting in Paris and discussing the same issue that April. Unlike the United States, most countries in Europe never recommended mammography screening for women under 50. The European Society of Mastology (EUSOMA) issued a statement that screening for women under age 50 should not be offered on a regular basis. Nicholas Wald, M.D., professor of environmental and preventive medicine at St. Bartholomew's Hospital Medical College, London, said, "It is clear that breast cancer screening is effective in women aged 50 years or older; there is uncertainty about whether it leads to a significant reduction in breast cancer mortality in younger women."[15]

Rumors were circulating in late summer and early fall 1993 that

NCI would, after all, change its guidelines. In November, the National Cancer Advisory Board (NCAB) noted that there was great controversy over the question and recommended that NCI defer making any changes in its guidelines until better data were available. That would mean that the current guidelines recommending regular mammography screening for women 40 to 49 would remain. It was assumed that NCI would follow the recommendations of the NCAB, and many women breathed a big sigh of relief. But to the surprise of many that did not happen and, in early December, NCI changed its mammography screening guidelines and issued the following statement:

> There is a general consensus among experts that routine screening every 1 to 2 years with mammography and clinical breast examination can reduce breast cancer mortality by about one-third for women ages 50 and over. Experts do not agree on the role of routine screening mammography for women ages 40–49. To date, randomized clinical trials have not shown a statistically significant reduction in mortality for women under the age of 50.[16]

The NCI statement did not end the controversy. Far from it. It only succeeded in further confusing women as to whether they should be getting mammography screening.

In January 1994, House and Senate subcommittees held hearings on mammography in the context of health care reform. Disagreements over who should be screened and when were rampant. The Congressional Caucus for Women's Issues had been trying to forge a consensus between advocacy groups and the administration, but even caucus members were not in agreement. The caucus did call for a broader coverage of mammography in any health care package, including mammography for women between the ages of 40 and 49, who would have to make a copayment for a mammogram. Caucus cochair Pat Schroeder worried about restricting mammograms to women 50 and older. "Sending women the message that some mammograms may not be covered sends the message that mammograms are not important — and that's a dangerous message." Congresswoman Olympia Snowe (now a senator), cochair of the caucus, said, "I think we should adopt standards that are consistent with those of the American Cancer Society." Senator Barbara Boxer (D-California) vowed that she would not sit still while the administration abandoned mammography as a screening measure for younger women. Katherine Alley, M.D., a surgeon at George Washington University, testified for ACS and said, "Until we have the answers . . . access to mammography should not be limited."[17] The bottom-line question for many members of Congress appeared to be, should the health care plan err on the side of saving money or err on the side of saving lives? The hearing afforded Congress an opportunity to question NCI on its decision in 1993 to withdraw from the 1989 consensus guidelines on mammography screening for breast cancer.

At a House subcommittee hearing held on March 8, 1994, Congressman Edolphus Towns (D-New York) lectured Dr. Samuel Broder, who was then director of NCI, on what he characterized as the mission of the NCI, saying, "Like it or not, you are the National Cancer Institute. Women are looking to you to tell them whether they should or should not have mammograms. You are the ones that set the tone." Towns also charged that minority women were insufficiently represented in the eight clinical trials that NCI used in the meta-analysis, which led it to conclude that screening mammography does not save the lives of younger women. "Only one trial was conducted on American women, and that was the oldest trial in the group with the oldest technology," Towns said. "I fail to understand how NCI can make this unprecedented move based on a science that evaluated Swedish, Canadian, and English population groups, which are lacking the ethnic and minority makeup of American women."[18]

Schroeder said the change in the guidelines "fits in with how the federal government has been treating women's health all across the board." She said there still were not enough women working in key positions at NCI, the National Institutes of Health (NIH), and the entire scientific world. "It's been a great all-boys club. It really has been a cultural thing."[19]

Breast cancer advocate and surgeon Susan Love described the old guidelines as "more the product of wishful thinking than good science, [which] became etched in stone." She supported the NCI decision that, she said, gives women under 50 the opportunity to weigh the benefits and risks and decide for themselves if they want a mammogram. As to ultimately who will benefit from mammography, Love says, "In some women cancer is so slow-growing that it doesn't matter whether it is found this year or next; they will live, either way. In others, the cancer is so aggressive they will die no matter when diagnosed."[20]

Critics of the change in the guidelines charged that the changes were brought about as a result of pressure from the administration as it sought ways to contain costs under the proposed health reform plan. The original Clinton health reform plan provided no coverage for mammograms on women under the age of 50.

Broder denied that charge, saying, "There is no political imperative or momentum to what we were doing. . . . This process has been slow and deliberate and it started in 1991 [before the current talk of health care reform]."[21]

Fran Visco, of the National Breast Cancer Coalition, called for an end to the debate and enough money so that a scientific answer could be obtained. She testified that NBCC wanted every woman [between the age of 40 and 49] enrolled in a national system of randomized clinical trials, testing different modalities of screening to determine what works best for this age group. As new techniques were developed, they would be folded into the trial design.[22]

Also calling for additional investigation into the efficacy of mammography screening in younger women were the International Union Against Cancer and ACS. The organizations proposed a large, international randomized study that would enroll 1.5 million women aged 40 to 42 and follow them until they turned 50. The U.S. arm of the study would include one million women.

But would a time-consuming and costly study actually be useful? Russell Harris, M.D., at the Limberger Comprehensive Cancer Center in North Carolina, has serious doubts. He points out that enormous efforts are under way to come up with alternatives to mammography, such as chemoprevention and identifying genetic markers. Harris says, "It is unlikely that screening mammography will be the long-term vehicle for controlling this disease."[23] By the time any study is completed, mammography may no longer be used.

Broder as well has doubts as to the long-term use of mammography. He said that mammography is a technology that has nearly reached its limit in the detection of breast cancer. "We do believe that some new technologies, such as digital mammography and magnetic resonance imaging, will improve imaging capabilities."[24] He sums up the issue of the studies and guidelines as follows: "There is extreme polarization and controversy in the scientific community. Many individuals of goodwill and of comparable intellect have looked at the data and have come to opposing conclusions."[25]

The critical report, "Misused Science: the NCI's Elimination of Mammography Guidelines for Younger Women," was published in October 1994 by the House Committee on Government Operations. It charged that NCI failed to follow procedure for consensus conferences, had an advisory board comprised of experts known to oppose mammography for women under 50, misinterpreted data from studies, and failed to provide documentation for crucial decisions. The report came out of the House subcommittee hearing held in March. The American College of Radiology praised the report and supported its findings. It was one of the most vocal opponents to the guidelines change. The report also criticized NCI's statement that "randomized clinical trials have not shown a statistically significant reduction in mortality for women under the age of 50," saying that most people "will probably interpret the statement to mean that mammography screening is not beneficial for women between 40 to 49." The report said that the statement caused confusion among all women, not just those under 50, and gave a message to younger women that they "do not have to think about early detection until they are in their fifties."[26]

In March 1994, the National Cancer Advisory Board recommended that NCI get out of the guidelines business altogether. The following December, it was reported that NCI was considering a conference to "reevaluate" the available scientific wisdom on mammography for women aged 40 to 49. To avoid any appearance of impropriety, NCI recommended transferring funds to the Agency for Health Care Policy and Research so that that agency could conduct the conference.[27]

Common sense dictates that the earlier breast cancer is found and treated, the better the chances are for a cure or long-term survival. And although some studies suggest that this is the case, most studies do not. If a woman chooses to start getting mammograms at age 40, maybe the prudent thing would be to get them yearly, since premenopausal breast cancer appears to be more aggressive. It is also probably prudent for any women who are at greater risk of breast cancer than women without any known risk factors to get mammograms starting at age 40, or even earlier. Unfortunately, there is no clear-cut answer as to whether women between the ages of 40 and 49 should get a mammogram. What is painfully clear is that mammography, with so many false positives and false negatives, is in the end a poor means of breast cancer detection.

15

Quality Control

Many mammograms will be read as negative when there is, in fact, a tumor. . . . Other mammograms are read as suspicious, leading to X-rays and unnecessary biopsies.

Susan Love, M.D., *director, UCLA Breast Center*[1]

Women will now have the peace of mind that when they get a mammogram, it will be the highest quality possible.

Senator Barbara A. Mikulski (D-Maryland)[2]

A mammogram is only as good as the machine it's taken on, the technician who takes it, and the radiologist who reads it. If any of these elements is less than optimal, the mammogram is likely to be as well. Besides being a waste of time, money, and anxiety, and causing unnecessary exposure to radiation, a less than top-quality mammogram can have more dire consequences. An incorrect interpretation or poor-quality mammogram can result in a false negative (cancer is present but does not show up or is not seen by the radiologist) giving a woman a false sense of security. If cancer is present and missed, by the time it is found it may be at a later stage and much less likely to be successfully treated. A mammogram that is false positive (in which it appears that cancer is present, but isn't) can result in an unnecessary biopsy in addition to extreme anxiety.

Testifying before a congressional subcommittee in 1994, Dr. Samuel Broder addressed the problem of a high false-negative rate in younger women.[3] Some studies have suggested that false-negative rates may be as high as 40 to 50 percent in women under 50, while in women over 50 the rate is about 10 percent. False positives are also a problem. According to Lawrence Bassett, M.D., director of UCLA's Iris Cantor Center for breast imaging, false positives range between 60 and 70 percent.[4]

It is not uncommon for mammograms to be misinterpreted and/or of poor quality. In the Canadian study, after looking at previous mammograms, it was found that 17 percent of the women in the study diagnosed with breast cancer had mammograms that showed the presence of cancer two to five years before those women were diagnosed and treated. Twenty-five to 50 percent of the mammograms taken during the first five years of the study were of unacceptable quality.

A study reported in December 1994, in the *New England Journal of Medicine*, found large discrepancies in the interpretations and recommendations of ten different radiologists examining the same 150 mammograms.[5] While one radiologist might recommend an immediate biopsy, another might recommend waiting several months and then getting another mammogram, and a third might tell the woman to come back in a year. The radiologists disagreed on the diagnosis 20 percent of the time. The study, done at Yale, suggested that it may be necessary to have specific criteria for the interpretation of mammograms by radiologists. It also questioned whether the training of radiologists to read mammograms might be improved. In the study, the radiologist who detected the most cancers recommended biopsies for patients, while other doctors told the women to come back in three months or a year. The radiologist with the highest detection rate also had a high rate of biopsies that turned out to be benign. Daniel Kopans, M.D., a leading radiologist at Harvard Medical School, said that improved cancer detection could be achieved by having two radiologists read every mammogram. He noted breast screening in Sweden that showed that "even among highly expert radiologists, double reading increases the rate of cancer detection by 15 percent."[6]

A false negative for any reason can have some very serious consequences. Betsy Lambert can testify to that. She was 48 when she was diagnosed with breast cancer in 1991.

> I'd had a baseline mammogram about three or four years before I discovered something in March 1991 and went immediately to have a mammogram. It showed nothing. I had an ultrasound and there was nothing. And I was really aggravated when the surgeon insisted that I go for biopsy [when nothing showed up on either test], which I thought would be needless surgery. . . . I really thought, "Well, a mammogram, it'll pick it up." . . . In the interim I had moved and everyone would ask "Have you had a mammogram?" and I would say "Yeah." I was just reading a book and rubbing my breast and felt something that felt hard, as if it were a bruise, but there was no bruise. . . . It took me about two months to go to a doctor. After having a clean mammogram, you just weren't in the same kind of rush. . . . It took me six weeks to get an appointment with a surgeon. Then it took me another couple of weeks to decide what to do. . . . [meanwhile] I did what they told me to do, not worry, so I didn't worry. But I'm sure they were worried, since they wanted me to have a biopsy. The thing that is terrifying is that I'm sure I could have walked away and procrastinated much longer.[7]

Fortunately she didn't. She had the biopsy, because by then she was getting worried, too.

Mary Strupp was also told not to worry. She had her first mammogram when she was 57. When she felt a small lump in her breast a few months later, she waited until she was due to have another mammogram to get checked, since the first mammogram had been "normal." Again, the mammogram was normal. When her breast skin dimpled, she went to her internist, who felt the lump, read the report from the two previous mammograms, and told her there was nothing to worry about. At her next annual mammogram there was a suspicious-looking lump. Two days later her breast, which contained a lemon-sized malignant tumor, was removed. When the first two mammograms were reread by another radiologist, they showed clear evidence of abnormalities that looked suspicious. Because her mammograms were not correctly read, she was diagnosed three years later than she should have been and with dim prospects of survival.[8]

The Food and Drug Administration (FDA) first took notice of

mammography following a report in 1974 by Henry Bicehouse, a Pennsylvania state inspector who had done some mammography surveys in the state measuring women's radiation exposures at different facilities. The report showed a few extremely high doses. "This was the first time there had ever been any real attention paid to mammography — how it was being conducted and what was happening," said Richard Gross, the assistant director in the FDA's Office of Training and Assistance.[9]

In 1976, the United States Bureau of Radiologic Health (BRH) started a free, nationwide service to ensure that mammography equipment being used was meeting standards in terms of radiation dosage. To use the dosimetry calibration service, the radiation facility simply had to notify the BRH. BRH would send a specially treated square to be exposed to the machine at the facility. All the radiologist had to do was mail back the square in a postage-paid envelope supplied by the BRH. The radiologist would be notified of any problems after the square was analyzed by experts at the BRH. It sounds simple enough, but in her book *Alternatives*, Rose Kushner said that the head of that program, Roe Jans, told her that relatively few radiologists made use of the service and added that in 1981 many mammograms were still being performed on all-purpose equipment rather than dedicated machines designed and built solely for the purpose of performing breast X-rays.[10]

In 1975, the Center for Devices and Radiological Health at the FDA started a national program in cooperation with the states called the Breast Exposure Nationwide Trends (BENT). The program's objective was to locate facilities giving excessively high radiation doses and to help them reduce the exposures. As a result of the program, radiation doses started to decrease. Richard Gross says, "Since 1974, the FDA has had performance standards for special-purpose mammography equipment so that mammography X-ray machines had to meet specific requirements, but quality and patient issues were left to state programs."[11] In 1985, the FDA conducted a survey under the Nationwide Evaluation of X-ray Trends (NEXT) program. Gross says that a wide range of image quality was found. "We found some images so bad that it would have been very difficult to detect anything. The problem was not with the equipment; the machines were performing accurately." The findings were given to the American College of Radiology (ACR). It was suggested to ACR that it should handle the problem.[12]

Ferris Hall, M.D., a surgeon at Beth Israel Hospital in Boston, talks about the great degree of training and experience necessary to do mammography and interpret it correctly. He says if all the women in the United States who fell under the screening guidelines went for mammograms, there simply wouldn't be enough skilled technicians and radiologists experienced in reading the mammograms to handle the demand.[13] (That was in 1986. A decade later it is still questionable just how many radiologists and technicians have the training and experience necessary to do state-of-the-art mammography.)

In 1985 and 1986, ACS and ACR formed a Joint Committee on Mammographic Screening. The ACR came up with an accreditation program in 1987. The goals of the program were as follows:

- Establish quality standards for mammography equipment, personnel, and performance.
- Provide a mechanism for mammography sites voluntarily to compare their own performance to national standards.
- Promote quality-assurance practices at accredited sites.
- Ensure reproducible high-quality images at low radiation doses to the patient.

The ACR accreditation program strove to ensure that the equipment used for a mammogram was dedicated, that the technologists were qualified and properly trained, that the radiologist interpreting the mammogram was qualified, trained, and experienced in evaluating mammograms, that the quality of the image and the radiation dose met national standards, and that quality-control practices were consistent and effective. As of 1992, ACR-accredited sites were required to perform and document the quality-control tests described in the ACR mammography quality-control manuals.

However, the ACR program was not mandatory. Facilities had to apply and pay a fee to be considered for accreditation. Accreditation was by unit rather than by site. The inspections of facilities were limited. And the only penalty for not meeting the criteria was loss of ACR accreditation or not getting it in the first place.

There have been startling and frightening exposés in the media on the quality, or lack of quality, of mammography. The headline in the

New York Times on February 17, 1993, read, "Mammograms Called Faulty in Nassau."[14] According to the story, a year and a half earlier, more than 200 women on Long Island had unknowingly received faulty mammograms from Padma Ram, M.D., an internist. Three hundred eighty-six violations of state procedure were filed against Ram for using a machine that exceeded the legal dose of radiation, produced mammograms of unacceptable quality, and was not registered in the state, and for using an unlicensed technician, who performed at least 255 mammograms between June 1990 and September 1991 after flunking the state's licensing test five times. The county could not notify the women who'd gotten the mammograms to get new ones until the case against Ram was resolved. At the time the article appeared in the newspaper, the women who had received the mammograms had still not been notified that their mammogram might not have been accurate. The radiation safety inspector who first saw the way the tests were conducted in Ram's facility in 1991 was appalled. At that time, he wanted to contact the women who had had mammograms there immediately. Officials told him it would require legal action.[15] So it was about a year and a half later that women got the news that their mammogram might have been useless, or even worse! Experts expressed a concern that a delay in telling the women could pose a health threat. Robert Kulikowski, director of the New York City Bureau of Radiologic Health, stated the obvious: "If there was a problem and the mammograms were not good, women need to be notified immediately. Time is of the essence."[16] In March 1993, Ram was found guilty and fined $170,000. She was also ordered to notify the patients she treated that they might have received a flawed mammogram and should be checked by another doctor. Mary Anne Harvey, Chief of the Radiation Equipment Section of the New York State Health Department, said at that time that the state was considering a proposal that would require doctors to get in touch immediately with patients when mammography machines fail to meet state standards.[17] The guilty ruling had no real impact on Ram's right to practice. In September 1991, she had obtained a mammography machine that met state standards and she continued providing mammograms.[18]

The highest percentage of medical malpractice cases in the United States are brought for the delay in diagnosing or the failure to diagnose breast cancer. In a review of 45 such lawsuits from 1971 to 1990, Patrick Borgen, M.D., director of the Surveillance Program at Cornell University Medical College, found that in 82 percent of the cases patients found a painless lump themselves with BSE. Only 50 percent of the patients were seen by the doctor for follow-up after they expressed concern. Eighty percent of the lawsuits filed by the patients who were referred for mammography after a lump was felt were a result of an incorrect reading of the mammogram.[19]

Most of the lawsuits escape public notice because women are in a hurry to settle and physicians want to avoid visible trials. Settlement agreements range from $50,000 to more than $2 million. In the past it was frequently difficult to win lawsuits because the doctor would say the patient would have died anyway. But lawyers say advances in treatment make it tougher for doctors to make that case. At the very least, patients can show that a disfiguring mastectomy could have been avoided if the breast cancer had been detected in an early stage.[20]

At a House subcommittee hearing in 1990, Congressman John Myers (R-Indiana) told of his wife, who had had annual mammograms. When she had a mammogram in December 1989, the radiologist called her gynecologist and told him she was okay but that she should return in six months. "My wife didn't wait six months, and in January a biopsy revealed a nine-centimeter tumor," says Myers. "The technician or radiologist who read those mammograms didn't know what he or she was doing. I brought her last two mammograms to someone here in Washington. An oncologist looked at them and said that we should have had her in here at least two years ago." Myers added that the facility where his wife had been going every year was not certified by the American College of Radiology.[21] That year, a Breast Cancer Screening Safety Act was drafted and introduced in Congress. It failed to pass.

The Breast Cancer Screening Safety Act was reintroduced in Congress in 1991. At a Senate hearing that November, testimony was given on the need for federal quality standards in mammography. A spokesman for the ACR testified that there was "still no comprehensive oversight of mammography." He said that in some facilities "untrained personnel" take X-rays with little professional support and "with equipment that is improperly used and inadequately maintained."[22] For the second year in a row the act did not pass.

In the fall of 1992, Congress finally passed the Mammography Quality Standards Act (MQSA). The legislation requires enforcement of federal standards for all mammography facilities. The standards were to be formulated by a special advisory committee. MQSA criteria is a combination of the ACR guidelines set up in 1987 and the standards set up by the Health Care Financing Administration for facilities to meet in order to receive Medicare reimbursement for screening mammography.

In December 1993, the FDA announced interim standards for facilities performing mammograms, subject to a 60-day comment period. The standards make it mandatory that each of the 12,000 mammography units in the United States pass inspection and become certified, have specialized, dedicated equipment and specially trained technicians, keep complete records of performance, and undergo annual audits. In addition, doctors must have read a minimum of 40 mammograms a month for six months, keep records of their mammogram results and post them, post information to let patients know where to go with complaints, respond to complaints within 90 days, and submit to annual auditing visits. The FDA estimated that the cost of compliance would be about $19,000 a year for each site, raising the possibility that some facilities might go out of business. Of course, that also raises the very likely possibility that the money needed for compliance will eventually come out of our pockets in the form of higher fees for mammograms or higher insurance premiums.

The new regulations also include standards for approval of the accrediting bodies that will evaluate the facilities and review films for image quality. The ACR is the main resource for accreditation, but states can set up their own accreditation programs. As of September 1994, 36 states had laws addressing quality control of mammography.[23] A much smaller number had their own certification programs: Arkansas, California, Maryland, Massachusetts, Michigan, New York, Nevada, Texas, and Iowa. Facilities in those states must still meet all the FDA requirements. The only mammography facilities that will not have to be accredited are those of the Department of Veterans Affairs. The FDA also established a National Mammography Quality Assurance Advisory Committee, which advises the agency on developing quality and personnel standards, and on monitoring the entire program.

The FDA will not do the actual accrediting but will oversee the agencies doing it — either the ACR or a state health agency.

On October 1, 1994, MQSA went into effect, requiring all mammography facilities in the country to meet the interim standards announced by the FDA in December 1993. As of October 1, almost 90 percent of the mammography facilities had taken steps to meet the deadline. At that time over 5,300 had been fully certified and over 4,400 had gotten provisional certificates good for six months.[24]

Joanne Mott, of the Public Citizen, an advocacy group, acknowledged that standards would improve but warned women they should not expect to see improvements overnight. The organization said it surveyed mammography facilities in Washington, D.C., that voluntarily followed standards similar to those under the new guidelines with some distressing results. They found radiologists who were not properly trained and a lack of quality control. Some of the facilities had machines in which the radiation was either too low to work effectively or too high, above the suggested maximum dose. Recommendations included making public the results of inspections of facilities so that women could rank the facilities themselves.[25] R. Edward Hendrick, Ph.D., who helped develop the guidelines, said, "We don't know how much sensitivity [of mammography machines] will improve with these guidelines."[26] Florence Houn, M.D., director of FDA's Division of Mammography Quality and Radiation Programs, noted that the FDA did not know what percentage of mammograms are currently not of acceptable quality. The information it does have is from quality studies performed in 1958, 1988, and 1992.[27]

In October 1994, the Department of Health and Human Services (DHHS) announced clinical practice guidelines on mammography that Secretary of Health Donna Shalala said would "empower women . . . literally save lives." The guidelines recommend that clinics notify women of their mammogram results within ten days, that follow-up be by the woman's health care provider or by the mammography clinic if the woman does not have a health care provider, that mammograms be performed only with modern, dedicated equipment, and radiologists and technicians be properly trained and licensed. The guidelines recommend that medical providers inform women that they should have a clinical breast exam as part of screening. However, the guidelines did not specifically say which women should get mammograms, saying only that mammograms decrease mortality for women 50 and over.

The FDA said it will use the clinical guidelines for its final set of regulations, which were to be issued by the end of 1995. The current Mammography Screening Quality Assurance (MSQA) certification requirements are interim.[28]

It is astounding and inexcusable that for so many years women went to mammography facilities that did not have to answer to anyone, other than an occasional attorney filing a malpractice lawsuit. The fact that there are finally recognized, enforceable guidelines is progress. However, it is now important to make sure that women know that the guidelines exist and that those guidelines are enforced.

16

Future Projections

I believe that if we can image missiles 15,000 miles away in outer space, then surely we should be able to see small lumps in women's breasts right in front of us.

Susan J. Blumenthal, M.D.,
Department of Health and Human Services[1]

We have great hope that [magnetic resonance imaging] will prove to be a very important adjunct tool for problem solving and evaluating breast cancer patients.

Beth Deutch, M.D.,
National Research Council of the National Academy of Sciences[2]

Digital mammography is the most promising technology for early detection of breast cancer.

Faina Shtern, M.D.,
head of the Diagnostic Imaging Research Branch at NCI[3]

Although mammography is far from perfect, it is still the best tool around for detecting breast cancer that cannot be felt in the breast. According to Beth Deutch, M.D., director of breast imaging at the Comprehensive Breast Center at Monmouth Hospital in New Jersey, four out of five patients sent for a biopsy after having an abnormal mammogram turn out to have benign breast disease.[4]

Research is under way to come up with a more effective way to screen for breast cancer. Dr. Deutch is involved with research into whether magnetic resonance imaging (MRI) could be that way. The pictures produced by MRI are many times clearer than those produced by X-ray mammography. Deutch says that radiologists who do mammography are excited about the possibilities of the new technology. In trials at Georgetown Hospital in the District of Columbia and Fairfax Hospital in Virginia, MRI appeared to be useful in women with very dense breasts, fat breasts, and breasts with silicone implants. In general, the younger the woman, the more dense her breasts are. MRI could define multifocal and multicentric disease better, as well as give better definition to the extent of disease, showing which women are candidates for breast conservation. It appeared that MRI has the potential of saving money by reducing unnecessary or unsuccessful surgery. Patrick Byrne, M.D., says a patient he saw had a negative mammogram and negative ultrasound. She was given an MRI and "a 1.5 centimeter breast tumor lit up like a Christmas bulb."[5]

NCI announced early in 1994 that it would fund a study to see if MRI could be used for the definitive staging of breast cancer and eliminate unnecessary breast biopsies and surgery. In 1995 a Request for Applications went out for institutions interested in being part of the MRI study. Funding for the four-year study was estimated to be $1.5 million a year.[6]

One new MRI procedure being investigated is called Rotating Delivery of Excitation Off-Resonance (RODEO). In a study of 30 patients, the sensitivity of RODEO was 94 percent, compared to 55 percent for conventional mammography. Seventy percent of the patients had multicentric disease that would not have been adequately treated by quadrantectomy (removal of a quarter of the breast). RODEO may be able to determine which patients with a presumed single tumor actually have multifocal disease. It can be used on breasts with silicone implants and in highly suspicious breasts in which mammography and/or ultrasound has not shown anything. Silicone-specific MRI may be useful in the absolute identification of silicone leaks suspected by other, less-specific imaging methods. Dr. Steven Harms, professor at Baylor University Medical Center, which developed RODEO, believes that in the short term it can be very useful in avoiding additional surgery by determining the real extent of the disease that was detected on a mammogram or by physical examination. He is optimistic that in the long run, with further technological advances, low-cost MRI will be available for breast cancer screening.[7]

Another technique being studied is digital mammography, which uses a computerized technique that displays images using an infinite scale of gray tones. Digital images could potentially enhance the quality of an image and even magnify the view of specific areas of the breast. Radiologist Daniel Kopans, M.D., at Massachusetts General Hospital and a leading authority on mammography systems, is optimistic. "Potentially because of digital mammography, we may be able to find more cancer and find those cancers earlier."[8] It is expected that digital mammography will improve the sensitivity of mammography, especially in dense breast tissue, and at the same time decrease the radiation dose of each mammogram.

In March 1992, NCI and the National Aeronautics and Space Administration (NASA) set up the joint NCI/NASA working group to investigate digital mammography. Joan Vernikos, Ph.D., director of Live and Biomedical Sciences and Applications for NASA, says it's not an unusual match, because NASA has been studying the effects of microgravity of space on the health of human beings. Many of the technologies being studied were orginally developed for aerospace and defense use. In the fall of 1994, a briefing called "From Missiles to Mammograms" was held on Capitol Hill. Doctors, government officials, members of Congress, consumers, and industry executives discussed breast imaging and early detection for breast cancer and explored how new technologies from defense, space, and intelligence programs might be used to improve breast imaging. One possible new technique is the adaptation of a high-speed method of detecting military targets to detect breast cancer. Curtis R. Carlson, Ph.D., executive director of the National Information Display Laboratory (NIDL) in Princeton, said, "Intelligence technologies have great potential to help with women's health." NIDL, which is managed through the CIA's Office of Research and Development, is investigating several possibilities, including the use of "computer-assisted" change detection to examine mammograms taken over a period of time and a technology using pattern recognition tools that could detect very subtle cues of cancerous tissue. That technique is derived from one used to detect small targets in reconnaissance imagery.

Speakers at the briefing said that the development of new, improved imaging and detection methods depends on the interest of industry. However, according to one industry executive, the financial incentives may not be there. Walter Berninger, Ph.D., at the General Electric Company, called the total mammography market a "peanut" commercially and estimated its worldwide market potential at $250 million. He pointed out that if companies involved in mammography put 10 percent of their sales into research and development, the total would be just $25 million.

Kopans, who moderated the briefing, said the money issue was "one of the things that has worried me for years. . . . There's not a lot of money in mammography." But he expressed hope that even though the big dollar payoff wasn't there, partnerships would find ways to do the research.[9]

The development of a computer that can potentially spot breast cancers on a mammogram that doctors have missed was announced in April 1995 at an ACS scientific conference. According to Dr. Maryellen L. Giger at the University of Chicago, it might find as many as half the cancers that radiologists failed to detect. She said, "It's like a second opinion," adding that it might be most useful to radiologists who do not routinely interpret large numbers of mammograms. It was to be put into regular use on an experimental basis at Chicago University. On the downside, the computer, called the intelligent mammography workstation, has a high rate of false positives.[10]

Researchers with a $3.28 million grant from the Department of Energy were looking at a plan to use a laser-based X-ray source, formerly used to inspect Star Wars components, to examine women's breasts. The project has been hailed by Senator Barbara Boxer as a prime example of how defense-conversion programs can apply military technology to productive civilian uses in the post–Cold War era.[11]

Another screening procedure being studied is scintimammography (SMM), in which an injected radioactive substance can show areas of rapidly dividing cells. Scintigraphy has been used in the diagnosis of cancer in many different organs, such as the bones, brain, kidney, and thyroid. In a pilot study using SMM to detect breast cancer, it was found to have improved the specificity of conventional mammography. It was concluded that further study should be done of SMM for the screening of breast cancer in the hopes that it will reduce the number of mammographically "indicated" biopsies that turn out to be negative.[12] The cost of the procedure is about $600, far less than a biopsy, which can cost anywhere from $1,500 to $3,000, and the equipment needed to perform scintimammography is already in the radiology department of virtually every hospital. At the annual meeting of the Radiological Society of North America in late November 1994, Dr. Iraj Khalkhali, associate professor of radiology at the University of California at Los Angeles, reported that in 147 consecutive patients who required biopsies for suspicious masses, scintimammography correctly identified cancer in more than 90 percent of cases. Khalkhali says, "If results are negative, we recommend that the patient be followed with periodic mammography or physical exam." Dr. Stephen Larson, at Memorial Sloan-Kettering Cancer Center in New York, said that the results looked good but that "it remains to be seen whether others will have a similar experience." Fifty hospitals in the United States and Europe started studies of the procedure in April, 1994. Results were expected in mid-1995.[13]

Positron Emission Tomography (PET) is a relatively new scan being investigated for use in the detection/diagnosis of breast cancer. A small study published in the *Annals of Surgery* suggested that PET scans could detect the breast cancer of some women better and earlier than other methods of detection. The study was funded by the U.S. Energy Department and Revlon. John Glaspy, M.D., a UCLA assistant medical professor and author of the study, said the preliminary results show that PET scans may prove to be useful as a supplement to mammography.[14] Randall A. Hawkins, M.D., Ph.D., at UCLA, is optimistic about its use in breast cancer detection but does not expect it to be used in general screening for breast cancer. In 1994, PET cost about $1,500, which makes it much more expensive than a mammogram.[15] PET measures emissions from a radioactive isotope injected into the blood and produces a three-dimensional image. As of 1995, PET was primarily used to examine brain and heart function.

Another possibility being investigated for the early detection of cancer is a blood or urine test. Laurie Locascio-Brown and Steven Choquette, at the National Institute of Standards and Technology (NIST), are trying to find a quick and inexpensive way to measure tiny amounts of estrogen by-products, which could be a marker for breast cancer risk or the disease itself. In July of 1994, Locascio-Brown got a patent on the device she invented that compares normal and abnormal amounts of estrogen by-products in a woman. Dr. Michael Osborne, director of the Strang-Cornell Breast Center, in New York City, said that the NIST test could play a crucial role in preventing breast cancer, if it is accurate. Although this early testing of the blood or urine can be done using radioactive material or sensitive analytical intruments, it is very costly and not practical.[16]

It appears that conventional mammography has gone about as far as it's going to go. If all the women 50 and over in the United States got regular mammograms, the mortality rate in women over 49 could drop 30 percent. But what about the women who could benefit from mammography but can't afford to get it? And the women who get one mammogram but never go back because they have a low tolerance for the pain they experienced while getting a mammogram? And what about the women under 50 whose breast cancer, generally premenopausal, is thought to be more aggressive?

Many women want to know when are we going to have a simple blood test to screen for breast cancer — as men have for prostate cancer — which would detect cancer long before it shows up on a screening device. It sounds like the perfect solution. It's cheaper and certainly easier on the woman. However, that solution just generates further possible problems. If breast cancer is discovered at such an early stage, how should it be treated? That question has been already raised by the "in-situ" cancers now being detected by mammography. It is not known which in-situ cancers will eventually become invasive and deadly. How would we know which women would benefit from treatment and which women would live out their life unaffected by breast cancer and die of other causes? That issue, of course, would be eliminated if we knew how to prevent breast cancer or how to cure it once it's been diagnosed.

Part IV

Treatment: Slash, Burn, and Poison

17

In the Beginning

A summary of the history of breast cancer has been a series of controversies.

— George Crile, Jr., M.D.[1]

Breast cancer has been known and recognized for thousands of years. The first known reference to breast disease was in the "Edwin Smith Surgical Papyrus" named for an archaeologist who discovered the ancient scrolls. They were written in Egypt sometime between 3000 and 2500 B.C. Described in these scrolls were cases of "bulging tumors." Some 1500 years later, another Egyptian papyrus described the treatment for the tumors as "with the knife" and by fire. In Mesopotamia, which is thought to have been the site of the earliest civilization, there were recorded references to breast disease. It was apparently routine procedure to cut out the diseased portion of the breast. Patients were given opium to relieve pain.

Hippocrates (460 B.C.–370 B.C.) thought the cause of breast cancer was menopause. Once the menstrual discharge was being suppressed, the breast would become engorged and eventually the cancer would develop. Hippocrates felt that it was "better to give no treatment in cases of hidden cancer." He thought that treatment brought on a speedy death, whereas omitting treatment would allow the person to live longer. So an ulcerated cancer in the breast would be removed, but a woman with a hidden cancer in the breast would be sent home.

De Medicina, written by the Roman Aulus Cornelius Celus in the first century A.D., was the first work to give a clinical description of cancer. "This disease occurs mostly in the upper parts of the body, in the region of the face, nose, ears, lips, and in the breasts of women. . . . There is a fixed irregular swelling. . . . Sometimes there is also numbness. . . . In certain cases they are even hidden from view; and in some the part is painful to the touch, in others there is no feeling. And at times, the part becomes harder or softer than natural." He also named four stages of the disease: malignancy, carcinoma without ulcer, ulcerated cancer, and a growth that resembled the flowers of the thyme and bled easily. And he concluded that the only patients who might benefit from treatment were those in stage one.

Early in the Christian era, the treatment of breast cancer was determined by the extent of the disease — whether there was or was not ulceration. The cancer that was not ulcerated was described as a bulky swelling, hard, and uneven, sending its roots inward over a great distance. Ulcerated tumors were steadily corroding and could not be stopped and therefore could not be removed. It was believed that women with breast cancer were doomed. The only time that surgery would be performed was when the tumor was smaller than half the breast and was not ulcerated.

The Greek Galen, who was born around 130 A.D., described a "carcinoma" as a malignant, very hard tumor which was a result of the congestion and buildup of black bile at a site within the body. This accumulation could take place anywhere in the body but was more likely to gather in the breasts of women who were no longer menstruating. Galen described the appearance of breast cancer as a swelling and distended veins — like the feet of a crab. He said that it could be treated conservatively or with surgery. The treatment for women under 50 who had stopped menstruating was to take hot baths, walks, and other external measures to start menstruation again so that the black bile could leave with the blood. Local treatment consisted of the application of various derivatives of plants and minerals. Galen claimed to have experienced some success with this treatment. If the tumor was a large mass, surgery was considered the only treatment that offered the possibility of a cure.

In his book *A Short History of Breast Cancer*, published in 1983,[2] Daniel De Moulin writes about the French surgeon Henri de Mondeville (1260?–1320), who also spoke of black bile in relation to breast cancer. According to de Mondeville, surgery for breast cancer was possible only if the entire tumor could be removed — and he generally advised against it, preferring instead purging and diet. He said surgical treatment of breast cancer should be performed only at the urgent request of the patient — and not until the surgeon had received a "substantial" fee.

The German surgeon Wilhelm Fabry (1560–1634) believed that breast cancer started with a drop of milk curdling in the breast. His treatment was surgical. He would remove bulky swellings in the armpit and cancerous lymph nodes as part of the treatment for breast cancer.

The sixteenth-century Italian surgeon Gabriele Falloppii, the discoverer of fallopian tubes, was very conservative in his treatment of breast cancer. He said that "quiet" tumors should be left in peace and that mastectomy was indicated only in some cases of ulceration. He recommended many medicines for local application. One he particularly recommended was mounds of marine fresh-water crabs, burnt to ashes or cooked in milk. If the pain could not be alleviated, he said, the good Lord should be asked to take the patient's life.

During the seventeenth and eighteenth centuries, a number of different theories emerged on the derivation of cancer. Pierre Dionis, an outstanding Paris surgeon, attributed breast cancer to the stagnation of lymph in the breast. Because most patients were between 40 and 60 years of age when diagnosed, he accepted the ancient view that the uterus played some role in the development of breast cancer. He also believed that the mind could influence the disease and its course. Since sorrow or anger were thought to bring about coagulation of humors, sufferers were encouraged to have a cheerful attitude.

During that time, there was some thought that cancer was contagious, especially cancer that was ulcerating. The Amsterdam physician Nicolas Tulp (who was immortalized in Rembrandt's famous painting *Anatomy Lesson*) cited the case of one of his patients who was suffering from open (ulcerated) breast cancer. It was thought that she passed the disease on to her housemaid. This served as positive proof that cancer could be caught from a person with cancer, and in some places cancer patients were not allowed in hospitals. This view persisted until well into the nineteenth century. Even today, late in the twentieth century, there are people who believe that myth.

During the eighteenth and nineteenth centuries, the treatment of breast cancer continued to be either conservative (purging, specific diets, bloodletting, and medicines) or surgical. Conservative treatment was generally the rule in early stages, as neither patients nor physicians liked the idea of surgical intervention. An example of this was the treatment, in 1664, of Queen Anne of Austria, mother of King Louis XIV of France. She sent for her personal physician to examine a small solid nodule in her left breast. He recognized its true character immediately but apparently followed the advice of Hippocrates, who felt that it was "better to give no treatment in cases of hidden cancer." The queen mother then followed the advice of her maids and applied compresses saturated in the juice of hemlock to her diseased breast. But the lump kept increasing in size, and the queen mother grew weaker. The king's personal physician was then called. He substituted ointments for the compresses. But that did no good and not long after, the breast burst open and a huge ulcer appeared. Another doctor treated the queen mother with arsenic and the necrotic parts were cut off daily. Queen Anne suffered enormous pain and died some twenty months after the first symptom of the disease had appeared.

In the eighteenth century, local causes of breast cancer were considered to be mainly of a mechanical nature — for example, a bruise resulting from a fall or blow, pressure caused by garments like the tight bodice introduced by Madame de Pompadour, the application of medicines or compresses or, as the well-known Paris surgeon Jean Astruc hypothesized, the compliance with which women allowed their breasts to be taken and handled, exposing them to compression that could result in breast cancer.

There were many points of view as to how a tumor became malignant. In the eighteenth century, theories about the causes of malignancy included menopause, psychic influences, family predisposition, childlessness, a sedentary life, bad dietary habits, late nights, and the consumption of alcohol and coffee. Some of those theories have a familiar ring and are still being investigated today.

Although there was not much support from surgeons for the heredity theory, that was not necessarily the case among women. A nineteen-year-old French nun refused treatment for breast cancer because her grandmother and great-uncle had both died of cancer, and she assumed that surgery could be of no help, since she carried the cancer poison.

The idea of cancer being able to metastasize (spread to other parts of the body) appeared in the early eighteenth century. According to le Dran, the cancerous fluid in the breast could find its way to the blood and lymph systems and travel to other places, such as the lungs, brain, and bones. Le Dran thought that although breast cancer developed locally, its presence might cause general irritation resulting in a cancerous disposition in the body that eventually resulted in cancer elsewhere.

There were virtually no statistics kept on breast cancer during this period, although le Dran wrote that it was a common disease. There were case studies, especially of women who survived longer than expected. The explanation of one surgeon was that differences existed between bodies and between cancers.

Diagnosis of breast cancer during the eighteenth century usually consisted of simple observation. A woman would come in with a foul-smelling and ulcerating breast and experiencing excessive pain. A physical exam would be confined to the affected breast and the area right around it. If the tumor was smooth and movable, and the woman was having no problems with menstruation, then it would be diagnosed as noncancerous. However, the Dutch surgeon Petrus Camper warned that this method could never really differentiate between a benign and malignant tumor.

The English novelist Frances (Fanny) Burney, who underwent a mastectomy in 1811 in France, described what she went through in a letter to her sister in England. At first, she said, the small tumor caused her no concern. But after a year, her husband insisted that she seek medical advice. Doctors made house calls in those days and saw indigent patients only in the hospital at free clinics. Antoine Dubois was called, and while he tried to reassure Burney, he told her husband of the gravity of the disease. He prescribed some medicine and left. After consultations and delays, surgery was performed by Dubois at Burney's home. Burney's description of her experience — hiring women who could care for her after surgery, making a will, suffering extreme anxiety caused by the three-week delay after she had consented to surgery, the excruciating agony of the surgery — is a moving, subjective account of what a woman had to go through before the existence of anesthesia. Burney probably survived the surgery because it was done at her home and not in a hospital in which infections ran rampant. The fact that she survived 30 years after the mastectomy leaves some doubt as to whether she actually had cancer.

Because fatal infections were so common after surgery and the lack of anesthesia precluded real research into new and better surgical techniques, the surgery being performed in the nineteenth century was virtually the same surgery that had been performed for a thousand years.

Later in the century, the Viennese surgeon Theodor Billroth described four kinds of breast cancer. He used his own names for the different types — and also included the names in common use that had been given to the same type of tumor by others. This eliminated much of the confusion that had resulted from different terminology being used for the same condition. Billroth used fine woodcuts to show in detail each kind of breast cancer. He believed that it metastasized by way of the lymph system, which would transport corpuscular elements throughout the body. In all cases in which breast cancer had spread to other parts of the body, he found that the regional lymph nodes were involved. And although he could find no anatomical evidence, he believed that cancer could also be spread through the veins. At that time, it was generally accepted that cancer was a local disease that started in one site and then invaded and infected other parts of the body. Billroth found that breast cancer most frequently spread to the liver first, followed by the pleurae and lungs, the bones, and the brain. These findings were primarily a result of statistical data. (Quantitative data had begun to be used along with qualitative assessment toward the end of the eighteenth century.) Billroth had his huge number of cancer cases analyzed statistically. Among his findings regarding breast cancer were that:

- Medullary carcinoma has the most rapid course and is more apt to occur in younger women in their late 30s.
- Carcinoma simplex occurs most frequently and has a very varying clinical course.
- Fast-advancing neoplasms, growths which can be malignant or

benign, occur particularly in young women between the ages of 30 and 40 in good general condition, first appearing as an infiltrative induration, extending rapidly and fairly quickly occupying the greater part of the breast.

Although he didn't have much to say about the cause, he wondered if the fact that breasts undergo functional changes during puberty and pregnancy might at least contribute to their being more prone to the development of autonomous growths.

In 1842, a provincial surgeon in Verona, Italy, collected data from death registries for the 80-year period from 1760 to 1839, which covered over 150,000 deaths. As to cancer, his findings included that:

- The incidence of cancer increases with age.
- The increase is mainly due to a rapid increase in uterine cancers.
- The frequency of breast cancer is inversely related to the incidence of uterine cancer for different age groups.
- Unmarried persons generally have a greater chance of contracting cancer, especially breast cancer in women.

In 1854 the Congress of the Académie de Médecin discussed whether there was any benefit at all to treating breast cancer. One surgeon, Joseph-François Malgaigne, deemed cancer to be an incurable disease. Alfred Louis Velpeau, who believed cancer had a local inception, favored surgery and felt it was important to operate as early as possible. Most of those at the congress shared that view. Velpeau claimed to have seen more than one thousand breast tumors over his 40 years of practice. And although there was little follow-up after a tumor was removed, Velpeau was convinced that he had saved more than a few lives. However, other statistics contradicted that. Jean Leroy d'Etiolles sent out a survey to which he received 174 responses. According to the data he collected, of 1,192 patients with breast cancer who had not had surgery, 18 had lived for more than 30 years, while the remainder lived from two to 25 years. Of the 804 women surgically treated, 4 were still alive after 30 years, 15 survived for 30 years, and 88 for 6 to 20 years. From his findings, he concluded that surgery was more dangerous than beneficial.

In 1844, in the United States, a Philadelphia surgeon named Joseph Pancoast recommended that the breast and glands be removed in one piece. Over 10 years later, the London surgeon Charles Hewitt Moore laid down the general principals of surgical treatment of breast cancer. Moore said the entire breast must be removed, as well as any tissue adjoining the breast involved in, or even approaching, the disease, including the skin, lymphatics, fat, and pectoral tissue; and diseased axillary lymph nodes in the armpit should be removed during the same procedure.

In 1880, another Philadelphia surgeon, Samuel Gross, reported the results of surgery on over 200 women with breast cancer. Of the first 55 women he treated, all died in a short period of time from recurrence. In those women he had not removed the entire breast. When he performed more extensive surgery on the other women, removing the entire breast, pectoral tissue, and axilla (the armpit, including vessels, nerves, and lymph nodes), he reported a three-year survival rate of nearly 20 percent.

Enter William Stewart Halsted. This American surgeon, who worked at Roosevelt Hospital in New York City, started routinely removing the pectoral muscle. He reported briefly on his procedure in 1894 at the new College of Medicine at Johns Hopkins University in Baltimore. Halsted recommended that all suspect tissue be removed in one piece to avoid the spread of any cancerous tissue. Just ten days after Halsted's paper was published, Willy Meyer, a surgeon at the New York Graduate School of Medicine, described a similar technique. The radical mastectomy, which became known as the Halsted mastectomy, had arrived. (This radical mastectomy is virtually the same procedure performed by Moore in the mid-eighteenth century.)

Although by the standards of some, tremendous progress has been made, others see the progress as minimal. There is still no treatment for curing breast cancer.

18

Surgery

I think it's crazy to go on with mastectomies as a routine. The problem of breast cancer is not in the breast.

—Gianni Bonadonna, M.D.,
Instituto Nazionale Tumori in Milan[1]

When they started discussing treatments, I realized they were offering me the same therapies my mother received when she was diagnosed in 1949.

—Ellen Crowley, *breast cancer survivor*[2]

I think that surgery, chemotherapy, and radiation are very crude ways of dealing with disease. They really show that we don't have any insight into this disease at all.

—Susan Love, M.D., *director, UCLA Breast Center*[3]

"Slash, burn, and poison" is how breast surgeon Susan Love, and many others, describe the current treatments for breast cancer. The official medical names are surgery, radiation, and chemotherapy. Love says that chemotherapy does help some women, but with tremendous side effects. It's not known who will be helped, so "we end up poisoning everybody in the hopes that it will help a few." Love says a minority of women with breast cancer are being truly helped and that a massive change of direction is needed.[4]

Maryann Napoli, associate director of the Center for Medical Consumers in New York, thinks that we are overtreating the majority to save a minority.[5] For example, since few of the women with node-negative breast cancer would ever have a recurrence, few of those receiving adjuvant chemotherapy actually benefit. But since it is not known which women will benefit, all women are treated.

Although changes in the treatment of breast cancer have been made during this century, the mortality rate has remained relatively stable. Controversy is rampant in terms of which treatment is best. There is also controversy over other treatment issues, such as why so many women diagnosed with breast cancer are having their breasts removed when there are data establishing the fact that the breast can be saved with much less radical surgery. A recent controversy revolves around who should be getting high-dose chemotherapy with autologous bone marrow transplant (HDC/ABMT), if anyone, and who should be paying for it.

Dr. Larry Norton, chief of the breast and gynecologic medical service at Memorial Sloan-Kettering Cancer Center, insists that progress has been made in the treatment of breast cancer. He acknowledges that the progress has been modest but says, "We're moving in a positive direction. We're not stymied. We've made some advances and we're working on several important leads."[6]

The first major improvement in the surgical treatment of breast cancer was eliminating the grossly deforming and debilitating Halsted radical mastectomy, which removed the breast as well as the underlying muscle in the chest wall, or pectoral muscles. The Halsted was the primary treatment for breast cancer for years. However, as early as the 1930s, there were surgeons who thought the radical mastectomy was too radical — that it was of no use in patients whose cancer had spread and that it was much too extensive for women whose tumors were small when found.

By the mid-1970s, Halsted's radical mastectomy had been replaced by the modified radical mastectomy, a much less debilitating surgery in which the breast and axillary lymph nodes are removed, in most hospitals. In March 1975, an article in *Ms.* magazine discussed preliminary findings in a study comparing types of mastectomies.[7] The early results indicated that the Halsted radical mastectomy was no more successful in preventing a recurrence of breast cancer than a total mastectomy (removal of just the breast). It reported that Dr. Bernard Fisher, professor of surgery at the University of Pittsburgh and chair of the National Surgical Adjuvant Breast and Bowel Project (NSABP), was proposing studies for even more limited surgery, while at the same time stressing that if such surgery (for example, a lumpectomy) was adopted, it must be carefully monitored. At that time, Fisher said that he believed that an ongoing problem in cancer research was the unwillingness of physicians to try new procedures, and that if there had been less medical resistance to the evaluation of new or alternative procedures to the century-old radical mastectomy, a study like the one the NSABP had undertaken could have begun ten years earlier.

Four years after *Ms.* magazine reported the preliminary results of the NSABP trial, in June 1979, breast cancer specialists at the National Institutes of Health (NIH) recommended that the Halsted radical mastectomy no longer be the standard primary treatment for all cases of breast cancer in the United States. In spite of this, a 1982 survey of 757 hospitals by the American College of Surgeons found that nearly 3.5 percent of the estimated 110,000 women diagnosed with breast cancer in 1981, or more than 3,500 women, had undergone a radical mastectomy. Since then some states have passed laws to prevent the railroading of women into unnecessarily extensive surgery. Testifying at a 1984 House subcommittee hearing, the late Rose Kushner, a major figure in the breast cancer movement, said that Medicare could help women over 65 by refusing to reimburse surgeons who remove the muscles unnecessarily [in the Halsted mastectomy].[8]

An unconventional surgical treatment for breast cancer was introduced at Massachusetts General Hospital in Boston in 1956. Physicians there started using a minimal surgery as an alternative to the mastectomy as a last resort for women who simply refused to undergo mastectomies. A "team approach" was instituted, with surgeons, pathologists, radiologists, and oncologists working together. In the alternative therapy, only the tumor would be removed, and both internal and external radiation would be given, depending on each woman's case.[9] Between 1956 and 1960, Oliver Cope, M.D., and colleagues at

Harvard Medical School treated 12 women with limited excision of the tumor and excision of some lymph nodes followed by heavy doses of radiation. Four of the women who had that unconventional treatment were still living with no spread of disease 19 years later. Says Cope, "This is what would have been expected if they had had a mastectomy. . . ." In his book *The Breast: A Health Guide for Women of All Ages*, Cope concluded that in 75 percent of cases, removing the breast will not stop the disease, since the cancerous cells have already disseminated by the time the cancer is recognized and treated. (The rate of cell growth in breast cancer is sometimes slow compared to other cancers, so that the cells can grow in a breast unnoticed for many years. It can take years for a tumor to reach the size of one centimeter, the size which can be felt by a woman examining her breast. It can also be years before cancers are detected elsewhere in the body.) "It's outrageous that we've been going to a surgical cure to such an extent," Cope said.[10] After 1960, Cope never performed a radical mastectomy again.

In 1973, Nisar Syed, M.D., a radiologist and surgeon at the Southern California Cancer Center and the Los Angeles County USC Medical Center, started using limited excision with internal and external radiation and sometimes chemotherapy. After seven years and having treated more than 100 patients aged 23 to 90, he found that Stage I patients had 100 percent local control of the cancer with no signs of metastases. In the more advanced stages, close to 80 percent local control was achieved.[11]

NSABP studies were started to evaluate the new alternative treatment. Studies comparing three surgical treatments — mastectomy, lumpectomy with radiation, and lumpectomy without radiation — were under way in the United States in the late 1970s. Dr. Oliver Cope, for one, was convinced that the radiation research already done was strong enough evidence that mastectomy had seen its day. In the January 1979 issue of *Ms.* magazine, Cope was quoted as saying, "We now have a nine-year follow-up and the information is coming out. All doctors have to do is read the literature." Cope said he doubted that most surgeons had even read the published report on his findings.[12]

A major complaint of women was that when they sought alternative treatment, a lumpectomy rather than a mastectomy, it was hard to get information and then it could be even more difficult to find a doctor who would cooperate. *Ms.* magazine offered to send interested readers a list of hospitals and clinics that provided the alternative treatment. One woman who benefited is Lee Miller, a survivor of breast cancer and one of the founders of SHARE, a breast cancer support group for women in New York. She says:

> I discovered the lump myself. I was forty-nine. I had just read an article in *Ms.* magazine that said if your breast dimples, it could be a sign of malignancy. I did a breast self-examination and when I raised my arm it dimpled. My husband had read the same article. It was January 6, 1975, I remember the date. When I ran in to show him, his face turned white and I knew then that I had breast cancer. So I went to Guttman [mammography facility in New York City] for my normal mammogram. The first doctor thought it was nothing. Then he called in another doctor and he said, "My dear, I'm afraid you're going to need a radical mastectomy." I didn't even know what that meant. I knew mastectomy but I didn't know what a radical was. Why would I? My husband asked about the possibility of lumpectomy. The doctor said, "If you want a lumpectomy, find another doctor." [She did!][13]

In Europe, researchers were also looking into alternative treatments. In the late 1960s, surgeons at the Milan Institute in Italy became interested in conservation surgery, which would remove the cancer and at the same time allow the woman's breast to be saved. There were several reasons for thinking that might be effective. Because of mammography, breast cancer tumors were being discovered earlier in their development, but aggressive surgical treatment was not improving the prognosis of women with breast cancer.

The breast-saving surgery developed in Milan was cautious. Its purpose was to have good local control over the disease combined with good cosmetic results. The procedure that was developed was called a quadrantectomy. In an extensive surgical excision, the tumor would be removed as well as the entire ductal tree in which the cancer had been found. It was thought that one of the ways breast cancer spread was through intraductal permeation, so that all the ductal branches connected with the involved duct should be removed. That meant that a quadrant, or quarter, of the breast was being removed. A total axillary dissection (removal of the lymph nodes under the arm) was also performed. The procedure, which preserved the breast, was considered to be very radical and was performed only on women with small tumors (under two centimeters).[14]

In 1969, at a meeting of investigators called by the World Health Organization (WHO) on diagnosis and treatment of breast cancer, the Milan Institute presented a plan for an international trial that would compare the quadrantectomy with mastectomy. It was approved as part of an international clinical trial, but it never happened. However, WHO's approval paved the way for the Milan Institute to conduct such a trial, in opposition to the wishes of the more senior surgeons there, who considered the trial risky and unethical.[15]

The first Italian trial, in 1973, compared the Halsted radical mastectomy with the quadrantectomy in 700 patients. Early results, published in 1981, showed clearly that the two procedures had similar survival rates of over 90 percent. The eventual big impact this had on breast cancer treatment came about slowly. Many surgeons felt that longer follow-up might show a difference in survival after many years. A final evaluation in 1990 confirmed the original findings in Italy.[16]

In the United States, the NSABP, funded by the National Cancer Institute (NCI), organized a clinical trial in 1971 to compare radical mastectomy and total mastectomy with and without radiation. More than 1,650 women in 34 institutions in the U.S. and Canada participated in the trial. Ten-year results were published in 1985. As hypothesized, the dissimilar treatments got similar results. The study provided unequivocal support for the new concept of breast cancer as a systemic disease that can spread and affect any part of the body. The study showed that the five-year results had accurately predicted the outcome at ten years and raised the question of whether it is ever necessary to remove a breast.[17]

Another NSABP study compared total mastectomy and lumpectomy with and without radiation. Researchers reported in 1985 that radiation therapy following lumpectomy (breast conservation therapy [BCT]) greatly reduced the number of recurrences in the same breast over five years. Although most patients receiving a lumpectomy did fine without radiation, there was no way to know which patients would. Hence, radiation was recommended for everyone and is now the standard treatment.[18] A conference convened by NIH strongly supported the research evaluating BCT but stopped short of endorsing it. Opponents expressed concern that there might be remaining cancer cells in the breast, and pointed out that if the entire breast is removed, a second tumor cannot form in that breast. There was more substantiating data in March 1989 with the announcement of the results of another NSABP study, which concluded that women who had had lumpectomies had virtually the same chance to be cancer-free in eight years as those who had undergone a mastectomy.[19] There was additional confirmation in April 1995, when ten-year results were reported which found that BCT with lumpectomy and radiation offered the same survival benefits as a mastectomy.[20]

A little over a year later, in June 1990, an NIH panel of 15 experts concluded that breast conservation performed in the early stages of breast cancer gives as good a survival chance to women as a mastectomy. Ten years after an NIH expert panel proclaimed mastectomy to be the standard of care, and after 20 years of clinical trials on the efficacy and safety of BCT, the conclusion reached by the panel was that in stage I breast cancer with cancer-free nodes and a tumor smaller than one centimeter, a woman had a 90 percent chance of cure with either mastectomy or BCT, and that BCT was the preferable treatment. This was based, in large part, on the findings in the two large NSABP trials that were conducted on patients in the United States and Canada. The committee drew the line at saying BCT was the preferred treatment. As Dr. William C. Wood, chief of surgery at the Emory University Medical Center in Atlanta and chair of the panel, put it, "The therapies appear to be equivalent in survival. We believe it is preferable to preserve an organ."[21] Arthur Holleb, M.D., an official with the American Cancer Society, called the results "reassuring for women who have had lumpectomies."[22]

If there were any doubts about the preference of most women, a study done by Gerald J. Margolis, M.D., at the University of Pennsylvania School of Medicine in Philadelphia, published three months later, found that most women who had had a mastectomy would not make that choice if they had a chance to choose again, whereas those women who chose BCT would not alter their original decision. Margolis said, "The most important thing that came out of the study is that women should be given a choice."[23] Wood said for some women the choice would be a mastectomy. "There may be individuals who prefer to have the breast removed rather than undergo six weeks of radiation. For that individual, mastectomy would be a very appropriate choice."[24]

There are women for whom BCT isn't recommended, including

those women with multicentric breast cancer (in which malignant cells are found in more than one quadrant of the breast), diffuse intraductal breast calcification, certain collagen-vascular diseases, or tumors that are large relative to the size of the breast. It was estimated that 70 percent of newly diagnosed cases of breast cancer could be adequately treated with BCT. A study in 1983 showed lumpectomy being performed about 13 percent of the time on women in the United States.[25] In an effort to change that, some states passed laws protecting a woman's right to be informed of all her treatment options. In 1988, some 16 states had passed such legislation. Two years later, a study conducted in 1,000 hospitals with about 24,000 patients showed lumpectomy being performed just 25 percent of the time.[26] The most common surgery was the modified radical mastectomy which removes the breast and the pectoralis minor muscle. Disturbed by the fact that surgeons still appeared to be relying on the mastectomy, in October 1990, an NIH federal advisory panel issued a strong recommendation in favor of BCT.[27]

A woman's chance of getting conservative breast-sparing treatment appears to depend more on where she lives than on the stage and other conditions of the disease. A study published in 1993 found the lumpectomy rate ranged from 20.6 percent in the region encompassing Kentucky, Tennessee, Mississippi, and Alabama to 40.2 percent in New England.[28]

In a study conducted at the University of California at Irvine, Anna Lee-Feldstein found that lumpectomy was used most often at teaching hospitals. Published in 1994 in the *Journal of the American Medical Association*, the study showed that between 1988 and 1990, 50 percent of the patients with localized breast cancer and 40 to 50 percent of women with regional disease received breast conservation therapy at a teaching hospital, whereas during the same period of time 30 percent or less of patients at nonteaching hospitals received lumpectomies. In an editorial in the journal responding to the study, several reasons for the findings were advanced:

- Doctors at teaching hospitals may be better informed and thus more inclined to participate in clinical trials.
- The older generation of doctors may not be convinced that the reported results are valid.

- Some male physicians may not understand that women value their breasts as part of their person and not because of vanity and sexuality.

Many women still find themselves in the difficult position of having to confront the physician over the choice that the physician has made for them.[29]

Elizabeth Belden, a founder of a support group in Cedar Rapids, Iowa, was 54 years old when she was diagnosed in the late 1980s. When I spoke with her in 1993, she told me she started to go for mammograms when she began estrogen replacement therapy. On her second mammogram, a half-centimeter cancerous lesion was found. She did her homework to find out what would be her best treatment option:

> Five years ago lumpectomies were very rare [in Iowa]. I did research to find out if lumpectomy [with radiation] was as effective as mastectomy. Surgeons discouraged me. Some years earlier my general practitioner showed me horror pictures of radiation to the breast, where the breast was shriveled. I simply said to my surgeon, "We're doing a lumpectomy." He said something about mastectomy being the traditional treatment but readily agreed to do a lumpectomy. I had chosen a young surgeon because I thought he'd be most likely to be knowledgeable and experienced in the latest surgical procedures. When I got to the radiologist, he said, "You got the right treatment." Just in the last six months there appear to be more women having lumpectomies. All of a sudden I've had visits with women who have had a lumpectomy. They're slowly increasing.

Dr. Marc Lippman, director of the Vincent T. Lombardi Research Center at Georgetown University, finds the limited use of breast conservation surprising. "I am puzzled as to what combination of educational, prejudicial, financial, and historical issues have failed to get lumpectomies going." He contends that the problem is the doctors and says that "in most cases, what is happening is inappropriate encouragement to undergo a mastectomy from the first care-giver they see, the surgeon who does the biopsy." Lippman, a medical oncologist, notes that surgeons make more money doing mastectomies and radiologists benefit financially when lumpectomies are performed.

Lippman does not say that that is the reason, but the implication is there.[30]

The question remains: Why, when lumpectomy is as effective as mastectomy and so much less traumatic for the woman, is it still being used far less often than it could be? Some experts say that question reveals an overlooked aspect of medical practice, that data alone may not be enough to force a change in medical practice even when the statistics are supported by medical experts. As Cynthia Pearson, at the National Women's Health Network, says, "Many doctors are just not up with the times. They're going to stick with what they know."[31]

There are doctors who have psychological difficulty letting go of the method and philosophy they learned in medical school. Mastectomy is what they have been doing for years. They are comfortable doing it. There's also the issue of losing control. The surgeon is not completely in charge when the patient goes off for radiation.

Breast surgeon Susan Love says, "Very often what a surgeon does is say, 'You have two options. If I were you or you were my wife, I'd choose a mastectomy.' "[32] There is no question that a statement like that has a big influence on many women. In the early 1990s, Charles M. Abernathy, M.D., a surgeon at the University of Colorado Health Sciences Center in Denver, questioned some 175 general surgeons on their attitude toward surgery. About 25 percent thought mastectomy was preferable to lumpectomy, describing it as the "gold standard." Another third said the two were equivalent, but still described mastectomy as the gold standard.[33]

Unquestionably, there are women who prefer a mastectomy. Jeanne A. Petrek, M.D., assistant attending surgeon at Memorial Sloan-Kettering Cancer Center in New York, says, "According to recent studies from England, Italy, and the U.S., only one-half to two-thirds of patients who are given the choice choose breast conservation."[34]

Former First Lady Nancy Reagan was not one of them. When she opted for a mastectomy rather than a lumpectomy in the late 1980s, many women were enraged and disappointed, worried about the impact her decision would have on women who would be diagnosed with breast cancer down the line. Six months after her mastectomy, Mrs. Reagan explained her decision this way. "I couldn't possibly lead the kind of life I lead and keep the schedule that I do having radiation or chemotherapy. Maybe if I'd been 20 years old, hadn't been married, hadn't had children, I would feel completely differently. But for me it was right."[35] Eighty-eight-year-old Ethyl Feldmeyer, whose tumor was small, also chose a mastectomy. Her husband was ill. "I couldn't see myself being tied up for [radiation treatments], so I had a mastectomy."[36]

Umberto Veronesi, M.D., director of the Milan Cancer Institute, was quoted as saying that the reason Mrs. Reagan chose mastectomy for her 7-millimeter tumor was that she feared radiation. Whether or not that was a contributing factor to her decision, as Veronesi claims, it is not at all uncommon for women to be fearful of radiation treatments.[37]

Many women who choose mastectomy do so because they don't want to worry about additional breast surgery if the cancer recurs in the same breast. Generally, that would necessitate a mastectomy. They just want to be done with it.

A woman's options can shrink if she lives in an area where the nearest radiation facility is hours away and she has neither the time nor inclination to travel long distances for daily treatments. She may not be able to afford to stay at a hotel near the facility and, even if she can afford it, it may be just too great a disruption to her family.

Nancy Brinker, the founder of the Komen Foundation and a breast cancer survivor, looks at the issue from yet another point of view. "What a lot of physicians and scientists have never accounted for is that the fear of this disease has run so deep, and the treatment is so harsh, that women still have in their minds that the more you cut, the more you keep it from spreading. . . . I can't tell you how many women I talk to who say, 'I just want to get it out.' "[38] Even though the statistics do not support their feelings, many women believe they have a better chance of survival if they have their entire breast removed. What is particularly unfortunate is how many doctors believe it, too.

The earliest stage of breast cancer called "in situ" poses a different dilemma for both physicians and patients. There is some controversy as to whether in situ carcinomas are even real cancers. In situ means the cancer is contained and not invasive — it hasn't invaded any of the normal tissue. Tissue invasion is one of the characteristics of cancer and is required for cancer to spread. Removal of the breast is considered a cure. As Dr. Larry Norton puts it, "We are now in the bizarre position of sacrificing the breast to treat noninvasive disease and recommending that women save the breast when the cancer is invasive."[39]

There are two kinds of in situ breast cancers: lobular carcinoma in situ and ductal carcinoma in situ (also known as intraductal breast cancer). Lobular carcinoma in situ (LCIS) is found in the breast lobules and ductal carcinoma in situ (DCIS) is found in the ducts in the breast. As recently as the early 1970s, both were thought of as premalignant diseases and treated in the same way. It is now known that they differ significantly.

The earliest documentation of LCIS was in 1898. In 1941, it was called lobular carcinoma in situ by two researchers who found it in two of 300 mastectomy specimens. In 1978, it was suggested that it be called lobular neoplasia by researchers who questioned whether it was inevitable that LCIS would become invasive cancer. LCIS cannot be detected on a mammogram. It is usually found incidentally, during an unrelated biopsy by a diligent pathologist. Only about 33 percent of the women who are found to have LCIS will eventually be diagnosed with invasive cancer.

Today LCIS is considered to be a risk factor rather than a precursor for invasive cancer. A woman with LCIS faces a risk similar to the risk of having a strong positive family history of breast cancer. The risk is the same in both breasts, 1 percent a year after diagnosis. In the past, since the understanding was that LCIS would eventually become invasive, the treatment was mastectomy. Once it became known that LCIS was a risk factor rather than a precursor, and that both breasts were equally at risk, the standard treatment changed. Removing just one breast made no sense. And it was questionable whether surgery was even appropriate, since invasive breast cancer does not develop in as many as 66 percent of the woman diagnosed with LCIS. Many patients and physicians consider a double mastectomy far too aggressive and instead choose frequent observation as an alternative. Careful observation is the chief treatment choice for LCIS as it is for any woman at an increased risk of breast cancer. For some women, living with the increased risk is so anxiety-provoking that they opt for having prophylactic mastectomy of both breasts.

DCIS is more risky than LCIS. It was first described in the early 1900s and it was distinguished as a noninvasive tumor in 1946. Until fairly recently, it was treated the same as any other invasive breast cancer, with removal of the breast. Whereas in the past DCIS accounted for 3 to 5 percent of all breast cancers, it now represents as many as 20 percent of all the breast cancers diagnosed at some hospitals. It is believed that the huge increase is a result of more sophisticated mammographic equipment picking up cancers that in the past were too small to be felt. It is not really known how DCIS found by a mammogram will progress, since its detection in that manner is so recent. In the past most patients with DCIS were treated with a mastectomy, so that it was not possible to watch its natural history. One of the few studies that followed women who had only a biopsy was done in the late 1970s and early 1980s. Seven of 25 patients, 28 percent, who had been diagnosed with DCIS but had no further treatment were found to have invasive breast cancer within ten years of the original biopsy. In another, similar study, eight of 30 women, 27 percent, were diagnosed with invasive breast cancer within ten years.[40]

Although the development of invasive cancer is not inevitable after a diagnosis of DCIS, a significant number of those women will be diagnosed with invasive breast cancer within ten years. It is not known how to distinguish the DCIS that will become invasive and therefore require treatment from the DCIS that will not become invasive and therefore is not a threat. As with LCIS, in the past DCIS was automatically treated by mastectomy. However, while mastectomy does remain the gold standard, in recent years more conservative treatment has come into play. This can cause quite a dilemma for a woman diagnosed with DCIS. It did for Susan Pringle in 1991. She was 48 when microcalcifications seen on her mammogram were diagnosed as malignant. She called me in a panic.

"The radiologist told me to see a breast surgeon," she told me. I could hear the anxiety in her voice. "He told me he saw some microcalcifications. What is that?"

I explained, and Susan then went to a breast surgeon, who performed a biopsy. More questions quickly followed.

"The surgeon says the microcalcifications are malignant. And the surgeon told me I could wait and have another mammogram in six months or have a mastectomy, which the surgeon said would be a cure. She told me if it were her, she'd probably wait and see, but then she said she couldn't really say what she'd do if it really were her."

Susan went for a second opinion. The breast surgeon she saw at a comprehensive cancer center told her that many doctors didn't even consider what she had to be cancer. She went for a third opinion at another comprehensive cancer center. The surgeon there advised an excision to remove a part of the breast, just to make sure they got it all. Susan, whose breasts were relatively small, realized that if she were to have an excision, so much of her breast would be gone that she might as well have a mastectomy. She called me back again and told me the three opinions. "I don't know what to do. Isn't the whole purpose of getting a mammogram to find any cancer as early as possible, so that it can be cured? Doesn't this kind of defeat the whole purpose if I don't follow through with treatment? I'd rather wait and see, but would that be foolish since I've had this warning? Would that be tempting fate?" I had no answer. Susan finally decided to wait and see.[41]

Susan Pringle's dilemma is one faced by many women. There is no clear-cut answer as to which treatment would be of most benefit. In 1993, results of the first large scientific study of intraductal carcinoma were published in the *New England Journal of Medicine*. The study compared excision of the cancer with and without radiation. Of the 319 women treated with lumpectomy and radiation, only 10 percent had a recurrence in four years, and only 3 percent had serious cancer. That led Dr. Bernard Fisher, professor of surgery at the University of Pittsburgh and chair of the National Surgical Adjuvant Breast and Bowel Project, author of the study, to conclude that "the bottom line based on these results is that lumpectomy plus radiation for women with ductal carcinoma in situ is an acceptable strategy." The study also showed that radiation was an important part of the treatment. Of the women who received a lumpectomy without radiation, 16 percent of the women had a recurrence and half of their tumors were invasive.[42]

Susan Pringle faced yet another dilemma a short time later. More microcalcifications were found and this time a small number of malignant cells were found to be invasive. Her options were now changed. Her surgeon told her she could have a lumpectomy with radiation or a mastectomy, and that based on Susan's history, she was definitely recommending a mastectomy. She says that making the treatment decision was the hardest part of all.

I was stunned and shocked. I guess the two hardest things about making this decision was that I seemed to have such a small indication of disease and the recommended cure was such a radical procedure for such a minute cancer. My initial reaction was to want something modest because it would impact me least from a physical standpoint. Another doctor said my body was giving me a second warning. My breast surgeon was going away, so I had the luxury, if you could call it that, of speaking to doctors and speaking with people who had had mastectomies, lumptectomies, resections, reconstructions — even going to a plastic surgeon to find out about options for reconstruction. There were two very different readings of the pathology. It was almost impossible to get the two pathologists together. People told me a pathologist from one hospital won't talk to a pathologist from another place, so I had a third pathology done. I went through a tremendous amount of stress before I made the decision. The trauma wasn't the surgery. The trauma was making the decision. What was disturbing was that so little seems to be known. One doctor said radiation [that would follow a lumpectomy] might exacerbate the cancer if you had microcalcifications. That was tough. We don't know as much as we should or could about breast cancer, especially this new issue of microcalcifications.[43]

There are not many who will dispute that. Some leading breast cancer specialists still have many questions that they say weren't answered in the 1993 study. They acknowledge that the numbers were hopeful but said the results didn't justify an across-the-board change, since a mastectomy is virtually a guaranteed cure. They also suspected that more of the women treated with a lumpectomy would have a recurrence at some later date. Dr. William Wood called the publication of the research "a very important study that's going to be telling us a lot over ten years, but the most important part [now] is that it is preliminary." He pointed out that the study did not address the issue of how lumpectomy compares with mastectomy, which, he said, "we know . . . eliminates the issue." Wood emphasized that there was evidence to suggest that DCIS took an average of ten years to recur, but added the results of the study might encourage older women to go for lumpectomy with radiation.[44] Dr. Larry Norton agreed that the recurrence rate was likely to increase as the years went by.[45]

19

NSABP Datagate

Women feel they weren't being told information that affects their lives and are upset because they think someone made a conscious decision to hide it.

—Cynthia Pearson, *National Women's Health Network*[1]

I voted for medical research because I hoped it would lead to good treatments, not to give scientists sandboxes to play in.

—Congresswoman Pat Schroeder (D-Colorado)[2]

No woman who has relied on the results of modern clinical trials to select a breast-sparing procedure following a diagnosis of invasive breast cancer should feel that she has made the wrong choice.

—Samuel Broder, M.D., *former NCI director*[3]

In the fall of 1990, a strong recommendation in favor of breast conservation therapy (BCT) was issued by an NIH advisory panel. Unbeknownst to NIH, the National Surgical Adjuvant Breast and Bowel Project (NSABP) had found some problems with data in the studies comparing lumpectomy with radiation and mastectomy earlier that year. When the story finally became public in 1994, it made headlines, creating confusion, distress, anxiety, and anger among thousands of women with breast cancer as well as people in the general population and many medical professionals.

In June 1990, an internal memo at the University of Pittsburgh suggested that a thorough audit be done because a data manager had noticed discrepancies in data submitted by an institution in Montreal taking part in the NSABP. A second audit was done that September. Two months later, a statistician at the university told Dr. Bernard Fisher, who was chair of the project, that the data management practices were faulty. In December, the NSABP audited the Montreal institution and found that records of some of Dr. Roger Poisson's patients at St. Luc's Hospital had been altered.[4]

In January 1991, another audit was done. As a result of the audits, in February 1991, NSABP suspended accrual of patients to its trials at the Montreal institution and notified NCI for the first time, eight months after it learned of possible problems. NCI then notified the Office of Scientific Integrity (OSI) and the FDA. Both agencies started investigations. In May 1991, Poisson admitted to the FDA that he had falsified data. In September 1991, the OSI filed a formal complaint against Poisson.[5]

In March 1992, NSABP briefed NIH, NCI, and the successor office to OSI, the Office of Research Integrity (ORI), and said that after deleting the data from Montreal, the results were the same. ORI documented 115 instances of data fabrication or falsification involving 99 patients, or 7 percent of the 1,500 patients accrued by the Montreal institution, and recommended that all data from that institution be deemed unreliable. ORI recommended that NSABP publish a reanalysis of its studies without the Montreal data and that Poisson be barred from receiving federal funds.[6]

In February 1993, ORI asked NCI to study the impact of the faulty data on the study results. The following month, Poisson was barred from getting federal grants for eight years because of fabrication and falsification of data. In April, the ORI gave NSABP its final report. In September, the University of Pittsburgh detected another irregularity at a second Montreal hospital. During a period of the probe, NCI and NSABP officials were requested not to comment publicly on the issue.[7]

The results of the ORI investigation were published in 1993 in a paragraph in the *Federal Register*, but went virtually unnoticed. The fact that false data had been used in a study that was responsible for a major change in the way breast cancer was treated didn't come to widespread attention until the *Chicago Tribune* ran a story on it on March 13, 1994, three years after NCI knew that the data might have been faulty. NCI officials came under a storm of criticism for not disclosing the matter sooner.[8]

On March 18, 1994, NCI ordered NSABP to suspend Tulane and Louisiana State University from new patient accrual. Bruce Chabner, at that time director of NCI's Division of Cancer Treatment, explained that "because there was so much data missing [on patients in the study], we couldn't establish the eligibility of a majority of patients at these two sites."[9]

On March 27, NCI asked Pittsburgh University to replace Dr. Bernard Fisher as principal investigator of the trial. The following day Fisher said in a statement that he had asked for administrative leave as principal investigator of NSABP. On March 29, NCI called for a temporary halt to new patient accrual into 14 cancer studies, including the tamoxifen prevention trial (which was being conducted with women at high risk of getting breast cancer, to see if taking the hormonal drug tamoxifen could prevent breast cancer). It also demanded the resignation of Fisher as coordinator of the NSABP. In a letter to Pittsburgh officials, NCI said it now believed not only that "the credibility of the NSABP is at stake" but that "the integrity of the entire NCI-supported clinical trials program may be jeopardized" by the alleged malfeasance of Fisher and his top aides. Evidence emerged that Fisher and his colleagues had been deliberately ignoring NCI's increasingly urgent appeals that they correct the affected studies. Fisher insisted corrections were not urgently needed because nothing had changed. The NCI team's report and related documents portray the NSABP as an organization so intoxicated by its own reputation that its officials refused or simply ignored NCI's requests for copies of its unpublished re-analysis or information about the status of the patients at St. Luc's in Montreal.[10]

Congressional hearings followed shortly thereafter. Fisher declined to testify at the House Subcommittee on Oversight and Investigations hearing. At the same time an attorney for the University of Pittsburgh asked that the 75-year-old-doctor be excused from testifying because of his age.[11]

At the hearing, NIH head Dr. Harold Varmus and Dr. Samuel Broder, who was then director at NCI, faulted their own procedures in dealing with data that were falsified by scientists at the two Canadian hospitals. They accused Fisher of having an arrogant and cavalier attitude in dealing with federal officials on the falsified data, ignoring the guidelines of his own studies, and failing to publish a timely correction. Broder said the hearing could have been avoided if Fisher had listened to pleas from federal health officials that he quickly publish the re-analysis of the lumpectomy study. Broder testified that when the fraud issue was brought to Fisher's attention, Fisher responded, "Who are you to question me?" Says Broder, "We clearly understand the principle that we cannot allow a grantee's formidable reputation, history of prior accomplishments, or service in science stand in the way of prompt corrective action and oversight. We cannot, and will not ever again, defer or appear to defer to the timetable of a grantee in reporting fraud and fabrication to the public."[12]

Others testified as well. Fran Visco, president of the National Breast Cancer Coalition (NBCC), and cancer survivor Jill Lea Sigal said they'd lost faith in NCI and that the reports had terrified thousands of women. Sigal, who was 32 years old, had undergone a lumpectomy six months earlier. She said, "I take no comfort from the fact that the [National Cancer] institute that swept the fraud under the rug for three years now claims to have conducted a re-analysis of the study and maintains that the findings are still valid. For me the National Cancer Institute has forfeited any claim to credibility. . . . As a result of the National Cancer Institute's behavior in this matter, I now question other policies of the National Cancer Institute, including its policy that women under the age of 50 should not get a mammogram unless they are at high risk."[13]

Congresswoman Olympia Snowe (who was elected to the Senate in November 1994) said that in addition to the lack of inclusion of women in clinical studies, "we now have lapses in ethics."[14] Congresswoman Patricia Schroeder contended that the public's anxieties could have been allayed if government scientists had allowed more consumer representation in the planning and conduct of research, which breast cancer advocates strongly endorse.[15]

Another issue was raised at the hearings as well. Chair John Dingell (D-Michigan) described as "not too cricket" the partial endowment of a university chair at the University of Pittsburgh by the pharmaceutical company that makes tamoxifen, which is being studied as a possible breast-cancer preventative in a large NSABP-sponsored trial.[16]

In a letter from Dr. Bernard Fisher published in the *New England Journal of Medicine*, he explained that he had failed to anticipate the seriousness of public reaction to his delay in publishing a correction. He said that the delay resulted partly from his team's finding that even after excluding Poisson's data, subsequent re-analysis did not change the study's conclusions. Fisher did not apologize, admit to errors, or respond to the NCI's assertions that his team had failed to follow its own guidelines in the studies.[17]

In an editorial in that same issue, journal editors Dr. Marcia Angell and Dr. Jerome P. Kassirer wrote that Fisher had failed to live up to his responsibilities as chief investigator of the NSABP. They criticized all parties, saying there was no excuse for a four-year delay in publishing a re-analysis of the data. "It is not enough to establish guilt and stop the funding of a guilty researcher; it is also crucial to publish corrections or retractions of fraudulent data."[18]

In early April, NCI released a press statement on the results of the first independent re-analysis of a breast-cancer study, which excluded the tainted data. The re-analysis reaffirmed the study's main finding that lumpectomy with radiation and mastectomy are equivalent procedures in early breast cancer for all treatment outcomes, including overall survival. NCI had taken the unprecedented step of hiring an outside contractor to do the analysis. In addition, re-analysis was done in two other trials and the results, minus any tainted data, were the same as the original outcomes.[19]

In early June, federal health officials approved resumption of the trials on a limited basis. Three of six trials that the University of Pittsburgh coordinates at nearly 500 hospitals were allowed to enroll patients. Also in June, NCI announced that other institutions would be allowed to bid to take over leadership of the NSABP. Samuel Broder said that giving other institutions the possibility of running the research project was a way to restore the project "to its previous glory. We're trying to solve a problem and this is the way I think would be the fairest."[20]

In October 1994, NCI released a summary of a meta-analysis done on studies of survival after lumpectomy versus mastectomy. The tainted NSABP data from Canada were not included. The five studies, in America and Europe, had a combined total of nearly 3,000 participants. The results showed that breast-conserving therapy and mastectomy were equivalent in terms of overall survival.[21]

The Office of Research Integrity announced in October that it was starting an investigation into whether any possible misconduct of science occurred in the NSABP. The ORI had earlier conducted an investigation into the falsified data. Lyle W. Bivens, ORI director, said the earlier probe concluded that there was sufficient evidence to warrant the new investigation. He added, however, that "there is no determination that misconduct occurred, so there should be no presumption of guilt."[22] In November 1995, the *New England Journal of Medicine* published the results of an audit of the medical records of patients enrolled in the NSABP study comparing mastectomy and lumpectomy with radiation. Two different re-analyses reaffirmed the original findings.[23]

The impact of the falsification of data on women choosing lumpectomy with radiation over mastectomy won't be known for some time, even though re-analysis of the data has shown no change in the results. But even before those questions arose, far fewer women than expected and eligible were choosing breast conservation therapy.

20

Adjuvant Therapy

I believe chemotherapy is presented as a "cure" rather than a treatment. It isn't explained that it [only] extends life for several years.

—Maryann Napoli,
Center for Medical Consumers[1]

We have now conclusively shown that adjuvant systemic therapy, drug or hormonal, makes a major difference in the prognosis of almost all patients.

—Larry Norton, M.D., *chief of breast and gynecologic medical service,*
Memorial Sloan-Kettering Cancer Center[2]

Adjuvant therapy is treatment that is used after the primary treatment to cure, reduce, control, or palliate the cancer. In breast cancer, in which the primary treatment is generally surgery, adjuvant treatment may be one or a combination of the following:

- radiation (when given following a lumpectomy, it's for a cure; it's palliative when used to eliminate pain when breast cancer has spread to the bone)
- medical therapy (chemotherapy and hormonal)
- surgery
- biologic therapy (the newest treatment, primarily investigational)

In the first lumpectomies, performed in the mid-1950s on women who refused to undergo a mastectomy, both internal and external radiation were given depending on each woman's case. As results came in showing lumpectomy to be as effective as mastectomy, there was still concern about cancer cells remaining in the rest of the breast after lumpectomy. An NSABP study reported in 1985 showed that radiation therapy following mastectomy greatly reduced the number of recurrences.[3]

At a 1993 meeting of the American Society of Clinical Oncology, some researchers questioned whether a more extensive surgery than lumpectomy, such as a quadrantectomy, would be the equivalent of lumpectomy and radiation, thereby eliminating the need for the time-consuming and costly adjuvant radiation. Umberto Veronesi, M.D., director of the National Cancer Institute in Milan, said it could be, at least in women over 55. In his study, published in the *New England Journal of Medicine* on June 3, 1993, he noted that radiation had a significant effect in the NSABP study because lumpectomy removes only the primary cancer, whereas the quadrantectomy performed by his group removed two to three centimeters of healthy breast tissue around the tumor as well as the overlying skin and underlying muscle tissue. However, his view on the generation of younger women was different. Veronesi cautioned, "In younger women, even an extensive surgical resection offers only incomplete protection." He said it was "essential" that radiation therapy be given after the surgery to younger women.[4]

A Swedish study started in 1981 using women with Stage I breast cancer and published in 1994 found that adjuvant radiation therapy after a lumpectomy might not be beneficial for all patients. The women who did not receive the radiation treatment showed a five-year recurrence rate that was 20 percent higher than that of the women who had received the radiation. However, the five-year survival for both groups was the same. The 1990 NSABP study on women with Stages I and II found that after nine years of follow-up, 90 percent of the women who had received radiation treatment had not had a recurrence, while 60 percent of the women who did not get the radiation treatment had had a recurrence. As in the Swedish study, overall survival rates were the same. Other studies have offered similar results. The Swedish study suggests that "radiotherapy given routinely is over-treatment in

80 percent of patients in whom local tumor control has already been achieved by tumor resection alone." The authors of the study go on to say that further investigation is needed to determine which, if any, patients can avoid radiation treatment.[5]

Marc E. Lippman, M.D., director of the Vincent T. Lombardi Cancer Center at Georgetown University in Washington, says that the evidence does not warrant a change in the current practice of radiation following a lumpectomy. But Lippman views the new findings in a positive light, saying, "I would modestly say, this is good, this is encouraging. Maybe . . . we can begin to find those patients for whom the expense and toxicities of radiation may be omitted."[6]

Studies at the turn of the century found that adjuvant surgical removal of the ovaries benefited about one in three premenopausal women with advanced breast cancer. The first established use of hormonal manipulation in breast cancer was by G. T. Beatson, who published his findings in 1896. He had done an oophorectomy (removal of the ovaries, the primary source of estrogen) on a woman whose breast cancer had spread. In his paper, he said that "all vestige of the previous cancerous disease had disappeared postoperatively at eight months." Hormone dependency of at least some breast cancer was established. Removing the ovaries after a mastectomy became fairly common practice, although it was not understood why it worked in some women and not in others.[7]

In 1962, researchers discovered the estrogen receptor (ER), which enabled some breast cancer cells to grow. Tamoxifen, a hormonal or anti-estrogen drug, blocks the estrogen receptors and does chemically what an oophorectomy does but does not require surgery. It was first used in England in 1973 for the treatment of advanced breast cancer. It was approved for use in the United States five years later. In hormonal treatment with tamoxifen or oophorectomy, cells whose growth and division are estrogen-dependent are specifically targeted.[8]

Chemotherapy, which is the other medical adjuvant therapy for breast cancer, targets rapidly dividing cells in general. (The term chemotherapy frequently serves as an umbrella term including both chemical and hormonal treatment.)

In March 1991, the results of an NSABP trial were announced at a chemotherapy conference in Arizona. In that trial, about 1,900 women with breast cancer were divided into two groups — one group got chemotherapy and the other group got hormonal therapy (tamoxifen). It was found that the postmenopausal women who were estrogen receptor positive (ER+) with between one and three positive (cancerous) lymph nodes had half the recurrences when treated with tamoxifen as opposed to the women who were ER+ and received chemotherapy. Older ER+ women with four or more positive nodes did even better. Women under the age of 50, or premenopausal, did not benefit from the tamoxifen, regardless of their estrogen receptor status.[9]

Chemotherapy was used originally as a last resort in breast cancer patients who could no longer be helped by surgery and radiation. In 1958, the NSABP conducted a trial in which half of 826 women with positive lymph nodes were given a chemotherapy drug, thiotepa, and the other half were given a placebo. After five years of follow-up, there was a significant improvement in the survival of premenopausal women with four or more positive lymph nodes who had the chemotherapy. In 1961, a second study was started using the chemotherapy drug 5-fluorouracil (5FU). It produced similar results. The premenopausal women with breast cancer who had four or more positive lymph nodes did better than the women who did not receive the chemotherapy.[10]

In February 1976, the findings of an NCI-supported study in Italy were published in the *New England Journal of Medicine*.[11] The data showed that women who had one or more positive lymph nodes and were treated with chemotherapy following surgery had fewer recurrences and longer disease-free periods than untreated women. The premenopausal women fared better, but the postmenopausal women benefited as well. Those studies marked the beginning of regular use of adjuvant chemotherapy in node-positive women with breast cancer, in the hopes of wiping out any remaining cancer cells in the body. That, in itself, was a major step in the treatment of breast cancer. An Italian study published in 1995 with 20 years of follow-up further confirmed the advantage of adjuvant chemotherapy in node-positive women. It also showed a very small increase in length of survival.[12]

An even bigger step was the recommendation of adjuvant chemotherapy for women at the least risk of having a recurrence, those in whom no positive lymph nodes were found. In May 1988, NCI did just that. In an unprecedented move, it issued a clinical alert based on four studies that had not yet been published.[13] The studies, three of which were funded by NCI, indicated that some women with breast cancer who have no positive lymph nodes could benefit from adjuvant therapy after surgery. The NCI thought the findings so significant that it urged adjuvant therapy for virtually all women with breast cancer, the major exception being women with in situ, or noninvasive, breast cancer. The prognosis for women with node-negative breast cancer has always been better than for women with nodal involvement. Studies have shown that the majority of node-negative patients treated with a mastectomy or lumpectomy and radiation do not have a recurrence. But up to 30 percent of women with node-negative breast cancer will ultimately have a recurrence of their cancer. Those recurrences usually result in death. All the studies showed that the women who received the adjuvant therapy fared significantly better, remaining disease-free for three or four years (the years for which NCI had data), than the women who did not receive the therapy. However, at the same time that it issued the alert, NCI acknowledged that it was too early to know if the adjuvant therapy would also increase overall survival. The studies were published in the *New England Journal of Medicine* the following February. At that time, Samuel Broder said, "The extended disease-free survival we have found is itself an important benefit. Hopefully, it will also translate into a long-term survival benefit."[14] The studies did not include women with in-situ, noninvasive breast cancer and at that point did not recommend adjuvant therapy for them.

The studies also left unanswered a number of questions. One question, noted earlier, was whether adjuvant therapy would simply delay recurrence or result in longer overall survival. Another question was the role of therapy, if any, for women with very small tumors. It was also not known if using chemotherapy and hormonal therapy together would be more beneficial than just chemotherapy.

In 1992, Richard Peto, an English epidemiologist at Oxford University, did a meta-analysis of 133 trials conducted worldwide on 75,000 women. Thirty-one thousand of the women suffered a recurrence and 24,000 died. The much-quoted study concluded that for women over 50, and that accounts for more than three-quarters of the women diagnosed with breast cancer, adjuvant chemotherapy enhances the ten-year survival by 5 percent, compared with having no treatment other than surgery; two years of adjuvant hormonal therapy with tamoxifen increased survival 8 percent over just surgery; and a combination of tamoxifen and chemotherapy increased the survival rate 12 percent. Peto said that a lot of people, "especially in the United States, are getting chemotherapy, when in fact, hormonal treatments, or a mix, are more effective." (Hormonal treatments are much less toxic than chemotherapy and have fewer side effects.) In women over 70, hormonal treatment with only tamoxifen was found to be as effective as chemotherapy. In women under 50, the meta-analysis showed that surgical removal of the estrogen-producing ovaries is slightly more effective than chemotherapy in the ten-year survival rate when compared with surgery alone. And by using a combination of both, ten-year survival improved slightly more.[15]

The meta-analysis indicated that the effects of adjuvant therapy persist long after most women have stopped taking the chemotherapy or tamoxifen, and that the benefits are noticeable ten years after the primary surgery as opposed to only five years later. That finding surprised virtually everyone, as it had been assumed and expected that the benefits of adjuvant therapy would start to diminish after five years.

The study also showed that in node-negative women, those with the largest tumors derived the greatest benefit from adjuvant chemotherapy. According to Peto, for every 100 women with Stage II breast cancer treated with adjuvant therapy, there will be 12 additional survivors for ten years; in Stage I breast cancer, for every 200 women receiving adjuvant therapy, 12 additional women will survive an extra ten years. In the United States, adjuvant therapy in women with no positive lymph nodes could save the lives of at least 3,000 women a year.[16]

There is still uncertainty as to whether adjuvant therapy for women with the tiniest cancers, under one centimeter, is beneficial. As more and more of those tiny tumors are being picked up by mammography, more and more women are being faced with the dilemma of whether to go through adjuvant chemotherapy.

Dr. William C. Wood, chief of surgery at the Emory University Medical Center in Atlanta, says, "Since the average woman gets breast cancer in mid-life, benefits that go past ten years are no small thing . . .

to have a benefit that goes beyond ten years is really very exciting."[17] Peto, too, says the results are very positive: "The number of ten-year survivors that you can guarantee [with adjuvant breast cancer therapy] is bigger than can be guaranteed for any other cancer."[18]

In a review article in the *New England Journal of Medicine*, in 1992, the role of adjuvant therapy in breast cancer was evaluated. The article said that the effect of adjuvant chemotherapy on amount of time until the cancer recurs is generally larger than the effect on overall survival, that combination chemotherapy has a better effect in pre-menopausal women, while the hormonal therapy tamoxifen has a greater effect in postmenopausal women, and that the presence and extent of positive nodes is the best-established prognostic factor for recurrence.[19]

One of the most controversial aspects of the use of adjuvant therapy has been, and remains, its role in women who are node-negative. The rate of recurrence in those women is 10 to 40 percent. The larger the tumor, the greater the risk of recurrence. The studies have shown that adjuvant therapy is beneficial in at least some of those women. However, there is no way to tell who those women are. It is difficult to make individual risk assessments because the clinical course of breast cancer is so variable. The three most promising tests are the following:

- The gene HER-2/*neu* (also known as c-erbB-2). High levels of this gene mean a greater chance of recurrence. Preliminary studies suggest that women with this marker might benefit from more aggressive chemotherapy regimens such as those containing Doxorubicin (adriamycin). Tumors with HER2/*neu* are associated with fast growth, but they are also one of the most treatable breast cancers.
- The protein p53, which helps suppress tumor development. However, when mutated it can lead to cancer. Women with high levels of mutated p53 in their cancer cells have a worse prognosis and may benefit from more progressive chemotherapy.
- Angiogenic factors: The length of time it takes for the formation of microscopic blood vessels is another promising prognostic factor. Tumors that can stimulate the growth of new blood vessels are more likely than other tumors to sow seeds of recurrence by releasing daughter cells into the bloodstream. Research suggests

that measurements of tumor-secreted angiogenic factors that have overflowed into the urine may help identify patients most likely to relapse.[20]

However, the tests are not yet sufficiently accurate to assess who is at greatest risk. The results have not been reliable, at least in part, because of a lack of standardization of test methods. There is also no effective method of combining the results of multiple assays that might be conflicting.

There are no formal guidelines for the use of adjuvant chemotherapy in patients with negative lymph nodes. In general, many doctors do not advocate adjuvant therapy for patients whose tumors are under one centimeter and do favor treating women whose tumors are over two centimeters. As for the women in the middle, treatment is much more controversial. There simply is no way to determine who would stand to benefit most from adjuvant therapy. Debate continues as to whether many women are undergoing expensive treatments, with extensive and sometimes debilitating side effects, with dubious benefit.

In 1992, William L. McGuire, M.D., and Gary M. Clark, Ph.D., examined the downside of adjuvant therapy in node-negative women.[21] Of all women diagnosed with breast cancer, about two-thirds will be node-negative and about 70 percent of them will be cured with local surgical treatment alone. Recommending adjuvant therapy for all those women would result in a large number of women being subjected to the toxic effects of the therapy and possibly a few deaths from it. The benefits of the currently available regimens are small, so that only a minority of those destined to relapse would benefit. The dollar cost of treatment for women who did not benefit would be about $500 million a year, not to mention the physical and emotional toll. McGuire and Clark suggest what they call a more rational approach — treating the 25 percent of node-negative patients with tumors over three centimeters with adjuvant therapy, as their recurrence rate is 50 percent, and using only local treatment for the 25 percent of patients with a 1 to 10 percent risk of recurrence whose tumors are under one centimeter, and for ductal carcinoma in situ (DCIS), pure tubular carcinoma, papillary carcinoma, or typical medullary carcinoma. The NIH Breast Cancer Consensus Conference of 1990 recommended that few of those patients receive adjuvant therapy.[22] The question then is how to treat the remaining 50 percent of women diagnosed with breast cancer, who have a long-term recurrence rate of 30 percent. Most of them are cured without adjuvant therapy. However, a significant number, 30 percent, are not. Reliable prognostic indicators must be found that can help identify who in this group would be most likely to benefit from adjuvant therapy. McGuire and Clark do outline what should be done in making a decision about treatment for these women. The doctor and patient must examine the available prognostic factors to determine the likelihood that the breast cancer will recur without additional treatment; all the treatment options must be considered with evaluation of benefits; and the benefits must be weighed against the known short-term and long-term toxic effects.[23]

Surgeon Susan Love offers similar advice. She says that the decision to use adjuvant therapy should be made by the woman after she knows the risk of relapse without the treatment, the expected reduction of risk with the treatment, the toxicity of the treatment, and its impact on the quality of life. As long-term side effects of the many treatments are not known, she emphasized that it's important that oncologists not treat women with strong drugs just because they are available and *might* help. "It is now obvious that all we can hope to achieve by treating [just] the breast is local control."[24] It is not the lump in the breast that is the killer, but the micrometastases that have entered other parts of the body and have not been eliminated by the body's own immune system.

Oncologist Larry Norton uses estimates of recurrence risk based on the size of the tumor and nodal status when deciding which patients could benefit from adjuvant therapy. Norton is convinced of the benefits of adjuvant therapy for the right population. He notes that chemotherapy works better in younger people, while tamoxifen works better in older women and especially those women with estrogen-receptor-positive tumors. Norton says each patient must be assessed individually. "There's a broad spectrum of therapies to choose from and you have to choose the individual therapy in each individual case." Chemotherapy does help some older patients and hormonal therapy can help patients who are younger.[25]

The use of tamoxifen in node-negative postmenopausal women who are ER+ is becoming more and more prevalent. In addition to its apparent benefit of reducing the risk of cancer in the other breast, there is evidence that tamoxifen may also reduce the risk of osteoporosis and heart disease. It is also relatively nontoxic and, in general, has far fewer and milder side effects than chemotherapy.

At first tamoxifen was given for one or two years, then three years, then five years. In 1994 Larry Norton said he was keeping most women on tamoxifen for a maximum of five years.[26] The Early Breast Cancer Trialists' Collaborative Group assessment of tamoxifen in nearly 30,000 women indicated that long-term treatment with tamoxifen, two years or more, is effective.[27] In November 1995, the National Cancer Institute issued a clinical announcement to some 22,000 oncologists recommending that tamoxifen be used for a maximum of five years in the treatment of women with early-stage breast cancer. The advisory followed a decision by the NSABP to stop a trial that was comparing five and ten years of tamoxifen after surgery because no additional benefits were found after five years.[28]

The biggest remaining issue yet to be resolved about adjuvant therapy is who in the large group of node-negative women with breast cancer will actually benefit from it. Once again, the decision-making burden is on women, many of whom are overstressed by anxiety, and who have had to decide whether to have a lumpectomy with radiation or a mastectomy. As of now, there is simply no way to tell, in most cases of node-negative breast cancer, which woman would be most likely to benefit from adjuvant therapy and which would not.

21

High Dose/High Tech/High Cost Chemotherapy

I was told to get a bone marrow transplant at Stanford. I had to fight my insurance company. I also had to have a [unnecessary] mastectomy to fit into the protocol.

Ellen Hobbs,
breast cancer survivor[1]

Insurance companies say [HDC/ABMT] is an experimental treatment, and the longer they can say it's not a proven treatment, the longer they are off the hook. But every oncologist these days is prescribing this treatment.

Beverly Zakarian,
director of CAN ACT[2]

I think there are a lot of women getting bone marrow transplants inappropriately. If the doctor says you should get a bone marrow transplant, patients think they should. The area is ripe for profit making.

Kimberly Calder,
director of public policy, Cancer Care[3]

What is commonly referred to as a bone marrow transplant for breast cancer confuses the issue for many people. First of all, it is really an autologous bone marrow transplant (ABMT), which means the patient's own bone marrow is used. Second, ABMT isn't the treatment; it is really the vehicle that is used to deliver the actual treatment, which is a very high (large) dose of chemotherapy (HDC), so high that it is capable of destroying the blood's capacity to regenerate, resulting in a high rate of treatment-related toxicities and possibly death. As of late 1994, the term "bone marrow transplant" had, in most instances, become a misnomer, although it is still commonly used when talking about the procedure (and will be here for convenience).

George Raptis, M.D., assistant clinical attending physician at Memorial Sloan-Kettering Cancer Center in New York, says he would call the procedure high-dose chemotherapy with autologous stem cell support. He cites the use of peripheral blood stem cells instead of bone marrow stem cells for "rescue" after the administration of high-dose chemotherapy and says that as "more and more people are becoming familiar with the advantages of [peripheral] stem cells . . . the use of stem cells [rather than bone marrow] has become the standard." Those advantages include the fact that obtaining peripheral stem cells from the patient does not require hospitalization and general anesthesia, as does obtaining bone marrow, which decreases the cost substantially. In addition, a greater number of stem cells can be harvested from peripheral blood than from bone marrow. The peripheral stem cells also bring about blood count recovery more quickly, which means that there is less chance for patients to get sick, have an extended hospital stay, require lengthy treatment with antibiotics, or need blood transfusions. Furthermore, with peripheral blood stem cells, patients can receive multiple cycles of high-dose chemotherapy more rapidly, which theoretically is most effective. Last, peripheral stem cells may contain fewer cancer-contaminated cells than bone marrow, although the technology to detect this difference is only now emerging.[4]

Although BMT has been used in the treatment of cancer since the early 1970s and is considered standard treatment for leukemia and lymphoma, it made its first appearance in the treatment of breast cancer in the United States in 1982 when Duke University Medical Center started doing HDC/ABMT in patients with metastatic breast cancer as well as patients at high risk for recurrence because of the presence of positive lymph nodes. HDC/ABMT for breast cancer went from 265 cases in 1989 to more than 1,000 in 1993, making it the most common form of cancer treated in this way.[5] At a conference in 1992, William Peters, M.D., director of the program at Duke, said that studies have shown an improved disease-free survival and overall survival, as well as improvement in quality of life in those patients treated with higher doses of chemotherapy compared to lower doses.[6]

Early data on a relatively small number of patients — 307 treated at Duke — indicated that, of the women with metastatic breast cancer, approximately 15 percent of all patients treated with HDC/ABMT would achieve a complete remission, and 23 percent of all patients who achieved a complete remission would be alive and disease free five years later. The data also indicate that treating patients who have primary breast cancer with nodal involvement reduces risk of recurrence.[7] Raptis says that there are multiple small, nonrandomized, noncomparative studies that have followed patients from four to more than seven years; usually between 10 and 25 percent of those patients are without disease progression during that period of time. This appears to be a big improvement over treatment with conventional-dose chemotherapy. He points out that there's never been a good randomized trial comparing women with metastatic disease who have had conventional treatment with those who have had the high-dose chemotherapy with the transplant. There are several centers that are attempting to do so both here and in Europe, but results are not yet in.[8]

In April 1994, a preliminary report by the Emergency Care Research Institute (ECRI) (an independent, nonprofit institute specializing in technology assessment) was skeptical of HDC/ABMT, saying, "Current data suggest that it is highly unlikely that controlled trials will demonstrate any substantive improvement in the quality of life or survival times for patients with metastatic breast cancer." The report dealt only with patients with metastatic disease. It concluded that there is "insufficient data" for assessing HDC/ABMT in high-risk patients with Stage II or III cancer. Nelson Erlick, senior research analyst and chief author of the report, said, "I was absolutely floored by the consistency at which this procedure is ineffective." According to Erlick, individual studies that showed improved success against metastatic disease tended to be biased or flawed because they were small or lacked rigorous scientific controls, or the treatment was used in patients most likely to respond to chemotherapy. He says that there is no evidence that conventional chemotherapy wouldn't also achieve the same gains seen in those patients.[9]

Just one month later, a study was reported which found that women treated with standard or high-dose chemotherapy had a significantly longer disease-free survival and overall survival than the women treated with low-dose chemotherapy. The report concluded that the doses of chemotherapy to treat breast cancer, especially early breast cancer, should not be reduced if the maximal benefit was to be achieved.[10]

Another study, also published in May 1994, in women just diagnosed with breast cancer who had a high risk of recurrence, found no advantage to high-dose chemotherapy. Of 2,300 women with advanced breast cancer randomly assigned to standard, higher, or double doses of standard chemotherapy, survival was the same in all groups. Lawrence Wickerham, M.D., a breast cancer specialist at the University of Pittsburgh, who directed the national study, said, "I don't think, based on these data, that there is justification for using higher doses of chemotherapy at this time. One should not confuse the desire to improve women's outcomes with the ability to improve outcomes."[11] John Bailes, M.D., at the University of Texas Health Science Center in San Antonio, said that although the new findings "raise the question of whether more is better, I don't think this closes the question."[12] Researchers said the findings may indicate a threshold effect; that there is only so much good that chemotherapy can do, and once you reach that dose, giving more won't make any difference. However, it is important to note that even the highest doses in that study did not approach the level used in autologous stem cell support.

David M. Eddy, M.D., who was acting as a consultant to the Medical Advisory Panel of the Blue Cross/Blue Shield Association in Chicago, Illinois, looked at all the published studies on HDC/ABMT and said that firm conclusions could not be made because of the lack of controlled studies and the presence of numerous biases. He did note evidence that indicated a higher complete and overall response rate in women with metastatic breast cancer treated with HDC/ABMT than with conventional treatment. However, there is no evidence that these rates imply longer overall survival or a higher probability of a cure, which is considered by many researchers to be the real test of the effectiveness of a treatment. Existing evidence does not demonstrate that high-dose is superior to conventional-dose chemotherapy for the treatment of metastatic breast cancer. What Eddy did acknowledge was that on a short-term basis it appeared superior to conventional-dose chemotherapy. Eddy notes that observation of cases with longer-term disease-free survival are promising but not conclusive and that the best that can be said is that the effect on survival is unknown.[13]

Amitabha Mazumder, M.D., director of the bone marrow treatment program at the Vincent T. Lombardi Cancer Center, which had treated more than 60 patients as of April 1994, says that the patients they treated with HDC/ABMT tended to feel better and require less follow-up care. But he also acknowledges that it currently is not known if HDC/ABMT actually prolongs survival. He tells patients, "I don't know that high-dose chemotherapy will cure you. But I do know that we've brought it to a point where it's easier on a patient than conventional chemotherapy and can keep you disease-free longer." As for patients at Georgetown entering a clinical trial of HDC/ABMT, he says, "Most of our patients either aren't eligible [because they don't meet the trial criteria for entry] or don't want to be randomized. . . . They want control of their lives. It's very hard for them to come in and be randomized."[14]

Testifying before a congressional subcommittee in August 1994, Bruce Cheson, M.D., head of NCI's medicine section, said that "high-caliber institutions supported by NCI . . . have provided encouraging results for the efficacy of ABMT in women whose breast cancer has either spread to sites other than the breast or who are at a high risk of recurring following their initial surgery."[15] Highly publicized, potentially favorable study findings combined with a lot of media hype have resulted in a big demand for this type of treatment by breast cancer patients, many of whom see it as their only hope.

When Terry MacKinon was diagnosed with breast cancer at 43, she had a mastectomy. She had a recurrence two years later. The breast cancer had metastasized to her lungs. It wasn't only the glowing news reports that convinced Terry to go for HDC/ABMT:

> The doctors told me a bone marrow transplant was the only way I'd have any long-term survival past five or six years. The decision to have bone marrow transplantation was easy. I wanted to live. I had to read

a list of all the side effects from the medicine. I almost had second thoughts, but I wanted to do it. Some people said, why do you want to do all that when maybe you could live out your remaining five or six years without going through that? But I'd rather have more. My insurance finally paid for it. I went to one lawyer in Lexington [Kentucky], a woman, who wanted to charge me $20,000 to sue the insurance company. We found a guy in New York who does this for people at a minimum fee of $500. And he did it all by telephone and now my insurance company pays for it for everybody.[16]

Insurance companies will often back down when threatened with a lawsuit and agree to pay for the treatment. They are reluctant to spend the time and money it takes to fight the lawsuit. And there's also the possibility that they'll lose.

In 1991 NCI approved four randomized trials of HDC/ABMT. Two of the trials were for women with advanced breast cancer (metastatic disease) and two were for women with Stage II disease, who have a high risk of recurrence. The transplant was a combination of stem cells and bone marrow, because at that time it had not been established that peripheral stem cells could produce new blood cells forever, as could bone marrow. (Dr. George Raptis says that now evidence is plentiful that stem cells are as effective as bone marrow.)[17] In an unprecedented move, Blue Cross and Blue Shield Association agreed to support four NCI trials financially under a national demonstration project and encouraged its affiliated health plans to pay at least part of the costs incurred by patients in the trials. Some agreed and many didn't. U.S. Healthcare also agreed to support the trials financially.[18]

Some of the insurance companies involved put an unrealistically low maximum on what they would pay for the procedure, so that hospitals which could not afford to perform HDC/ABMT at such a low reimbursement could not take part in the trial. Recruitment efforts into the four trials were disappointing. As of March 1993, one study had just 25 participants when its goal was 300; another with a goal of 429 participants had just 81; the third trial, with a goal of 340, had 279; and the fourth trial, with a goal of 550 patients, had 150. At some point, one of the studies was closed because of the small number of participants.[19] According to Dr. Bruce Cheson, some 1,000 women were enrolled in the trials in September 1994.[20] In October 1994, the study with a goal of 429 had just 173 participants. Stressing the importance of the trials in the development of future breast cancer treatment, NCI threatened to close the poorly enrolled trial if there was not a significant increase in patient participation by January 1995.[21]

There are many reasons for the surprisingly small response. Some doctors are uncomfortable recommending the randomized trial when they believe that the high-dose treatment offers the best and only hope for some women. They consider it unethical. Other doctors contend the possible advantages are not proved and the acute dangers (death as result of treatment) are clear. With the ambivalence and controversy surrounding the treatment — whether high-dose chemotherapy is beneficial, harmful, or in the end only as effective as conventional-dose chemotherapy — many doctors find it hard to persuade a patient to take part in a randomized trial. It is easier for a patient, who sees this as a life-or-death decision, to enter a trial if the doctor is encouraging and supportive and emphasizes that it is not known which treatment is better.

Another deterrent is the fact that some cancer centers are not taking part in the HDC/ABMT trials because of a failure to reach reimbursement agreements with insurance companies. One insurance company will pay for the treatment only at hospitals that agree to accept their reimbursement limit of around $65,000. That excludes a number of large cancer centers, which consider that amount far too low.[22] There are also cancer centers running their own trials. For example, in California UCLA and the City of Hope have nonrandomized research protocols. They contend that their job is to pioneer potentially better treatments rather than to compare known ones.

It is not unusual for patients to go to their doctor knowing exactly what they want. They have heard of the promise of HDC/ABMT and don't want to be randomized and risk not getting it. As breast cancer survivor Ellen Hobbs puts it, "I understand the scientific justification for the trials. But when it's life and death, you don't feel it's that important to do something for humanity."[23] Another factor hampering recruitment into the four HDC/ABMT clinical trials is a lack of awareness that they exist and of where they are being done. Also, in many cases, potential participants do not meet the specific criteria needed to enter the trial.

The bottom line is that as HDC/ABMT is becoming more available outside of the clinical trials, and with insurance companies providing coverage to avoid costly and time-consuming lawsuits, fewer patients are entering the trials. The result is a delay in getting definitive answers on the overall efficacy of this treatment.

A growing number of patients are suing their insurance companies to get reimbursed for the high-dose treatment. Ricky Stouch in Lancaster, California, is one of them. She was diagnosed with breast cancer when she was 40. She not only had to fight the cancer, but she had to use precious energy to fight the system:

> The first day I went to my doctor, he told me, "You have to have a bone marrow transplant." I'd never heard of that and neither had my family. . . . It was hard for them to understand that I had to go through this to save my life. I didn't find out for several months that the insurance denied it. The doctor at City of Hope [hospital] had notified my doctor. There was a really long delay. I always thought that my doctor would work this out. It never happened. And finally I found the name of a lawyer who I could use. He filed the lawsuit. In the meantime I went to three or four other places to see about getting into a clinical trial, but ultimately they said I would have to pay for it or my insurance would have to pay for it. They wouldn't take me. After I finished my radiation and saw my oncologist, he said, "You have to go back to City of Hope and see if there's any way they can get you in." I went back. They'd just opened a protocol that didn't use bone marrow. It used growth factors to bring back bone marrow. So that's what I had. I wasted a whole year of my life. It was terrible thinking that the insurance was just holding up my treatment. And I still don't know if my odds would be better if I'd had the bone marrow transplant up front. I hope my odds are fifty-fifty.[24]

As was the case with Terry MacKinon, Ricky Stouch did not decide on her own to go through this treatment. She was following the advice of her doctor, whose job was to treat her breast cancer in the best way he knew.

In 1991, two women in New Hampshire filed a lawsuit to get Blue Cross and Blue Shield to pay for their treatment. Fifty-five-year-old Margaret Terninko, a first-term state legislator, and 42-year-old Brenda Miller were both challenging the refusal of the insurance company to pay the $100,000 that the treatment cost. Paul Barbadoro, a

Concord, New Hampshire, lawyer who represented the women, said, "We brought these cases because these women need this treatment to survive. It is more effective than any other treatment."[25]

In December 1993, a jury in California awarded an unprecedented $89.3 million to the family of a woman whose HMO, Health Net, refused to pay for HDC/ABMT. Nelene Fox died at the age of 40. Lawyer Mark Hiepler charged that Health Net had violated a promise in its contracts to pay for bone marrow transplants. He also contended that Health Net had financially rewarded its executives for denying coverage of costly procedures. Hiepler called the case a warning to any HMO or other insurer that offers such incentives. Dr. Sam Ho, the medical director of Health Net, called the incentives charge "preposterous."[26]

Charlotte Turner was in her mid-40s when she was diagnosed with breast cancer. In May 1993, her cancer recurred in her bones. Her oncologist gave her under a year to live and the following three options: let the disease run its course, receive conventional chemotherapy to control her pain, or try HDC/ABMT. Turner's HMO, in Massachusetts, refused to pay for the transplant, saying that it was too experimental. Turner says the HMO's board of appeals was interested only in statistics when her case was heard in June. Three months later she found out her appeal had been denied. "I was shocked they wouldn't give me a chance," said Turner and described appealing her case like "begging someone for your life."

Massachusetts state lawmakers credit Turner for propelling a bill out of committee and into law to force health insurers to pay for HDC/ABMT for women with advanced breast cancer. As a result of hearing her story, women in the state legislature organized a public forum at the State House. Turner was too ill to attend, but her husband went and told her story. An intense lobbying effort was undertaken, and in the last days and hours of the 1993 session, women fanned out, lobbying and passing out pink ribbons. The bill passed on the final night of the legislative session, which was gratifying to Turner. "We wanted other women to be free from what we went through."[27]

Two doctors at Duke University, William Peters and Mark C. Rogers, looked at the way insurance companies decided to reimburse for HDC/ABMT and reported their findings early in 1994. The frequency of approval for patients enrolled in the HDC/ABMT clinical research trials appeared to have little relation to available medical or scientific information, and often seemed "arbitrary and capricious." Of two requests to the same insurer by similar patients in the same protocol, one request might well be approved and the other denied. The doctors stated, "It's generally accepted that by requiring that treatments meet minimally acceptable standards in the medical community, insurers will avoid providing coverage for worthless treatments. . . . The finding that with many insurers the outcome of the predetermination process varies from request to request is particularly disconcerting." They said that waiting for a decision from the insurance company was a time of great anguish for many women.[28]

Of 533 women enrolled at Duke in grant-supported clinical trials of HDC/ABMT from 1989–1992, 77 percent were approved for insurance coverage. Insurance was denied to the other requests primarily because the therapy was considered experimental. Of the patients denied coverage, 51 percent eventually underwent HDC/ABMT. In some instances the patient had to hire a lawyer to gain coverage. Peters said that 19 of 39 women who had been denied payments persuaded their companies to pay after they hired a lawyer. It was not uncommon for a denial of coverage to be reversed when an attorney stepped in.[29]

Another person who took a look at the way insurance companies decide who and what procedures to reimburse is Arthur Caplan, director of the Center for Bioethics at the University of Pennsylvania. He says the process favors the rich over the poor, the assertive and articulate over the reticent and reluctant. "Squeaky wheels get rewarded." Caplan said he often asked insurance companies how they decide when to refuse payment. He says they use these four criteria: "Does this person have a lawyer? Is the person articulate? Have we already tried to say no once? Is this a person who can muster sufficient resources to give us a hard time by getting media attention or starting a letter-writing campaign?"[30]

In 1988, representatives of eight major oncology organizations, including NCI and the American Society of Clinical Oncology, issued a consensus statement recommending third-party coverage for the costs of patients in research protocols of cancer treatment: "Policy restrictions that limit access to clinical trials are likely to delay the evaluation of therapeutic programs and to result in the relegation of patients to outdated and inferior treatments." Not surprisingly, some in the insurance industry disagreed, saying that it's not the insurance company's responsibility to cover the cost of research. And to make that statement even clearer, some insurers have put in a specific clause that they do not cover HDC/ABMT for women with breast cancer.[31]

In August 1994, a congressional hearing was held on HDC/ABMT coverage for federal employees, chaired by Congresswoman Eleanor Holmes Norton (D-District of Columbia). Testimony was given by breast cancer survivors, doctors, and government officials. Rebecca Perez-Ford, who worked for the IRS for 17 years, said she tried unsuccessfully, and at great cost, to get her Federal Employees Health Benefits Plan (FEHBP) to pay for the $175,000 transplant. She spent her life savings on chemotherapy treatments and lawyers' fees. With no money, she qualified for Medicaid, which meant U.S. taxpayers ended up paying for her transplant.[32] Catharine B. McKulsky testified that when she found out that the insurance would not cover the treatment, "I literally felt like someone had kicked me in the stomach. Tears were streaming down my face."[33]

Arlene Gilbert Groch, who represents women trying to get coverage, charged that the government was using the breast cancer issue to try to establish a precedent so that insurance denial of any benefit by the FEHBP would not have to undergo judicial review. She called that a patent injustice to all people covered by insurance carriers under the government's health plan.[34] Congresswoman Norton pointed out that Virginia has passed a law requiring every health insurance company in the private sector to cover HDC/ABMT. The policy does not apply to federal workers covered by FEHBP.[35]

Dr. Bruce Cheson, at NCI's Division of Cancer Treatment, said that standard treatment for breast cancer had improved, making it difficult to say that HDC/ABMT is always superior. He added that the women who have been in the trials tend to be highly motivated and generally in otherwise good health, and the researchers are extremely qualified to provide the therapy. "This therapy," Cheson said, "is being increasingly delivered by inexperienced physicians outside of clinical trials who are far less familiar with dealing with the life-threatening complications of this treatment, which threatens patient safety and reduces the likelihood of benefit."[36]

At the end of the hearing, the head of the federal government's

Office of Personnel Management (OPM) reviewed data from clinical trials of HDC/ABMT and reviewed its policy as well. In September 1994, OPM announced that all plans in the FEHBT must, at a minimum, cover HDC/ABMT in nonrandomized clinical trials for the treatment of breast cancer, stating, "Our position with respect to coverage for ABMT is based on general acceptance in the medical community for each particular diagnosis."[37]

Kimberly Calder, director of public policy at Cancer Care, says a lot of calls the agency gets are from women with breast cancer who are seeking help in obtaining HDC/ABMT and are worried that they won't be reimbursed. Calder is pleased with the response Cancer Care has obtained. "Overall we've been pretty successful in getting insurance companies to reimburse HDC/ABMT, because the [transplant process] is a procedure and not drugs." The chemotherapy drugs used are FDA approved. Calder's concern is that there's no FDA process that will give approval to the ABMT part of the therapy, which is the way of administering the treatment, and that it will always be a matter of scientific debate as to how effective it is.[38]

Despite the lack of conclusive evidence, HDC/ABMT is getting gut-level acceptance from many physicians for the treatment of breast cancer. A survey of oncologists published in 1991 found that 71 percent would offer it in nonrandomized trials to patients with locally advanced disease. The way it's been presented in the media as the only worthwhile treatment for a woman with metastatic breast cancer, it's no wonder that a lot of women, even those who are in a trial, think that one treatment is better than another.[39]

Dr. Larry Norton, regarded by many as one of the top breast oncologists and breast cancer researchers in the United States, is convinced that high-dose chemotherapy is the best treatment around for some women. "There's no question there are patients who have received this who are disease free, who would not be disease free if they'd received any other treatment. I'm convinced of this. The percentage of patients entering what we call durable complete remission in high-dose programs is much higher than anything we'd see with anything short of such treatment. Patients with conventional therapies do achieve durable complete remission in a very small percentage of cases [but] they never come close to as high a percentage of patients who receive a high-dose regimen. So I think that's really established in my mind. What isn't established is the way to give high-dose therapy, the least noxious way to give it, the most cost-effective way to give it, and the most effective [medical] way to give it." Norton adds that high-dose chemotherapy is not more expensive than kidney dialysis, some cardiac surgery, or a variety of other medical procedures that are routinely performed.[40]

Susan Love is not nearly as confident as Norton. She feels that the intuitive feeling on the part of many physicians that HDC/ABMT is the best treatment is based on the notion that more must be better. "That was certainly the notion we used with the radical mastectomy, but it turned out not to be true." She thinks that there's a good possibility that some women have cancers that are resistant to chemotherapy and you can give them higher and higher doses and they are not going to do any better. She intuits that ultimately it will turn out that in one group of women more is better; there will be another group of women who are resistant and it doesn't matter what you do; and there will be a third group of women in whom standard dose is plenty and more doesn't really add anything. "We really need to have everyone who's getting a transplant or high-dose chemotherapy to be getting it in the setting of a clinical trial." Many women are not willing to take the chance that they'll be randomized into the group getting conventional treatment. But Love says that women can't have it both ways. If they want new and improved treatments, they must be willing to take part in clinical trials so that those new and better treatments, such as HDC/ABMT, can be shown to be effective.[41]

Many physicians, researchers, and others involved in breast cancer agree that HDC/ABMT should be performed only in clinical trials. I. Craig Henderson, M.D., director of clinical cancer programs at the University of California, San Francisco, supports the HDC/ABMT program but says it is still experimental. At the congressional hearing in Washington in August 1994, he said that there was no evidence that the procedure prolonged life. Citing the NCI randomized trials, he said, "It would be unethical to run these trials if it were already known that high-dose chemotherapy and bone marrow transplant were better than conventional treatment."[42] Henderson also stressed the need for HDC/ABMT to be done only in clinical trials. "If we don't test them, if we don't find out if they work or not, we inflict a therapy that causes misery with no real benefit and we could drive the cost of medical insurance up."[43]

Sharon Green, executive director of Y-ME, a national support group, says, "We don't have evidence that BMT works." She adds that the treatment should not be funded outside of clinical trials. "We're now seeing hospitals putting pressure on their physicians to do HDC/ABMT outside of the trials. It's a big moneymaker for hospitals." Green says that women call Y-ME and say that it's the only thing that's going to keep them alive. "So she [a woman with breast cancer] should get money for it because she thinks so?" Green asks. She says that if a woman wants to get HDC/ABMT outside a clinical trial, she should raise the money to have it, because, as Green puts it, "if society as a whole has to pay for HDC/ABMT for anyone who demands it, it affects all of us."[44] The high costs of this treatment eventually get passed on to all of an insurance company's subscribers.

The debate over HDC/ABMT is not confined to the United States. In Belgium, Allen van Oosterom, M.D., professor of oncology at Antwerp University Hospital, says there is insufficient data on the efficacy of the treatment and that until there is a 10 percent increase in survival or a one-year survival improvement, he is not convinced of the benefits. He acknowledges the response rate has been high but says that survival data is questionable. He calls its use outside of clinical trials "malpractice and an unjustifiable economic burden."[45]

In the early years of HDC/ABMT for breast cancer, the treatment could cost as much as $250,000. The economic burden faced by patients and insurance companies in the United States is not as great as it once was. At the cancer centers most experienced in doing HDC/ABMT, the cost of doing the procedure has been dropping. At Duke, which pioneered HDC/ABMT for breast cancer, the price tag has gone from $200,000 to $65,000, which approaches the cost of conventional chemotherapy for breast cancer. The biggest savings are from the reduction in length of stay required in the hospital. At Duke, most breast cancer patients are treated as outpatients once they undergo the treatment. "We've cut the cost in half in the last two years," says Peters, "by learning how to cut corners safely." He predicts the cost will eventually be $25,000.[46]

Whatever the eventual cost, the real question is whether this treatment will result in longer lives for women. That can only be definitively determined through clinical trials. Dr. George Raptis is optimistic. He says that the data is accruing rapidly and believes future questions will focus on how the treatment can be offered to more women at a lower cost and to women who do not have access to large medical centers. "I think we're going to find that a certain percentage of women may be cured, but in the majority of patients this will only be a tool that can reduce a patient's metastatic disease to a microscopic amount. . . . The question will then be how we can use this in concert with other treatments . . . to drive that minimal disease to the cure threshold."[47]

22

Alternative Treatments

The cancer establishment has characterized the alternative and adjunctive cancer therapies as the work of quacks preying on desperate and credulous cancer victims, while the proponents of alternative therapies have depicted established therapies as the 'cut, burn, and poison' therapies of a cynical and profit-driven conspiracy.

— Michael Lerner, Ph.D., *Commonweal Cancer Help Program*[1]

Once we understand [the Chinese and Indian] medicine systems, I guarantee you, our confidence in natural remedies will increase and someone will capitalize on them in the United States.

— J. Paul Jones, Ph.D.,
vice president for R & D of Procter & Gamble[2]

A Harvard University study released in 1993 found that 30 percent of people who sought care from a general practitioner also looked to alternative medicine for cancer treatment.[3] Unconventional treatments include psychological/behavioral approaches, dietary manipulation, and the use of herbal, pharmacologic, and biologic substances. Since psychological/behavioral treatments such as relaxation, imagery, hypnosis, and biofeedback are generally used in conjunction with traditional treatment, many doctors do not have a problem with them and they will not be discussed.

In 1990, the Congressional Office of Technology Assessment (OTA) released its report *Unconventional Cancer Treatments,* which had been requested by the House Committee on Energy and Commerce.[4] It concluded that none of the treatments reviewed supported a finding of "obvious, dramatic benefit that would obviate the need for formal evaluation to determine effectiveness, despite claims to that effect for a number of treatments." The OTA report recommended that the federal government provide technical assistance to alternative physicians in undertaking scientifically credible studies of unconventional treatments, saying that NCI has a "mandated responsibility" to pursue information about and facilitate examination of widely used conventional treatments. Following are brief descriptions of some of the more well-known and controversial alternative treatments (none of which is specifically targeted against breast cancer), and their current status:

Antineoplaston therapy was developed by Stanislaw Burzynski, M.D., in the late 1960s. The antineoplastons are peptides produced by the body. Burzynski claims the peptides are produced in individuals as part of a "biochemical defense system" that inhibits cancer cell growth. He says that if the system breaks down in the body, cancer will develop. His treatment consists of restoring this cancer defense system. From 1974 to 1976 Burzynski received funding for research from NCI. In March 1989 approval was given for a clinical trial of antineoplaston A10 in a small number of women with advanced, refractory breast cancer. However, the study was "delayed," according to a public notice from Burzynski's staff, "due to the high cost" of conducting a trial in the United States. NCI subsequently reviewed seven cases of patients with primary brain tumors who were treated with antineoplastons A10 and AS2-1 and concluded that antitumor responses did occur and in 1994 was conducting a phase II clinical trial using antineoplastons to treat adults with refractory brain tumors.[5] In August 1994, Burzynski was put on probation by the Texas state medical board for violating various portions of the Texas Medical Practice Act by selling or giving away his drug.[6]

Biologically guided chemotherapy is a treatment developed by Dr. Emanuel Revici, which he describes as nontoxic, individually guided chemotherapy using lipid and lipid-based substances. Revici wrote that his treatment "when correctly applied . . . can, in many cases, bring under control even far-advanced malignancies." A main component of his treatment is selenium, a nonmetallic mineral of the sulfur family. Revici has been using organic selenium in the treatment of cancer and other illnesses since the 1940s. A relatively high intake of selenium has been linked to some lower-than-usual incidences of cancer. In Yugoslavia, scientists studied 33 breast cancer patients. They reported in 1990 that the level of selenium in the blood of the women with cancer was found to be only half that of healthy volunteers. There have also been reports of selenium's toxicity and the possibility that it can cause cancer. In 1965, nine physicians evaluated Revici's treatment and concluded it was without value in the treatment of cancer. Their findings were published in the *Journal of the American Medical Association*. In 1988, the New York State Board for Professional Medical Conduct recommended that Revici be placed on probation for five years. There has not been a controlled clinical trial to evaluate the safety and efficacy of biologically guided chemotherapy in the treatment of cancer. It is still being used by some cancer patients seeking alternative treatment.[7]

Cancell is a mixture of chemicals intended to treat cancer by depriving cancer cells of their ability to obtain energy. It was developed in the 1930s by James Sheridan, a former researcher at the Michigan Cancer Center. Sheridan charges that when clinical trials were set to begin in 1953, they were blocked by representatives of ACS. Preliminary tests were done by NCI in 1990 and conducted twice for verification. The results indicated that Cancell did not demonstrate a biologic effect worthy of further study. The FDA has issued a permanent injunction prohibiting the sale of Cancell across state lines.[8]

Essiac is an herbal treatment developed in Canada, where it was reported to have originated in Native American folk medicine. It was developed by nurse Rene M. Caisse ("essiac" is the reversal of the letters of her last name) while she was working at a medical clinic in rural Ontario in the early 1920s. She claimed that the formula was given to her by a patient whose breast cancer had been cured. Thousands of cancer patients have been treated with it. Essiac was tested at Memorial Sloan-Kettering Cancer Center in New York and NCI in the 1970s and was said to have no anti-tumor activity in animals.

Although Essiac cannot be marketed freely in the United States or Canada, a company in Ontario is allowed to provide it to Canadian patients under a special arrangement with health officials there.[9]

Gerson therapy was developed by the German-born doctor Max B. Gerson, M.D., and is based on claims that a natural diet would restore the human body's resistance and healing power lost through years of artificial nutrition. It is one of the most widely known unconventional cancer treatments. Gerson started using his diet on cancer patients in 1928. His natural diet is low in fat, low in animal protein, and high in carbohydrates and is obtained through organic fruits, vegetables, and grains. Some specific elements include over a dozen glasses a day of freshly extracted vegetable and fruit juices (mostly carrot); a daily vegetable soup; and a low-salt, high-potassium regimen with potassium supplements, among other things. Gerson also advocated coffee enemas, which appeared in the medical literature as early as 1917. He used them as part of his general detoxification regimen. Only a few clinical trials have been done on the Gerson diet. An Austrian doctor, Peter Lechner, M.D., reported that "the patients treated with the adjuvant nutritional therapy are in a better general condition with less risk of complications, and they also tolerate radiation and chemotherapy better than patients who do not follow the diet." In 1990 the English medical journal *Lancet* published a report that examined case histories of 149 patients of the Gerson clinic. Although they wrote that they "could find little objective evidence of an antitumor effect," they noted "the high degree of control the patients felt they had over their health, and perhaps, as a consequence, their high ratings for mood and confidence." In the late 1940s, NCI reviewed ten cases submitted by Gerson but found no convincing evidence that it worked. They asked Gerson for additional data, but he did not provide it. NCI does not believe further evaluation is necessary. One big proponent of Gerson's therapy was Albert Schweitzer, M.D., who wrote, "I see in him one of the most eminent geniuses in the history of medicine."[10]

Harry Hoxsey's herbal tonic treatment was offered at a number of clinics in the United States from 1924 until the late 1950s, when a federal court issued an injunction to stop the sales of the "ineffective cancer treatment." That followed ten years of litigation. The treatment consisted of ten different herbs that Hoxsey claimed corrected a chemical imbalance in the blood. Hoxsey said the treatment was discovered by his great-grandfather, Harry Hoxsey, whose horse was cured of a cancer in its leg after eating some herbs growing in a field. In 1956 Hoxsey explained his belief that cancer was a systemic disease, although he never claimed to know its fundamental cause. He did say that it "occurs only in the presence of a profound physiological change in the constituents of body fluids" and that it leads to a "chemical imbalance in the organism." Although he couldn't say how or why his herbal treatment worked, he maintained that it corrected the "abnormal blood chemistry and normalized cell metabolism" by stimulating the elimination of the toxins that were poisoning the system. No objective, scientific data supporting his claims of success have ever been published. Hoxsey charged that the American Medical Association had organized a widespread conspiracy against him. He also said that it was the responsibility of NCI to verify his case records and that their failure to do so was deliberate. In 1947, Senator Elmer Thomas of Oklahoma asked the U.S. Public Health Service to investigate Hoxsey's treatment, but he was turned down. In 1951, Senator William Langer of North Dakota sponsored a resolution under which a subcommittee would have been organized to study Hoxsey's treatment, but the resolution was never reported out of committee. In 1953, after examining records of Hoxsey's litigation with the AMA and the federal government, attorney Benedict Fitzgerald reported to a Senate committee that NCI "took sides and sought in every way to hinder, suppress, and restrict [the Hoxsey Cancer Clinic] in their treatment of cancer." No longer available in the United States, the treatment can be obtained in Mexico.[11]

Immunoaugmentative Therapy (IAT) was developed by Lawrence Burton, Ph.D., and is one of the most widely known unconventional cancer treatments. It consists of daily injections of processed blood products. According to IAT patient literature, IAT acts as an immunologic control that causes most types of cancer to either stabilize or regress. Burton first offered it to cancer patients in the 1970s in New York. He left New York in 1977 to start the Immunology Researching Centre in the Bahamas. In 1978, the Bahamian government asked the Pan American Health Organization (PAHO) to review the treatment. The organization unanimously recommended that the center be closed. The clinic remained open but only for the treatment of non-Bahamians. A second clinic was opened in Germany in 1987 and a third in Mexico in 1989. In 1984 NCI examined sealed specimens provided by five patients who had returned from the clinic in the Bahamas. The analyses revealed the samples to be dilutions of blood proteins with no evidence of the immunologic components described by Burton. Bacteria was found in all the samples and four of the samples had indications of contamination with hepatitis. Those results were confirmed by subsequent analyses of more than 70 samples by the Centers for Disease Control and Prevention (CDC), NCI, and other independent laboratories. In 1985 the Bahamian Government closed the clinic after being advised to do so by CDC and PAHO. However, when Burton promised sterile conditions at the clinic, he was allowed to reopen the clinic several months later. In July 1986, the FDA imposed a ban prohibiting the importation of IAT to the United States "due to the direct hazards that have been associated with IAT." There are currently no reliable data on the efficacy of IAT as a cancer treatment.[12]

Laetrile is a substance containing the poison cyanide. It is made from apricot pits. It became a cancer remedy in France in 1840 after a French country doctor reported that he had cured six cancer patients. He based his conclusions on the fact that the six patients were still alive after two months. Laetrile was first used to treat cancer patients in California in the early 1950s. In his book *The Cancer Industry: The Classic Exposé on the Cancer Establishment*, Ralph Moss claims that studies done at Memorial Sloan-Kettering Cancer Center (MSKCC) from 1972 to 1977 by chemist Kanematsu Sugiura showed that laetrile stopped the metastases of cancer in mice and improved their well-being, but that the cancer center had engineered a cover-up.[13] MSKCC said that further investigations did not support the original findings of Sugiura. In 1980 cancer researchers conducted a study to determine whether laetrile was effective against cancer cells and found that it killed just as many normal cells as cancer cells. In an NCI study of laetrile conducted at the Mayo Clinic, 54 percent of the 178 patients enrolled in the study had measurable cancer progression after 21 days of intravenous treatment. After three months, 91 percent had disease progression, and after seven months all patients' tumors had grown larger. Half of all the patients in the study died within five months after starting the treatment; within 8 months 85 percent of the patients had died. The findings were published in the *New En-*

gland Journal of Medicine in January 1982. Laetrile supporters criticized the study, claiming that a degraded form of laetrile was used by NCI.[14]

The macrobiotic diet, which has its origen in Buddhism dating back to twelfth century China and Japan, consists primarily (50 to 60 percent) of whole grains, including brown rice, barley, millet, oats, corn, rye, wheat, and buckwheat; and vegetables (25 to 30 percent) such as cabbages, broccoli, watercress, onions, turnip, squash. Some vegetables that are avoided are white and sweet potatoes, eggplant, peppers, asparagus, spinach, zucchini, and avocado. Fish is allowed in small amounts one to three times a week. Sugar, meat, and animal products are not allowed. Macrobiotic diets are among the most popular unconventional approaches used by cancer patients. Some supporters say the macrobiotic diet is an effective primary treatment for cancer, while other supporters claim it can be effective when combined with other forms of treatment. Few studies have been done on the benefits of macrobiotic diets for cancer patients, and there is no scientific evidence that it can be effective when used alone or in combination with conventional treatment of cancer. NCI and ACS believe that a strict adherence to the diet can pose a serious health hazard.[15]

Shark cartilage is another alternative treatment that has gotten a lot of media attention. The substance purportedly contains a protein that inhibits the angiogenesis (growth of blood vessels) needed for tumor growth. In the book *Sharks Don't Get Cancer*, authors I. William Lane and Linda Comack call shark cartilage a "breakthough in the prevention and treatment of cancer and other degenerative diseases." However, according to John Harshbarger at the Smithsonian Institution in Washington, D.C., sharks do indeed get cancer. He has records of at least 20 cases of sharks with cancer that orginated in their cartilage as well as in kidneys, liver, and blood cells. Judah Folkman, M.D., who does research in angiogenesis at Harvard Medical School, says there is no evidence that ingesting shark cartilage can treat cancer. On the basis of what is known, he says that "a patient would have to eat hundreds of pounds of cartilage" to have any chance of experiencing any effect. Folkman adds he has been trying to stop Lane from using his name to promote a shark cartilage product.[16] In February 1993, the television news show "60 Minutes" did a segment on shark cartilage as a promising treatment. The segment, which focused on a trial of 29 patients in Cuba, was updated and aired in July 1993. Mary McCabe, of NCI's Division of Cancer Treatment, said, "The data we did review [in the Cuban study] was incomplete and unimpressive." John Renner, M.D., a member of the ACS Subcommittee on Questionable Methods expressed concern about the shark cartilage pills being sold in health food stores for upward of $100 a bottle. "The '60 Minutes' show," says Renner, "has done the nation a great disservice. . . . The Cuban study was presented to the public as reliable research, which it is not."[17] In the United States, Charles Simone, M.D., of the Simone Protective Cancer Center, in Lawrenceville, N.J., presented preliminary results from his shark cartilage trial with 20 cancer patients. He says that half the patients reported less pain and a better appetite. In August 1993, Daniel Eskinazi, M.D., of the Office of Alternative Medicine (OAM) at NIH, said that while Simone's work was promising, the OAM was far from ready to recommend it for treatment.[18]

Because of growing interest in unconventional treatments, the Office of Alternative Medicine was created through a Congressional mandate in 1992. In 1994, the OAM awarded 30 grants, most in the amount of $30,000, for the investigation of different alternative therapies. The ones that could affect breast cancer include electrochemical treatment of tumors, imagery, relaxation, macrobiotic diet, hypnotic imagery, and massage therapy.[19] Not everyone was pleased. The "ad hoc advisory board," comprised of people from the alternative medical community, says it had been told by then OAM director Joseph Jacobs, M.D., that it would have final approval over the selection of all grants. However, input from the advisory board was not solicited in the awarding of the grants.[20] In early August, after serving just 20 months, Jacobs announced his resignation as OAM director.[21] Jacobs said the $2 million annual budget was ridiculously small and that he felt stymied by the demands of numerous politicians, each with his or her own story of a miraculous alternative treatment. Critics had complained that Jacobs wasn't moving fast enough and was a poor administrator. Ralph Moss, a frequent critic of the medical establishment and a member of the OAM advisory committee, said, "[Jacobs] seemed very uncomfortable with the job. I wasn't happy with the direction of the office. I see it from the point of view of N.I.H. wanting to do things the way N.I.H. usually does." But Brian M.

Berman, M.D., an assistant professor of family medicine at the University of Maryland, and also a member of the advisory board, regretted Jacob's resignation, saying, "He did an excellent job of bringing the concept of alternative medicine to the conventional medical community." Early in 1995, OAM named Wayne Johnson, M.D., of Walter Reed Medical Center, as its new director. In its latest budget report, a Senate Appropriations subcommittee proposed increasing the yearly budget for OAM to $6 million. OAM was granted $5.2 million for fiscal year 1995 — a big improvement over its original budget of $2 million but in relative terms still a small amount.

As an indication that alternative therapies are becoming part of the mainstream, in February 1994, the Columbia University College of Physicians and Surgeons opened the Rosenthal Center for Alternative/Complementary Medicine. It is headed by Dr. Fredi Kronenberg, a physiologist who hopes to get grants from NIH's new Office of Alternative Medicine. The center will collect and evaluate existing data on alternative medical practices and eventually offer an information clearinghouse for physicians and the public. The center is the first of its kind at an Ivy League university.[22] There is also a new center for alternative medicine at Brigham Young University.

23

Mind Matters

I didn't belong to a support group which was a big mistake. I would tell anyone, seek them out, join.

— Loretta Fields, *breast cancer survivor*[1]

It is not simply a case of mind over matter; rather, it is now clear that mind indeed matters.

— David Spiegel, M.D., *Stanford Medical School*[2]

I owe my sanity, my return to life, to Expressions [breast cancer support group].

— Jan Kutschinski, *breast cancer survivor*[3]

Years ago there was no such thing as a support group for women with breast cancer. A woman diagnosed with breast cancer rarely talked about the disease. It was something to be ashamed of. Michael Sarg, M.D., associate director of oncology at St. Vincent's Hospital in New York City, remembers growing up in the late 1940s. He says, "I can recall my family whispering about the disease to avoid using the word. They referred to 'it' in hushed tones with looks of dismay. To me, those afflicted with it seemed doomed, the ultimate unfortunate ones. Their illness was itself unspeakable, treatment was mysterious and thought to be ineffective, and their future was to confront unspeakable horror until they finally died."[4] With attitudes like that predominating, it would not be surprising that a woman diagnosed with breast cancer would feel utterly alone.

Roz Kleban, C.S.W., a social work supervisor at Memorial Sloan-Kettering Cancer Center in New York, says that women diagnosed with cancer have "a tremendous sense of isolation and alienation . . . [and that] coming together in a group immediately alleviates that isolation." Seeing other women going through the same thing, they realize that the feelings they are having are normal. "Women get a tremendous amount of support and validation from the group," says Kleban, "and they realize they are not alone in the struggle." She calls participation in a support group "the single most important intervention."[5]

One of the first breast cancer support groups was started in New York City in the mid-1970s. Sandy Warshaw was an original member of the group, which became known as SHARE, for Self-Help Action Rap Experience. "We talked about the emotional issues of cancer, the inability to get insurance, job discrimination, the high cost of insurance, and the attitude of surgeons."[6] Lee Miller was another founding member of SHARE. In 1987, when she was president of SHARE, she testified at the Surgeon General's Conference on Self-Help about what she and others had learned during the eleven years of "groping pain, trial and error, sharing, and laughter" that had taken place as SHARE grew. Following are the ten conclusions she came up with as a result of the support group experience:

- Fear, anger, and depression are normal responses to serious disease.
- There is solace and validation in sharing with peers.
- Grieving is healthy because it frees up your energy to get on with your life. But grief comes in layers, and each layer must be worked through or it goes underground and emerges in undesirable ways. One woman told us that after mourning the loss of her breast she was able to grieve for the loss of her father, then her divorce, and finally, the loss of her pet.

- Facing the possibility of death means losing your feeling of invulnerability. It is much like losing the innocence of childhood. But facing reality can enhance the good times, change your perspective, and establish your priorities. You become able to ask questions like, "If not now, when?" and the social hypocrisy most of us indulge in from time to time seems superfluous.
- We need to feel in control again, even if we know it is an illusion in the grand scheme of things. We need to feel we can take charge of our own bodies, be informed medical customers, and participate fully in decisions regarding our health. An uninformed choice is not a real choice.
- We are more alike than different, but we need to appreciate and respect our differences.
- There is a difference between enlightened self-interest and selfishness.
- Living with uncertainty is difficult, but it is possible. Having cancer taught us what was always true, that life is uncertain.
- There are many kinds of courage, and though we cannot absorb courage from others, we can be inspired by it.
- Each of us is a person of value, and when we respect our own essential humanness, we can bring that respect to others.[7]

Today it would be unusual for a woman with breast cancer not to find a support group. But it can still happen. Dusharme Carter, a Miss Oklahoma, was just 20 when she was diagnosed with breast cancer. She found the lump in her breast when she was trying on swimsuits for the Miss America competition. She had a hard time getting doctors to take her seriously because she was so young. And she had a hard time finding support.

When I sought support from agencies designed to help women like myself, I found once again that I was out of my league. There were agencies for older women. I was not only out of my league because of my age but because of my experience with the situation. I had not had children. I didn't have to put other things aside. . . . My femininity and my life were in jeopardy and no one was there to help me or fully understand. I felt terribly alone. I finally created my own support group at my university and discovered that there were several young women like myself ignorant of their disease and left to fend for themselves and face the fear of dying alone.[8]

Creating her own support group (which is how many of the support groups came into being) was probably helpful on several levels. It enabled Carter to talk with women her own age and share her experiences and feelings. It also empowered her, giving her some sense of control over what was happening to her and what she could do for herself. Psychologist Julia Rowland, Ph.D., at Georgetown University, says, "I feel that being involved in your care, being an active participant in what happens to you . . . makes the course easier."[9]

Studies done at Stanford Medical School support that premise. David Spiegel, M.D., and his colleagues have been evaluating support group interventions since the late 1970s. Spiegel says, "It is known that psychosocial support can affect the way patients and their family adjust to their illness." In a study conducted by Spiegel and others, it was shown that direct confrontation with fears of dying and death and venting of strong emotion in a supportive setting are effective in improving patients' and their families' ability to cope with the illness. In a study of 86 women with metastatic breast cancer, one group received standard medical care, while the other group had the same care along with one-and-a-half-hour sessions each week for a year of supportive-expressive group therapy. Patients in the control group suffered a substantial worsening of their mood, including anxiety, depression, fatigue, confusion, and loss of vigor. Patients in the support group had the opposite response, showing an improvement in mood. Spiegel was not particularly surprised by the results. The study confirmed his thinking that even a confrontation with death in the form of a terminal illness could be a period of growth and life enhancement rather than emotional decline.[10]

The growing belief that the right mental attitude or imaging could affect the course of cancer prompted Spiegel to look at the survival time of the women in both groups. "We reasoned that since we had demonstrated a psychological effect as a result of group treatment, the absence or presence of any difference in survival time between the treatment and control groups would be important." The death records of the 83 women who had taken part in the study and died (three were still living) were obtained. One finding was that after four years all the women in the control group had died, while one-third of the patients in the support group were still living. The mean survival from the time of study entry until death was 18.9 months for the control group and 58.4 for the intervention group, a significant statistical difference.

"We came to the conclusion," says Spiegel, "after three years of re-analysis of the data that something about the intervention had influenced survival time." That finding came as a surprise to Spiegel.[11]

While this is a potentially life-lengthening intervention, Spiegel has some concern that the mind-over-matter approach might lead some cancer patients to think that they have failed to exert the proper mental control if their cancer progresses. He cites as an example a woman with metastatic breast cancer who was told, "You caused your cancer, you can cure it." That may be effective with some patients, but for many it can add additional stress, distress, and guilt over not getting better.[12] That is also a concern of Julia Rowland, who says the fact that there is beginning to be some data suggesting that psychological intervention can affect outcome should not lead women to conclude that "if I can control the outcome, I should be able to control getting it." Rowland says that there are no data to suggest that stress or depression causes you to develop cancer, and how the psychological and physiological are tied together is still unknown.[13] A report in the *British Medical Journal* in May 1992 stated that "no evidence was found to show that stress is conducive in cancer." It concluded, "Most severe life events and social difficulties are not preventable. Psychosocial intervention, however skilled, can soften their adverse impact to only a limited degree. Women with a history of breast cancer who fear that unavoidable emotional traumas like bereavement may cause them to relapse should therefore find consolation in our results."[14]

Jimmie Holland, M.D., who founded the highly regarded psychiatric division at Memorial Sloan-Kettering Cancer Center in 1977, does not support the thesis that one causes one's own cancer or that with enough determination and positive thinking one can be cured. But she does say that there is evidence that the body's physiology may be altered by the intense anxiety experienced by some patients at high risk of getting cancer, such as women with close relatives who have died of breast cancer. Holland feels strongly that psychological counseling is an option that should be "part of regular medical care."[15] Unfortunately, these days, when psychotherapy is covered by a medical plan, it frequently is of very limited duration.

Marvin Stein, M.D., a psychiatrist at Mt. Sinai School of Medicine in New York City, noted that the longer life spans that Spiegel reported could have been the result of other factors — such as women in the support group getting more sleep or eating better or being more conscientious in following medical advice — rather than any effect psychological support had on the immune system. Stein acknowledges that support groups can have a positive impact on the body's immune system but says, "The question is whether these [support groups] have anything to do with health and illness."[16] Holland has her own questions. "The changes in immune cell activity are quite small. They are blips compared to the range that a clinical lab would report as an abnormal finding. We need more research to find out if there is any real clinical significance."[17]

Besides Spiegel's study, there is a small but growing body of literature suggesting that psychosocial support may have an influence on the rate of disease progression. In 1990 a study was published that showed a higher risk of cancer mortality for both men and women who were socially isolated. There is evidence that marital status is a strong predictor of a more positive prognosis. There is also evidence that psychosocial stress such as bereavement, job loss, forced relocation, and other life upheavals are associated with a higher risk of relapse of breast cancer. Therefore, data suggest that screening for psychosocially-at-risk patients (stressed or isolated) could be of benefit.[18] The role stress plays in cancer, if any, remains controversial and inconclusive.

Steven P. Hersh, cofounder of the Medical Illness Counseling Center in Chevy Chase, Maryland, calls psychological help "essential" in the treatment of breast cancer patients.[19] Julia Rowland says, "Psychological counseling should be a standard part of [breast cancer] treatment. . . . Increasingly, oncologists are recognizing that this is an important aspect of care."[20] Psychooncology has blossomed in the last 20 years. Patti Wilcox, a nurse practitioner at Johns Hopkins Breast Center, says, "In the beginning, most women are so consumed by information and the decisions they have to make that they have to turn the emotions off. Several months later a woman will suddenly be confronted with 'Oh my God, I've had cancer.' "[21]

Donna Sauer says she is the oldest member in her support group in California. When I talked with her in 1993, she was 59 years old. She was diagnosed with breast cancer in 1986 at the age of 52 and had a mastectomy in 1989. She says that the camaraderie and support that the group offered her is immeasurable.

The mistaken belief that some people have that this is a "boo-hoo" group, that we're all going to moan and groan, is a misconception that I would like to see lifted. Breast cancer groups are never that way. They're information groups that offer more than just hope, more than support. I think women are short-changing themselves by not attending, if nothing else but to give of themselves.[22]

Supportive counseling is being recommended for patients undergoing HDC/ABMT. Christina A. Meyers, Ph.D., associate professor of neuropsychology at M. D. Anderson Cancer Center in Houston, says, "Even a few minutes spent on counseling and providing information may have a tremendous long-term impact."[23] Dr. John Wingard, M.D., director of the bone marrow transplant program at Emory University School of Medicine in Atlanta, says that he has found patients who feel abandoned because their oncologist has not explained adaquately all that they would be going through. Meyers describes the procedure as an extremely traumatic experience. "I know that some people I talked to thought they were going crazy."[24] Meyers says, "If patients and their families understood that some symptoms — such as short-term memory loss — are fairly common and can be dealt with, this would go a long way to reducing further emotional complications."[25] Michael A. Andrykowski, Ph.D., associate professor of behavioral science at the University of Kentucky, stresses the importance of repeatedly informing patients about psychosocial issues. He says that patients who are undergoing HDC/ABMT are often in a very vulnerable state and don't really hear, or remember, what they've been told.[26]

With more research maybe we will eventually know for sure whether being in a support group can lengthen the survival time for a woman with cancer. What we do know, without question, is that supportive care and taking part in a support group can enhance the woman's quality of life.

24

Doctor/Patient Relationships

Doctors are sometimes intimidating unless you really do assert yourself. Sometimes with the doctors you just have to educate yourself when you get a disease.

— Betty Reed, *breast cancer survivor*[1]

I owe my life to the physiatrist. He took me seriously. I was starting to feel like a neurotic woman, all these pains I was having. . . . he said, "You know, you're not getting better. We have to see what's going on here."

— Pat Skowronski, *breast cancer survivor*[2]

The doctor patted me on the head and told me I was being paranoid because my mother had had breast cancer. She felt sure that this was just fibrocystic disease and that if it would make me feel better I could go have another mammogram. She said I was worrying just because of my mother and not to worry.

— Mary Katzke, *breast cancer survivor*[3]

A doctor's medical decisions and demeanor can have a major positive or negative impact on the extent and course of a patient's recovery. It seems as if not a week goes by without new findings or a change in the treatment for breast cancer. If a doctor is not up on the latest medical developments, it can be lethal to the patient. A woman diagnosed with breast cancer is usually anxious, frightened, and stunned. A doctor who takes the time to explain what is going on and answer questions patiently can be a calming influence. The doctor who is short, impatient, and patronizing can add stress to an already stressful situation.

It is not unusual for a patient to leave the doctor's office with many unanswered questions. Many times a newly diagnosed patient, under a lot of stress, will remember a small part of what the doctor says or will not understand everything. When someone is diagnosed with cancer, it is not unusual for her to undergo a psychological phenomenon called "shutdown," in which nothing else is really heard after the word "cancer."

There are doctors who do not want to be questioned, on any level, by a patient. They don't want their choice of treatment to be second-guessed or they carry such a large patient load, they simply do not have the time to spend with an individual patient. One woman told me her doctor always had his hand on the doorknob and was halfway out the door when he talked to her. Another woman said until she brought a friend along, her oncologist would talk on the phone as he gave her chemotherapy.

"Women should investigate who their doctors are," says Kimberly Calder, at Cancer Care. "They should be comfortable with what they're saying."[4] Certainly good advice, but easier said than done. Dr. Julia Rowland says older patients are more comfortable letting the doctor make the decisions, whereas younger patients are more aggressive. In general, the older a woman is, the more likely she is to want the doctor just to tell her what to do. Younger women tend to ask questions and demand answers. However, there are many younger women who do not like having all the options dumped in their laps and being told to make a choice.[5]

I had just one brief bad-doctor experience. When my cancer recurred in 1981, I was terrified and bursting with anxiety. I considered being treated at NCI, which was interested in having me take part in one of their clinical trials. The doctor who was then head of the breast cancer division looked at my records, did a cursory physical exam, looked me straight in the eye, and said, "If you'd gone on the vacation you were planning, you would have come back a very sick woman and you would have been dead in six months." My mother was with me and when we left his office we both burst into tears. I am compelled to add that his insensitivity, abruptness, and lack of compassion were the exception and not the rule at NCI. I was pleasantly surprised when all the other doctors I encountered were considerate and compassionate. Overall, I was luckier than many women. I had an oncologist who I knew cared about me, always treated me with respect, and was certainly competent. Many women, in big and small cities throughout the United States, have not been as fortunate as I was. Most of the women I talked with who had a bad experience with a doctor were able to turn it around, usually by going to another doctor. That is probably why they were able, and sometimes eager, to tell me what happened to them.

Just as I know there are many competent and caring doctors out there, I also know that there are many women who are silent and uncomplaining, accepting shabby medical treatment and emotionally damaging care. Following are excerpts from just some of the stories I heard from women with whom I spoke:

Ester Johnson, diagnosed with breast cancer in her late forties in 1985:

> I fired my doctor because he played God. He said, "You will do it my way or no way." I am my own woman and do my own thing. Educate me and let me make my own decision. . . . When he had diagnosed me, he asked me if I had any questions and I asked him when I could be reconstructed. He told me that couldn't be my first question, then proceeded to tell me why, and that I should rant and rave and scream and cry. I didn't have to. After the surgery I asked him again about reconstruction and he told me I had to wait a year. I left and called a plastic surgeon and had it done three months later. My surgeon got on my case real bad, and I said, "I don't think you and I need to be [in a] doctor-patient relationship." . . . I did not have adjuvant chemotherapy because my doctor didn't think it was necessary. I think he cheated me, because I will always have that little doubt; if it recurs, if I'd had chemo, would it have?[6]

Ruth Mendoza was diagnosed with breast cancer at age 38 in 1989. Her experience with an HMO physician is frighteningly common. These for-profit institutions do everything possible to cuts costs, often at the expense of the patient and good medical care.

Someone told me about the (800) 4-CANCER number at NCI. I spent over an hour on the phone being respected, and loved, and treated like a person who could learn. The experience was really exciting. I was a little angry and wanted immediately to talk to my HMO doctor provider. . . . I said, "It's a year since my surgery." I started asking questions. I insisted on being in his office, not the examining room. NCI suggested I talk to the doctor in his office. We needed to be equal and really communicate. When I'm in the examining room, undressed, I'm being a patient. I started asking inquisitive, pointed questions. He went behind his desk and never came out. He said come back in a week, when he would review my history, and then we could better talk. I went back a week later with my husband and NCI materials and the doctor had forgotten to read my history and had nothing to tell me. He asked if I perceived my body as being "cancer ridden," is that why I was there? Well, my husband held me back from climbing over the desk and the doctor said, "Let me do something for you," and he called an oncologist. I was to be satisfied with a conversation over an intercom to an oncologist about the findings I had in my hand from NCI comparing mastectomy with lumpectomy and radiation. . . . The oncologist said, "Oh, that report, oh, that's so new, I haven't even had a chance to read that report yet." I told my doctor I wanted a referral to USC [University of Southern California] that day. He insisted I see the oncologist first. . . . When I saw the oncologist, I was angry and bitter. . . . He apologized and said he was a contractor and HMO did not send patients to him, in their eyes you're done. It took me four months to get my referral. I called [my HMO doctor provider] and said, "If you won't give me my referral tomorrow, I will be on the phone to Channel 7 or be calling my lawyer." . . . When I went back to the surgeon to ask why there was no follow-up care, he said, "You have to understand, I was contracted out, I have nothing else to do with you. So I removed your breast and hoped you got care. I'm sorry that you didn't get care." That's all he said to me.[7]

Marlene Kessler was 36 when she was diagnosed with breast cancer in 1992:

He [the breast surgeon who did a biopsy] was three hours late and I was a nervous wreck and he comes in and I was sitting down and he says, "Marlene, you have cancer, so we have to take your whole right breast off." I was in shock just from the word 'cancer.' And then he said, "You can decide later if you want reconstruction, but in the meantime you can stick a sock in there." I left there and I went hysterical. My parents said I should go for a second opinion. . . . He [the second-opinion doctor] went over the report from the first surgeon and we talked about everything. I asked him his background. He said, "I don't know your background, so I don't have to tell you mine." My dad was in the room with me. I said, "Come on Dad, let's get out of here because I don't want this guy touching me, because I don't know his background." So I got dressed. I'll never forget this. I go out and the doctor called me back and I didn't understand what he wanted, so I went back. There was a lady in there wearing an examining gown. She was sitting up and the doctor says, "Marlene, this is what you're going to look like," and he pulled open the gown and the lady had no boob — all there was were big scars and I ran out of there. I cried and cried and cried and cried. My dad didn't know how to calm me down.[8]

Lois Joy Thomi was 55 when she was diagnosed in 1982:

The doctor came and told me I had a rare cancer called inflammatory carcinoma and that it was very aggressive. . . . He said I probably had six to eight weeks to live because this type of cancer can be all through your vital organs by the time it's diagnosed. He told me I'd be sick from the treatment and that I'd lose my hair. It didn't bother me as much as it might bother someone else. I was just interested in living. . . . My doctor came to see me and said, "Well, Lois, you've lived a good life and I could get hit by a truck going to the office," and I wanted to say, "If I were out there, you would!" . . . I finished chemo and started radiation. I was really scared but was happy. I'd lived the two months. I had stopped asking doctors questions because I guess I didn't want to hear their answers, they were so negative. At about the third week after the start of radiation, I asked my doctor if I'd lived that long if I was going to make it, and he told me not to start thinking like that because they'd never had anyone here who'd lived longer than two months. That really shot me down. It was the worst day of my life.[9]

Fortunately, for Thomi, at the time when she was feeling total despair, she received an unexpected phone call from the Kansas state attorney general. Her brother, who knew him and knew he'd survived cancer, had asked the attorney general to call. "He said, 'God gave us doctors and God gave us medicine and a brain to use.' It was so simple, but it was just what I needed to hear. He said, 'I believe God will bring you through this.' It was the first real encouragement any-one had given me." Thomi went on to start a support group in Wichita.

Lana Jensen was 32 when she was diagnosed with breast cancer:

I felt a lump under my armpit. The doctor sloughed it off. But I did say I'd like to have a mammogram. He wanted to know why and persuaded me not to have it at that time. He said, "Don't worry about it until you're forty." I always believed the doctors knew everything. Six months later they took twenty-five lymph nodes and some were posi-tive. I said, "Do you think if I had demanded a mammogram?" . . . They said, "We probably would have caught it at first stage and not at the second stage."[10]

In 1990, the Physicians Insurers Association of America chided doctors for not taking women seriously when they reported breast lumps they'd discovered. The association stated that in 69 percent of cases in which claims were paid in response to charges of unnecessarily delayed diagnosis, the woman had found the breast lump, but her physician had not taken it seriously.[11]

Breast oncologist Larry Norton believes that saying, "I'm the doc-tor and you should have breast conservation" is just as bad as saying "I'm the doctor and you should have a mastectomy." "Both are paternalistic. I think that people really have to be informed. I think we have to be very careful about dogma and making decisions for people."[12]

Unfortunately, we can't count on doctors learning this kind of sensitivity in medical school or picking it up on their own. It is our life and we must take charge — by making sure that we are taken seri-ously, that our questions are answered, that we are respected and not treated in a condescending manner, and that we are getting the best possible treatment. If you have cancer and are not sure you are getting the latest treatment, call NCI's Cancer Information Service at (800) 4-CANCER to find out what the National Cancer Institute says is the state-of-the-art treatment for your stage of breast cancer. Get a second opinion on your cancer treatment from a breast surgeon or medical oncologist. If you feel your doctor is not really listening to you, or is talking down to you, or is just plain rude, find another doctor. Call the local medical society or the nearest large hospital and ask for a referral to a doctor specializing in breast cancer or a medical oncologist. You can check the credentials of any doctor at your public library. There are plenty of competent and concerned doctors available. When you are fighting for your life, you don't want to be obstructed by a difficult doctor.

Part V

Psychosocial Impact

25

Sexuality

Since this is a country with breast fetishes, we are afraid of gender identity loss, so we avoid mammographies.

— Gloria Steinem, *feminist, breast cancer survivor*[1]

Every woman who goes through this will wonder about her femininity and sexuality.

— Ann Marcou, *co-founder Y-ME, breast cancer survivor*[2]

We live in a breast-oriented society. To the average woman, her breast is the badge of femininity, an important part of allurement to charm her male.

— Philip Strax, M.D.[3]

Bestselling novelist Jacqueline Susann died of breast cancer in 1974. In a 1975 article in the *Journal of Sex and Marital Therapy*, Mildred Hope Witkin, Ph.D., said that Susann had undergone a radical mastectomy 12 years earlier. When she was first diagnosed, Susann said she would not undergo a mastectomy but changed her mind after her husband pleaded with her to do it. She reportedly said, "I don't want to go through life with one breast. I'll be half a woman. How will I look in the mirror?" She swore her husband and mother to secrecy. Witkin says Susann "clearly identified with the breast-vaunting culture that characterizes America today." The formula is, according to Witkin, "A woman's worth depends on the approval of others, which in turn depends on physical attractiveness, on big breasts, [or], at the least, two breasts" and that Susann, like so many women, fell prey to that. The cultural emphasis on breasts with the subsequent internalization of "breast pride" can fill a woman with "fantasies of worthlessness." Says Witkin, "The mastectomy is a traumatic operation. It is made more traumatic by the cultural bias expressed in the media and echoed by some professionals."[4]

It is not possible to talk about the impact of breast cancer on a woman's sexuality and body image without bringing up the role of contemporary media. It wasn't until the middle of the nineteenth century that new technology made it possible to reproduce pictures of how women "should" look. Naomi Wolf, author of *The Beauty Myth*, says that at that time the first nude photographs of prostitutes appeared as well as ads featuring "beautiful" pictures of beautiful women.[5]

It is true that radio, television, and magazines have brought to the public a greatly needed awareness of breast cancer. At the same time, it is the mass media, run for the most part by white males, which have persistently promoted the young, beautiful, and generally "busty" woman as the most attractive, as the woman who gets the most desirable man capable of providing her with all that is important in life. Women's role, as defined by the media, has always been one of dependence on a male, and to get that male she must be more attractive than her competitors. Is it any wonder that some women are terrified of losing a breast, at times so terrified that they end up losing their lives instead?

According to sociology professor Allan Mazur, men place more importance on the way a woman looks than a woman does on the way a man looks. It is, therefore, important for women to look as close to the current ideal image of beauty as possible, so as to enhance her social opportunities. There is a lot at stake. Conformity to the latest body image is considered crucial to many women. Mazur says that places a lot of stress upon women to look like the latest media image, stress that can be deadly.[6] As women try to adapt to the image, there are some who overadapt. In recent years, women have literally starved themselves to death, becoming anorexic or bulimic, to be as thin as they thought was necessary. These kinds of behaviors are rarely seen in men. In a study of the ten most popular magazines read by young men and women, it was found that the women's magazines had 10.5 times as many ads and articles promoting weight loss as the men's magazines. The ratio of diet articles correlated almost exactly with the documented ratios of females to males having eating disorders.[7]

"The self-image of an American woman is not complete without her breasts, particularly in our society, where significant emphasis is placed on the female chest as portrayed on television, in magazines, and in newspapers," says Hal Bingham, M.D., a professor at the University of Florida College of Medicine. "We actually worship the female breast and when a woman has a breast removed, she loses one of her more important identifying features. This severely affects her body image."[8]

Rose Kushner also gives the media substantial credit for the obsession with breasts in the United States. She says the indoctrination starts early.

> The media were responsible for the long hours my sons spent discussing who was 32A or 34B and, wonder of wonders, the fifteen-year-old who had a 40D. The media are also the main reason my daughter and her girlfriends who, at the age of 12 or 13, stood before their mirrors trying to make the bumps in their training bras larger with the help of cotton balls, Kleenex, or ripped nylons (those worked best, by the way). . . . Male chauvinism plays an important role in all aspects of breast cancer, from the moment a sixth-grader's budding chest bumps make her popular, to the belief (many times correct) that breasts are vital to getting and keeping a boyfriend. The "importance" of breasts is constantly reinforced by the media.[9]

Janet Perkins, a breast cancer survivor, is one of many women whose self-image after surgery was affected by the cultural bias:

> I had this notion that now I was "damaged goods." My self-worth would be lowered. I would somehow be of less value. That threat to one's self esteem is always there. I think it's true if you're going to have

a leg amputated, but there's an extra loaded issue when it's a breast because we are women and it's a very important part of our anatomy and the image we present to the world.[10]

The issue of self-worth or self-esteem is also addressed by psychiatrist Christopher C. Gates, M.D., clinical instructor at Harvard Medical School. He says there are multiple injuries to self-esteem from both the diagnosis and the treatment of breast cancer. The woman's emotional life will be changed forever. "It is an outrage to have one's breast turn cancerous. The change in breast tissue from life-giving to life-threatening is a betrayal, a form of somatic treason. It is an outrage to lose a breast, lose hair, and undergo prolonged nausea, weakness, and vomiting from radiation therapy or chemotherapy."[11]

Linda Dackman was 34 when she had breast cancer. She says, "If you get cancer at a young age, you're still very caught up in the idea that as a woman you're attractive only if your body is perfect. I had to rebuild my self-esteem around the fact that my body was flawed. I had lost a breast and experienced a terrible sense of being disfigured and therefore less worthy." Dackman was able to work through her negative feelings and write the book *Upfront: Sex and Post-Mastectomy Women*.[12]

A study published in 1993 found many significant differences in the way women viewed themselves after they had breast surgery. Not surprisingly, women who had a lumpectomy were more satisfied than women who had had a mastectomy with reconstruction or just a mastectomy.[13] However, a recent study at the Center for Sexual Function at the Cleveland Clinic Foundation, in Ohio, on the effects of breast cancer on sexuality, body image, and intimate relationships, concluded, "The majority of women cope well with the stress of cancer surgery and the loss of a breast." Leslie R. Schover, staff psychologist, says the newer treatments like lumpectomy and reconstruction of a breast after a mastectomy give a woman the feeling of having more control and enable her to feel more comfortable with her body. Most of the married women questioned said their mastectomies had not harmed their marriages or sex lives. In many instances the effects of chemotherapy — hair loss, premature menopause, infertility, and weight gain — were as traumatic as the loss of the breast.[14]

The effect of breast cancer on sexual functioning has been rarely discussed and even more rarely studied. Julia Rowland says that many of the studies concerning the psychosocial effects of breast cancer "have looked at body image. Our appreciation of sexual functioning in breast cancer patients is very simplistic, in part because our understanding of sexual functioning in normal adults is also simplistic and old." Rowland's statement that the government has not supported research into sexual functioning also comes as no surprise.[15]

Richard Theriault, M.D., at M. D. Anderson Cancer Center in Houston, says, "Most of us are sexual beings and we are very concerned about our sexual function and yet we . . . haven't become aware enough to ask the question of most of our patients. . . . We have been remiss in that we have not been studying these . . . critical issues in women with a background of breast cancer." As a result, he referred to a study of some female leukemia patients who had undergone chemotherapy. He said of 36 patients, 80 percent reported vaginal dryness and 50 percent reported difficulty with sexual intercourse. The women also expressed concerns about "femininity, sterility, and the future regarding their sexual functioning."[16]

Psychologist Linda Bloom says that following breast cancer treatment, "Sex was just horrible, long after treatment ended and my energy returned." Bloom says that none of her doctors ever warned her about the sexual side effects.[17] Doctors are "uncomfortable with female sexuality, especially in older women," noted the late Helen Singer Kaplan, M.D., Ph.D., who was director of the human sexuality program at New York Hospital-Cornell Medical Center. It has been common to view any woman's problem with sexual functioning following breast cancer as psychological. A doctor will tell a woman, "It's all in your head" and give her the message that she is lucky to be alive. Kaplan said the problem is frequently physical, that the treatment a woman undergoes after the initial surgery for breast cancer can affect her sex drive. Chemotherapy can cause ovarian failure in both premenopausal and postmenopausal women, impairing "all three phases of the female sexual response cycle — desire, excitement, and orgasm." The ovaries secrete the female hormone estrogen and a small amount of the male hormone testosterone. Kaplan said testosterone is crucial for the libido in both man and woman, and without it, it is impossible to have a normal sex drive. "You can only feel hungry if the appetite centers in your brain are active. . . . Sex is the same. You can't feel erotic unless your sex centers are active, and they cannot operate without testosterone." After determining that a woman's loss of desire had been caused by a lack of sufficient testosterone, Kaplan prescribed a low dose of testosterone. "Invariably," she said, "when they get their testosterone, they call up and say, 'It's a miracle.' "[18]

James A. Simone, M.D., director of reproductive endocrinology at the Georgetown University School of Medicine, says that it is risky to give any reproductive steroid hormone to a woman with breast cancer unless she is considered clinically cured. Simone adds that it may not even be testosterone that sexually stimulates the brain. "There is an abundant and growing literature suggesting that the main mechanism for sexual stimulation in the brain is actually estrogen in both men and women."[19]

A side effect of the depletion of estrogen caused by the chemotherapy can be a failure to lubricate during sexual activity, which can make sexual intercourse painful. Women are advised to use nonestrogen vaginal lubricants, which are available over the counter in most drugstores. Another form of treatment is counseling to improve sexual relationships within the context of any physical limitations.

Now that breast cancer is finally out of the closet, the emergence and study of breast cancer's effect on sexuality, which is a major issue for women with breast cancer, is long overdue. When doctors discuss side effects of chemotherapy and hormonal therapy with patients, sexual side effects are rarely included. Many doctors, especially male doctors, will not address sexuality issues out of embarrassment or lack of knowledge. If a woman brings it up, they trivialize her concern. Many women do feel uncomfortable discussing how their breast cancer and its treatment will affect them sexually. It is up to the health care provider to afford a setting where women can voice their concerns and problems. More studies are needed and more education in dealing with sexual issues with patients is necessary for doctors.

26

Reconstruction or Deconstruction?

Advances in breast reconstruction and plastic surgery have played a valuable role in alleviating the physical and emotional consequences of breast cancer.

— Congresswoman Marilyn Lloyd (D-Tennessee),
breast cancer survivor[1]

They [breast implants] were supposed to be emotionally and physically a help, but they're time bombs . . . another poison in your body.

— Sheila Swanson, *breast cancer survivor*[2]

Reasonable people are not asking whether silicone causes disease, but how often.

— Eric Gershwin, M.D., *chief of rheumatology and allergy at the University of California at Davis*[3]

Since the early 1960s, about one million women have obtained silicone gel breast implants.[4] Most of those implants, about 80 percent, were for so-called cosmetic reasons, such as breast augmentation or reshaping of the breasts.[5] The cosmetic surgery was performed in otherwise healthy women who were often described as feeling physically inadequate and having doubts about femininity and desirability. The other 20 percent of the implants were used in the reconstruction of breasts for women who had had mastectomies as a result of breast cancer.[6] It wasn't until 1979 that insurance companies stopped classifying breast reconstruction after a mastectomy as cosmetic surgery and started to reimburse for it, although insurance companies never showed a similar reluctance to reimburse men for testicular implants.[7]

The use of silicone to enlarge breasts dates back to postwar Japan, when Japanese prostitutes had breasts injected with liquid silicone to make them bigger and more appealing to American men. It wasn't long before the practice spread to the United States. In the mid- 1940s, an estimated 50,000 women followed the example set by Japanese women and had silicone injected into their breasts. That included 10,000 waitresses and showgirls in Nevada.[8]

In 1965, Dow Corning got Food and Drug Administration (FDA) approval to conduct liquid silicone studies in animals and humans for medicinal use. Then, in the late 1960s, reports began surfacing about problems with the silicone. According to Edward Kopf, M.D., assistant professor of plastic surgery at the University of Nevada School of Medicine, thousands of women in Nevada "started hollering."[9] They complained of lumps, silicone cysts, and breasts that were hard as rocks. Kopf started lobbying to get silicone injections off the market in Nevada. In 1967, the FDA stopped the studies of injected liquid silicone and revoked the permission it had given Dow Corning. In 1969, the FDA gave Dow permission to test liquid silicone, but not in women's breasts. In the meantime, Dr. Kopf went to the Nevada attorney general and to the FDA and, in 1975, finally convinced Nevada legislators to outlaw all injectable silicone. Shortly after that, Colorado and California did the same. In Japan by the mid-1970s, doctors were reporting long-term effects of the silicone similar to those reported in the United States.

As early as 1962, Dow Corning researchers had invented a silicone breast implant in a silicone envelope.[10] By mid-1975, the company was selling its silicone gel–filled breast implants. According to Norman Anderson, M.D., a surgeon at Johns Hopkins Hospital in Baltimore, who was a consultant to the FDA on the issue, the company never tested its implants in, or just under, breast tissue. He came to that conclusion many years later after reviewing 10,000 pages of Dow Corning's submissions to the FDA when the silicone implants were the subject of a raging controversy. In a letter to FDA head David Kessler, M.D., Anderson said, "I find this omission a peculiar phenomenon which must be unprecedented in the history of device evaluation."[11]

Use of the silicone gel implant grew. In 1981, approximately 20,000 women in the United States had undergone breast reconstruction as a result of having had a mastectomy. Just four years later, it was estimated that 98,000 women in the United States had had breast reconstruction.[12] However, it is interesting to note that only a small percentage of the women who have a mastectomy opt for breast reconstruction. The FDA estimates that as of 1992, some 200,000 women had had breast reconstruction with an implant, whereas nearly two million women who had had mastectomies had not gotten reconstruction and either used a breast prosthesis or went without. Nevertheless, the availability of breast reconstruction was considered a big boon for women with breast cancer.

Wendy S. Schain, Ed.D., at the Memorial Cancer Institute in Long Beach, California, contends that "reconstructive mammoplasty may hold the key to psychological equanimity and provide a sense of security for the woman facing breast cancer surgery."[13] For many women it offers some reassurance to know that if they should develop breast cancer and have to have a mastectomy, rather than a lumpectomy, they can have their missing breast reconstructed. As to why the percentage of women who do get breast reconstruction has been so small, Schain says there can be any of a number of reasons, including not knowing that it is an option, lack of health coverage, not wanting to undergo any more surgery, or their general health status.[14]

Julia Rowland, Ph.D., an assistant professor of psychology at Georgetown University, says that "[with] reconstruction, women feel it improves body image and their sense of femininity."[15] Breast reconstruction can eliminate or at least reduce some of the negative reactions fostered by the mastectomy and restore a woman's feelings of wholeness, physical integrity, and body symmetry. A study in the Netherlands reported that more than 90 percent of the women surveyed described their reaction to reconstructive surgery as extremely satisfying.[16] The national breast cancer support group Y-ME did a survey in October 1991 of its own hotline counselors, all of whom are breast cancer survivors. Among the respondents who had implants, the overwhelming majority were satisfied with their implants and 87 percent believed the implant helped their emotional recovery.[17]

The most frequent reason that a woman gets reconstruction after having a mastectomy is to feel more like her former self and less self-conscious and sexually inhibited. Other reasons include: being able to get rid of the external prosthesis, which can be irritating and distracting; being less constricted in choice of clothing; and being less preoccupied with the reason she is missing a breast — the missing breast can serve as a constant reminder of the cancer as well as the possibility of its recurrence. Wendy Schain says, "For those women whose self-esteem is rooted mainly in physical attributes, breast reconstruction will help them maintain a healthy body image and a sense of psychological well being, and will also have a positive effect on quality of life."[18]

When Diane Zarafonetis decided, a year after her mastectomy, to have a prophylactic mastectomy on her other breast, she had breast reconstruction. "I had it to feel whole again. The prosthesis just didn't do it for me. I was young. That's how I felt. Other women don't necessarily feel that way."[19]

Rebecca Packer acknowledges some ambivalent feelings about getting breast reconstruction:

> Though I don't like to be captive to this culture, I am. I had potentially the right idea intellectually, but emotionally, I couldn't accept it. [We live in a] "culture of cleavage." Before cancer I always had feminist leanings, was aware of the inequities. I knew I lived in a society where women had to look a certain way. I learned sexism from other women as well as men. I was an ugly duckling who started to blossom as a teen. Boys always seemed to focus on "t and a.". . . I could speak in politically correct language, could express anger, but still wanted to be a "member of the club."[20]

When Mary Katzke was considering breast reconstruction, she spoke with seven women who had had reconstruction. Five of them regretted doing it; they didn't like the way it turned out. Some said it was painful and that they were unable to sleep on their chest or side because the implant was like a rock. And there was a lack of erotic sensation.[21]

When doctors advised Ann Marcou to have her other breast removed because of the very high likelihood of getting cancer in the second breast, she did so, two months after her first mastectomy. At that time she was offered the possibility of breast reconstruction, but she says the procedure was still relatively new and she wanted to wait until there was more information about it. Five years later she opted for bilateral reconstruction. She describes the results as "Barbie doll breasts, little round things. I wear a prosthesis over them."[22]

Jody Rogers was diagnosed with breast cancer in 1979 and had breast reconstruction a short time later. She is one of many women who had to have reconstruction done over again. She says when she got the implant, her doctor really didn't go into risks with her. But she quickly adds:

> I'm not sure they were known then. He did tell me there was the possibility of rejection or a hardening of the capsule around it. It never entered my mind that they could develop a leak and that formation of scar tissue could move it. I wish there had been more research then on the implant. I wish I had waited a while instead of being so anxious to do what I did. At that time, they didn't even have the saline implants. I did it because of my own vanity. My husband said he didn't care what I did as long as I was happy. . . . Breast reconstruction was just starting when I had it done. I don't know if I would have known about it, but my surgeon told me about it. He was a proponent of it and still is. I think there will always be a certain percentage of women who want to do all they can to come back to normal. With this recent [saline implant] surgery I feel more normal than I have in years and look more normal.[23]

Virginia Soffa did consider having breast reconstruction, but in the end decided against it. She says:

> I went through the process of looking at reconstruction. I felt comfortable with my decision. I didn't have reconstruction. In April 'ninety-one, there was a lot in the press on silicone implants. Doctors felt there was no problem with silicone. I knew there would be hearings on silicone. But doctors kept telling me it'd be fine and safe. I didn't feel the medical profession was on my side by giving me that recommendation when I was trying to do everything as holistically as possible. They didn't want to use saline. . . . I asked one doctor if he'd

just put nipples on my chest, but he was apprehensive because he was sure I would want, as he put it, bumps on my chest and he was afraid the nipples would then be in the wrong place. As it turned out, my scars are marks on my chest and I didn't want to have additional surgery. I'm only 5 foot 1. Not having breasts is not a big deal because I'm petite and having nipples would have given me that sexy feeling.[24]

During the early 1990s there was tremendous publicity about the safety of silicone gel implants and the problems they might cause. One of the first articles for the general public had appeared in the widely read women's magazine *Good Housekeeping* in April 1989. The article, "How Safe Are Breast Implants?" said that minor problems, such as loss of sensitivity in the nipple and scar tissue causing the breast to feel unnaturally firm, may occur occasionally. It also talked about the fact that an implant might make it harder to detect breast cancer in a mammogram.[25]

Suddenly, all kinds of problems were being attributed to the implants by women who had undergone reconstruction as well as women who had gotten the implant for breast augmentation. More and more women appeared in the media talking about their problems with the implant. Between January 1, 1991, and July 31, 1992, the FDA received numerous letters from women who complained of physical problems that they linked with their implants.[26] Here are excerpts from three of the letters from breast cancer patients:

> I am a breast cancer survivor with two breast implants. My first breast implant ruptured and had to be replaced. My second breast implant is now very hard and I am experiencing other medical problems such as joint pains for which I am being treated. My plastic surgeon has agreed to replace my two current implants with saline solution implants. At the time of my original surgery, I was never made aware of the many problems which could occur from breast implants. I am very upset and angry.

> I had bilateral mastectomies as treatment for breast cancer. My implants became firm, displaced, and distorted. I became ill, exhibiting various autoimmune symptoms, which increased over the years. I went to various physicians, told them of my symptoms, and never got any successful diagnosis or treatment until just recently. Prior to that time,

when I talked to the doctors specifically about the implants, I was told that mine were like everyone else's and that they could not be the cause of my problems.

I am a cancer patient and had double mastectomies. I decided to undergo surgery one more time for breast implants as an attempt to feel normal again. Since the date of my first implant, my health started deteriorating and continued to do so to the point that I lost my job. I have been unable to work and to conduct any kind of normal life. All along I have questioned the relationship of the implants to the way I've been feeling.

A study of 112 of the letters received by the FDA on the silicone implants — 46 from women who had breast cancer and 66 from women who had implants for augmentation — reached the following conclusions:

- The women were coping with illness and physical problems as well as the stress of having to prove that their problems were real and possibly related to the implants.
- Their physical problems had diminished the quality of their lives.
- They were desperately seeking help.
- They were particularly angry about the lack of information given them before the surgery.[27]

The women who described their problems felt strongly that their surgeons had minimized or denied altogether any risks before the operation and during the years when the women encountered difficulties.[28] The obvious question is why so many women needed to prove to their doctors that their symptoms were real and why the concerns of women were not taken seriously until all the publicity appeared regarding possible health problems associated with silicone gel breast implants.

Although the public only became aware of the problem in the 1990s, anecdotal evidence of trouble with silicone implants first started showing up in medical journals in the 1970s and 1980s. Dozens of case studies described many different problems that were possibly caused by the implants. In 1979 in the *Annals of Plastic Surgery,* Barry Uretsky, a cardiologist in Pittsburgh, described how a patient suffered fevers, sweats, swollen joints, and enlarged kidneys within days of getting silicone gel implants, and how she recovered within seven weeks after removal of the implants.[29] In 1986, Steven R. Weiner, a rheumatologist at UCLA, reported in the *Journal of Plastic and Reconstructive Surgery* on three breast implant patients who had joint pain, including one who lost partial use of an arm.[30]

Some researchers were having doubts as well. In 1976, Thomas Talcott, a chemical engineer who worked for Dow Corning, quit after trying to convince the company for over a year not to use liquid silicone for the implants. Talcott was the head of the company's technical services and development group, which was responsible for testing the implant components. He said that he could see no difference between the silicone Dow was putting into the gel and the liquid form the FDA had said should not be injected into women's breasts.[31]

James Rudy, the president of Heyer-Schulte, which manufactured silicone implants, became concerned when 140 ruptured silicone implants were returned to his company in a 13-month period from May 1975 to June 1976. He told plastic surgeons that they should warn patients of possible problems and complications of the silicone gel implant. For the most part, his warnings fell on deaf ears. Rudy contends that surgeons didn't want to criticize the implant because it could hurt their business, and silicone implants were a big business. A surgeon could make as much as $7,500 per procedure.[32] In 1986, oncologist Melvin Silverstein, M.D., presented his findings on implants to a meeting of plastic surgeons in Los Angeles. He told them that implants could interfere with mammography. His findings were called ridiculous and he was advised to do more research.[33]

When silicone implants were introduced in the 1960s, the FDA lacked the authority to regulate medical devices. In 1976, the FDA was granted that power. The implants were grandfathered. However, there was also a provision that the FDA could ask for safety data if it deemed it was needed. It wasn't until 1982 that the FDA moved the implants to Class III, a more stringent category that required the manufacturer to provide scientific proof that the implants were safe. It took another six years for the FDA to issue the final regulations regarding the reclassification and then start the process of asking for safety data. In 1988, the FDA notified the implant manufacturers that they had to submit data on the safety of the implants within 30 months. In 1990, the FDA actually requested that manufacturers file for formal approval. At the same time, the late Congressman Ted Weiss (D-New York), who was chair of the House Committee on Human Resources, which oversees the FDA, asked the agency what was taking so long. Finally, in April 1991, the FDA notified manufacturers that they had to submit their data on safety by the following July or their products would be taken off the market. In September, Bristol-Myers Squibb announced that it would no longer manufacture the implants because it could not provide the safety data by the FDA deadline.

The breast implant industry did not sit idly by as all this was happening. In October 1991, 400 women from 37 states flew to Washington, D.C., at the expense of the American Society of Plastic and Reconstructive Surgeons (ASPRS), to lobby congressional members to keep implants available. The multimillion-dollar media and lobbying campaign was underwritten by the nation's plastic surgeons and implant makers.[34] The ASPRS put together a $1.3 million fund for lobbying. The FDA received an unprecedented 20,000 letters generated, in part, by a $150,000 newspaper ad campaign. And while $1.5 million for lobbying may seem like a lot of money, compared to the $330 million a year that implant surgery generated for plastic surgeons, it could be characterized as a modest investment.

In November 1991, the FDA's General and Plastic Surgery Devices Panel (an outside advisory panel of medical and other experts) met to review the submitted data. It found the information provided by the manufacturers inadequate to establish the safety of the implants and recommended that the FDA require manufacturers to collect additional data on risks and benefits. It said that a strict deadline for delivery of the data should be set by the FDA. At the same time the panel also recommended that implants be available during the interim under certain conditions, with the requirement that doctors inform and educate patients about potential risks and the establishment of a national registry to provide data on adverse effects.[35]

In January 1992, FDA head David Kessler reviewed the additional documents and announced a 45-day moratorium on the sale of breast implants. The following month, Dow Corning released 800 pages of internal memos, documents, and letters at the demand of the FDA. At the same time, the company announced that chairman John S. Ludington was being replaced by Keith R. McKennon. (McKennon had been widely praised for his handling of Dow Chemical's problems with Agent Orange.)

In February, the FDA also held three days of emotional hearings on the safety and effectiveness of silicone implants. Data from manufacturers were reviewed and doctors, manufacturers, and women testified. Sue Richardson, a 50-year-old breast cancer survivor from Texas, had had two sets of implants that turned painfully hard. She was on her third set and said, if necessary, she'd do it again. "After I had the reconstruction, I didn't think about dying anymore. The reality in this world is that breasts are important to women."[36] Lynda Roth of Colorado also testified and asked why "they're up here saying you can't be a whole person without a breast? What's wrong with our society?"[37] Terry Davis of Florida had a similar question. "Why can't self-esteem start in your head, not your boobs?"[38] As the *Los Angeles Times* reporter Marlene Cimons put it, "The controversy has raised soul-searching questions about the values of a breast-conscious society."[39]

Many critics called the 30-year history of the implants a tragedy in which women had been used as guinea pigs for an unproven device.[40] The panel concluded that there was no "concrete evidence" that the implants can cause disease. Elizabeth Connell, M.D., chair of the panel and a medical school professor, said, "We're not ignoring the diseases, but we don't see a cause-and-effect relationship" based on current data.[41]

Some of the concerns brought up at the hearings included evidence that silicone implants rupture and leak at a higher rate than had been suspected earlier and the lack of data from animal and human follow-up studies proving the safety of the devices.[42] Researchers from Washington University in St. Louis and the University of Pittsburgh said that in their studies of women with implants, about 5 to 6 percent of the implants ruptured and leaked silicone into the body.[43] Frank Vasey, M.D., a rheumatologist in Florida, said that he had seen about 300 women with implants who had signs of autoimmune disorders or scleroderma, a hardening or contracting of the body's connective tissue. In an alarming statement, he alleged, "We are at the same position as doctors in Los Angeles and in New York in 1980 who were seeing immune-system disease in homosexual men."[44]

The panel agreed that more research was needed on what role, if any, silicone implants play in the development of immune-type diseases like scleroderma, lupus, and rheumatoid arthritis. The panel also said the rupture rate of implants and the rate at which the silicone bleeds into the body needed more study. It took several votes for the panel to come up with its recommendation that implants stay on the market but that every woman who got one would have to be part of a study to determine implant safety, and that the FDA should consider placing some limitations on the availability of augmentation implants intended only to enlarge breasts.

The recommendations came under fire immediately from several fronts. Kermit Campbell, Dow Corning group vice president, characterized them as "extremely confusing" for women with implants and women considering getting an implant.[45] Others said having the implants available only in clinical trials allowed even more women to be experimented on while the belated testing continued. Critics quickly pointed out that generally when a panel of experts cannot decide on the safety and effectiveness of a product, the FDA bans the product and does not give the manufacturer the benefit of the doubt.[46] On the other hand, Sharon Green, executive director of Y-ME, said, "To ban or severely limit silicone breast implants based on inconclusive data would be one more insult to women by taking away their right to make informed decisions regarding their own bodies."[47] Richard Krizek, M.D., a surgeon at the University of Chicago, said, "It is inconsistent to tell those who have implants that it's okay, but those who are candidates for them, you can't participate. It doesn't make sense scientifically."[48]

The suggestion that the implants be available only to women with breast cancer to limit potential risks to women who arguably have the greatest need for them was immediately shot down by Mary McGrath, M.D., a plastic surgeon at George Washington University. She said, "If there are dangers to implants, then these dangers apply to all users." In addition, she called allowing some women to have the implants "judgmental and paternalistic," saying that it's a "ruling on the validity of cosmetic surgery — and I don't think that's our business."[49] Marcia Angell, executive editor of *The New England Journal of Medicine*, said in an editorial that women should be allowed to have implants as long as they're aware of the possible risks. "Targeting a device used only by women raises the specter of sexism — either in having permitted the use of implants in the first place or in withdrawing them."[50] In the same issue, Kessler rejected what he calls the "fashionable" argument that women should be free to decide whether or not to take whatever small risks are involved in breast implants. "To argue that people ought to be able to choose their own risks, that government should not intervene, even in the face of inadequate information, is to impose an unrealistic burden on people when they are most vulnerable to manufacturers' assertions."[51]

Sharon Green, noting that the Y-ME hotline for breast cancer survivors had received thousands of calls from women with breast cancer as well as from women who simply wanted information about the implants, said, "For others to deny the right of women to implants because they fundamentally believe implants are unnecessary is arrogance in its ugliest form."[52]

In a letter to the editor in the *Wall Street Journal* on January 31, 1992, breast cancer survivor Edith H. Robinson said, "As a woman who has breast cancer and has silicone implants, I do not need David Kessler or Sidney Wolfe to help me make an informed decision."[53] Sidney Wolfe, M.D., who is the founder of the Public Citizen Health Research Group, opposes the use of any breast implantation, noting that cancers may develop 20 to 30 years after exposure to a toxin, so there is no way at this point to guarantee that the implants are safe.[54] The American Medical Association, the physician's lobbying organization, acknowledging safety concerns, said that until silicone gel implants were proved harmful, all women should be able to get them — whether for breast reconstruction or for cosmetic reasons.[55]

Some question whether breast reconstruction after a mastectomy isn't cosmetic surgery as well, since medically it is not really necessary. As for surgery to enlarge breasts, the American Society of Plastic and Reconstructive Surgeons (ASPRS) found a way to get around the "cosmetic" description. In 1982, it identified the "disease" that the silicone gel implants were treating as micromastia, or small breasts. It thereby medically justified the practice of breast augmentation by citing a "substantial and enlarging body of medical information and opinion . . . to the effect that these deformities [small breasts] are really a disease which in most patients result in feelings of inadequacy, lack of self-confidence, distortion of body image, and a total lack of well-being due to a lack of self-perceived femininity."[56] The ASPRS no longer endorses the view that small breasts are a "deformity" in need of a cure.

In the midst of the controversy, Dow Corning announced on March 19, 1992, that it would stop manufacturing silicone gel breast implants. On April 16, the FDA finally announced its decision on the use of silicone gel breast implants. The use of the devices was to be limited in a series of three stages:

- Stage one: only women with ruptured or leaking implants could get "urgent-need" reconstruction using the implants; their surgeon would have to certify that the implant was needed and the woman would have to sign a detailed consent form listing possible side effects; the women would be monitored and followed for years.
- Stage two: start-up would come months later when women with mastectomies, congenital deformities, or other breast injuries could have reconstruction with silicone implants; their surgeon would have to certify that a saline implant was not a satisfactory alternative; the women would be monitored and followed for years.
- Stage three: start-up in fall 1992, when intensive clinical trials would be set up; eligibility requirements established for implants for cosmetic reasons such as augmentation or to reshape the breast; the silicone implant would be available only under this investigational status; the size of studies would be limited to about 2,000 women.

The FDA's breast implant hotline, which began operating on February 18, 1992, received over 4,500 calls in the first four days, and ultimately 40,000 calls by July 10, 1992. By January 1993, the FDA was taking the heat. A House subcommittee accused the FDA of failing to monitor the use of silicone implants in the period since the restrictions had been placed the year before on their availability. Its report also expressed concern that physicians were able to define small breasts as a "deformity" in order to circumvent the restrictions and that the FDA had done nothing to prevent this. Kessler dismissed the charges as "patently false." He said that just 3,500 women had gotten silicone implants in 1992, down from 130,000 in past years.[57] Still, the subcommittee report stated that the fact that 3,500 women got the implants in a period of seven months "suggests that either there is 'business as usual' in breast reconstruction, or a very large number of women found ruptures." The FDA was also accused of watering down the consent forms at the request of surgeons.[58]

Although when the scandal broke initially, it appeared that virtually no research had been done on silicone implants, studies began slowly to surface as a result of all the publicity about the silicone gel implants, lawsuits that had been filed, and the FDA's demand for data. While the research that had been done was not extensive and was secret, its discovery shed light on the development and testing of the implant before it went on the market. Thousands of documents were released by Dow Corning in 1991 and early in 1992.

Internal memos obtained from Dow Corning strongly suggested that the company might have known or suspected for a long time the existence of major problems associated with implanting silicone. In a January 1975 memo, Arthur H. Rathjen, chairman of the Dow Implant Task Force, had a query as the company rushed the new silicone gel implant to market. "A question not yet answered is whether or not there is excessive bleed of the gel through the envelope. We must address ourselves to this question immediately. . . . The stakes are too high if a wrong decision is made."[59]

In a January 1992 article in the *Boston Globe,* Dan M. Hayes, Jr., CEO of Dow, said that in 1975 competition among implant manufacturers had been high and "there was market pressure [to move ahead with the new silicone gel implant], but you have to understand, the ingredients that make up this softer [more natural-feeling] implant were the same ingredients as before, so it was not as if we were introducing something new."[60] According to former Dow Corning officials, the company was under pressure to counter competitor McGhan Medical Corporation, which had seized as much as half of Dow Corning's market share.[61]

In a May 1975 memo, sales officials complained that the surface of the new silicone gel implants "became oily" during trade shows and was "bleeding on the velvet in the showcase." They were advised to wash off the implants periodically in the nearest restroom and dry them with paper towels.[62]

In May 1976, the concerns of a doctor in Florida complaining about "greasy implants" were discussed in a report. A plastic surgeon at Dow, Richard Phares, M.D., proposed animal studies. A month later, a response is recorded in a memo from Rathjen. "I don't necessarily agree with all that Dr. Phares proposes for animal work, but it should not be ignored. . . . I have proposed again and again that we must begin an in-depth study of our gel, envelope, and bleed phenomenon. . . . Time is going to run out for us if we don't get under-way."[63]

In 1976, over a year after the first woman received the new silicone-gel implant, Rathjen again questioned its performance and reliability. He wrote, "We are engulfed in unqualified speculation. Nothing to date is truly quantitative. Is there something in the implant that migrates out or off the mammary prosthesis? Yes or no! Does it continue for the life of the implant or is it limited or controlled for a period of time? What is it?"[64]

A memo to Rathjen from a scientist at Dow Corning on January 10, 1977, contained the line, "I am very surprised to find that we do not have any data on Si [silicone] levels in tissues or the distribution and fate of trace levels of polymer in the body."[65] The lack of data was a concern of Dow scientist Bill Boley in a September 1983 memo. "Only inferential data exists to substantiate the long-term safety of these gels for human implant applications." In a 1985 memo, Boley warned that more testing was needed to determine whether a particular formula of the silicone gel caused cancer.[66]

In 1973, Dow Corning published results of a two-year study of silicone implants in four dogs, in which they said the dogs remained in "normal health."[67] According to an article in the *Washington Post* on January 1, 1992, in actuality one of the dogs died during the study and another developed a large tumor known as a granuloma next to the implant.[68] Noel R. Rose, M.D., Ph.D., chairman of immunology at Johns Hopkins University, says the tumor seen in the dog could have been an early sign that silicone causes immune system disorders. Rose had previously testified on behalf of Dow Corning in other product liability cases. As to the actual findings in the study, he said, "Certainly you would want to know about that. Its significance is that one would want to look for other effects."[69] The alteration of the study findings was said to be one of the instrumental pieces of evidence in a case brought by Marianne Hopkins against Dow. Jurors in San Francisco, in November 1991, convicted Dow of fraud in concealing risks posed by the implants, despite the fact that Marianne Hopkins's doctors had testified that she had had symptoms before she got the implants. The jury awarded Hopkins, who contended that her autoimmune disease was caused by the implants, $7.34 million, of which $6.5 million was for punitive damages.[70]

Leia Zenderman, a Santa Fe, New Mexico, painter, was part of an experiment and didn't even know it.[71] As a teenager, she had Poland's anomaly, a condition in which only half the chest muscles and one breast develop normally. In 1965, a week after her high school graduation, she underwent surgery to reduce the size of the normal breast; at the same time she received a silicone implant on the other side. She also received liquid silicone injections because she had so little chest muscle. When the injections abruptly ended, she was never told why. She was left with asymmetrical breasts that were painful.

Zenderman's doctor was one of a handful of doctors working under the auspices of the Dow Corning Center to Aid Medical Research, which was set up in the early 1960s to explore medical uses of silicone. The center got FDA permission to pursue liquid silicone studies in animals and humans in 1965. Zenderman's parents say they were never told their daughter would be part of an experiment. Leia Zenderman found out years later when she saw Norman Anderson, M.D., a surgeon at Johns Hopkins Hospital in Baltimore and a consultant to the FDA on the silicone implant issue, talking about the implants on television and called him. According to Anderson, Zenderman is one of the many women upon whom doctors experimented without permission and whose records were never given to the FDA.

Anderson has been a critic of implants for years. He says that an article written by Zenderman's doctor in 1967, in the *Journal of Plastic and Reconstructive Surgery*, describes what happened when liquid silicone was injected into the breasts of Japanese monkeys and rhesus monkeys.In 13 monkeys the injections caused "marked fibrous response" and "destruction of anatomy." The same article stated that a "selected group of women" had been repeatedly injected with 5 to 10 milliliters of liquid silicone into the breasts. However, the results were never published, nor were they submitted to the FDA.[72]

In March 1993, Dow Corning reported that new studies on laboratory rats showed that the silicone gel used in breast implants was not inert and, in fact, had been found to be a strong irritant of the immune system in animals. Although it was the first time that the company had reported such a reaction to silicone, Myron Harrison, M.D., the chief medical officer of Dow Corning, acknowledged that scientists had seen something similar in research as far back as 1974. As for the possibility that Dow Corning scientists had hidden the earlier findings to avoid damaging sales, Harrison said, "I would hope that was not the case."[73] Days earlier, researchers at the University of California at Davis School of Medicine reported finding that among 100 women with silicone implants, 35 had antibodies against their own collagen (a protein that variously gives body tissues stiffness or elasticity), which meant that the women's immune systems were attacking their own bodies. In an interview, the scientists said that removal of the implants could nevertheless entail more risk than keeping them.[74]

Harrison called the report a surprise. "The significance of this finding is that it raises a concern on the part of people like me that silicone might play some role in autoimmune disease."[75] At the request of the FDA, Dow Corning set up a $10 million fund to investigate the health effects of silicone gel implants, even though it was no longer making them.

In 1994, Sydney Wolfe, of the Public Citizen Health Research Group, obtained a copy of a 1975 Dow Corning study from the FDA and gave it to reporters. The study showed that the silicone used in the implants harmed the immune system of mice. FDA spokesman Jim O'Hara said the report was not among the 21 volumes of internal documents that Dow had released in 1991, which at that time were believed to represent all the company's research findings on silicone's health effects. O'Hara said the FDA had received the report only the previous week, and that "we think it was relevant to the discussions the advisory committees were having in 1991 and 1992."[76] Dow scientists strongly disputed the relevance of the 1975 findings to human implant recipients.

At the hearings held in 1991 and 1992, the FDA examined questions regarding D4, a particular type of silicone gel that, in purified form, is highly toxic to the immune system and was used in the 1975 mouse study. At the hearings, Dr. Robert LeVier, a scientist with Dow, said that no "immunologic events" associated with D4 had been seen. In March 1994, he acknowledged under oath that he had received a copy of the 1975 report.[77] David Kessler testified that he'd seen nothing about the 1975 report. "The agency [FDA] has significant concern both about the findings and the manner in which they became available to us. . . . The report seems to suggest that D4, one of the compounds that we have been concerned about, is present in breast implants and does have adverse effects."[78]

Frederick Ellis, an attorney representing hundreds of women in a class-action suit against Dow, called the study the "nail in Dow's coffin." Ellis said, "Dow has always denied that such effects exist, contradicting what its own scientists found twenty years ago."[79]

In a February 1993 *Wall Street Journal* article, "Breast Implants Raise New Safety Issues," doctors expressed their concerns. Gary Solomon, M.D., associate director of the rheumatic diseases department at New York's Hospital for Joint Diseases, said, "I had been skeptical [about a disease-silicone link] but after seeing five or six patients, I was convinced."[80] His patients with silicone implants suffered chronic fatigue, inability to swallow, hair loss, and rashes on their upper chest. Many tested positive for antinuclear antibodies, entities that attack the body's own tissue. Alan J. Bridges, M.D., of the University of Wisconsin, said, "Even people who were skeptical are saying there's just too much scleroderma" in women with implants. "I believe there is a subgroup of women who will develop a disease if they have these things in long enough."[81] Eric Gershwin, M.D., chief of rheumatology and allergy at the University of California at Davis, says that children who were nursed by mothers with implants may get sick from the device, even years later.[82]

Meanwhile, new studies were emerging which suggested that the silicone was not as harmful as feared. A Canadian study published in the *New England Journal of Medicine* in June 1992 found that in 11,000 women who had had breast augmentation with the implant, about half the incidence of breast cancer that would have been expected in any normal group of women was diagnosed in a ten-year period.[83] The researchers cautioned that there was no reason to think that implants might somehow reduce the risk of breast cancer. In April, a study conducted at the University of Southern California found that women getting augmentation had about one-third less breast cancer than would have been expected for a group of women during ten years of follow-up. Hans Berkel, who directed the Canadian study, said, "Both of these studies are reassuring to women. We don't find an increased risk [of breast cancer]."[84]

A study done at the M. D. Anderson Cancer Center in Texas found no higher incidence of autoimmune disease among 250 breast cancer patients with implants than among 353 breast cancer patients who had reconstruction using their own tissue.[85] A Mayo Clinic study found no higher incidence of autoimmune disorders among 824 women with implants compared with 1,634 women who didn't have an implant.[86]

Still another epidemiologic study was done by Marc C. Hochberg, M.D., of the University of Maryland School of Medicine. He looked at women from four university settings and said he found no link between the implants and scleroderma. He did say that more study was needed to determine if implants are linked to symptoms like fatigue, low-grade fever, and atypical joint or muscle pain.[87]

In May 1994, the results of a $3.6 million study done by David Schottenfeld, of the University of Michigan, was reported by the Dow Corning Corporation of Midland, Michigan, which paid for it. An association between scleroderma and silicone breast implants was not found.[88] Schottenfeld found that fewer than one percent of the women with scleroderma had had an implant, suggesting that the implant could not be a leading cause of the disease. In fact, the women with scleroderma were slightly less likely than healthy women to have had breast implants. Richard Edelson, M.D., at Yale University School of Medicine, an expert on scleroderma, says no one knows what causes it.[89] Howard Ory, M.D., a private consultant in Atlanta, noted a similar study in Australia that failed to find an association between the implants and scleroderma.[90]

Attorney Stanley Chesley, who helped negotiate the settlement of a huge class-action suit brought by women with silicone implants, downplayed the study, saying it showed that Dow Corning "will do anything to try to save face." He said he continues to believe that with scleroderma and implants, "It's a direct cause and effect."[91]

The new studies did little to resolve the issues. For some, they just added to the confusion. Sharon Green, director of Y-ME, says breast cancer survivors are baffled and don't know what to do. "We originally took a stance to keep them on the market. We felt there were problems but we felt each individual had to determine what their risks were. But these studies, both national and international, are coming in and they are not showing definite [problems]. Now that there is a settlement on the table, what does that mean? I don't know what to tell anyone anymore."[92]

The findings in a third large epidemiologic study, published in the *New England Journal of Medicine* in June 1994, reinforced the findings of the earlier studies.[93] No evidence was found that silicone implants caused connective tissue disease or other diseases. The study of 749 women who had had breast implants between 1964 and 1991 was conducted at the Mayo Clinic in Rochester, Minnesota. The study was funded by the National Institutes of Health and plastic surgeons.

In an editorial in the same issue, executive editor Dr. Marcia Angell wrote, "The accumulated weight of anecdotes [implicating implants in causing immune diseases] was taken by judges and juries as tantamount to proof of causation. Multimillion-dollar settlements followed, along with poignant stories in the media and appearances by plaintiffs on talk shows. All this added to the weight of the anecdotes, which in a circular way became accepted by the courts and the public as nearly incontrovertible evidence."[94] Angell questioned the FDA's decision to restrict the use of the silicone implants two years earlier.

Bruce Burlington, M.D., director of the Center for Devices and Radiological Health at the FDA, said, "We are really glad to see this study published."[95] He called it one of the first pieces of solid scientific evidence on the risk of silicone implants. The lead researcher on the study, Sherine E. Gabriel, M.D., said, "We'd be happier if the numbers were bigger," but nonetheless hoped the results "will ease the minds of many women with implants."[96]

Sidney Wolfe immediately attacked the study, calling it "incredibly misleading." He said the study population was too small and that the incidence of problems could have been unreported. "To draw any comfort from [the study]," said Wolfe, "is to engage in misleading or delusional thinking."[97] Another critic of the study was Jane Sprague Jones, a medical sociologist who chairs the National Women's Health Network. She said, "Our experience is that problems seem to be related to the age of the implants."[98]

The question of who actually paid for the study was raised by attorney Stanley Chesley. He charged that the study was funded by the breast implant industry. In an Associated Press story, he is quoted as saying, "Almost all of the funding was put up by the breast implant manufacturers, particularly Dow Corning."[99] A Dow Corning spokesman said he did not have information on whether the company helped fund the study. Gabriel said the source of the funding was a nonissue. "No matter who gave us the money," she countered, "we would have conducted the study exactly the same way."[100]

In March 1995, researchers attended a workshop at the National

Institutes of Health in Bethesda on the effects of silicone on the immune system. Marc Hochberg, M.D., presented a meta-analysis on the studies of such diseases as scleroderma and rheumatoid arthritis. No association was found between silicone breast implants and increased risk for connective tissue diseases. However, another possibility was raised by Gary Solomon, M.D., and others, who contended that the implants are causing a new autoimmune disease. Says Solomon, "There is an atypical rheumatoid disease out there and that is what is not being picked up by epidemiologists [in other studies]. . . . You look at these [rheumatoid] diseases and try to get them to fit the criteria, but they don't."[101]

Three years earlier, in 1991, a jury in Manhattan Federal District Court in New York awarded $4.45 million to a woman after deciding that chemicals released from a breast implant caused breast cancer. The woman, who got the implants in 1983, had them removed 22 days later because her breasts were swollen and painful. Fifteen months later she was diagnosed with breast cancer. The jury found that her cancer was "promoted" by the release of the chemical TDA from the implant. TDA causes cancer in animals, but the Environmental Protection Agency says its carcinogenic effect in humans is undetermined. The jury also found that the woman lost her breast as a result of silicone that remained in her breast after the implant was removed, which caused chronic abscesses and infections that could only be treated by mastectomy.

Makers of the silicone breast implants and lawyers representing women who claimed to have been harmed by the implants negotiated a proposal in September 1993 to set up a $4.75 billion fund to compensate women with silicone implants. At that point, more than 11,000 lawsuits had been filed by women claiming health difficulties as a result of the implants. Under the proposal, $800 million would be used to remove silicone breast implants, compensate women whose implants ruptured, pay for medical monitoring of women with implants, and compensate women who had no adverse medical effects. Women who acquired one of the following eight diseases would be eligible for compensation:

- scleroderma — abnormal hardening and thickening of skin
- systemic lupus — an inflammatory disease of the connective tissue

- mixed connective tissue disease
- polymyositis — an inflammatory disease of the skeletal muscle
- dermatomyositis — inflammatory disease associated with skin inflammation
- primary Sjögren's syndrome — dry eyes and mouth in conjunction with connective tissue disease
- atypical neurologic disease
- atypical connective tissue disease/atypical rheumatic syndrome

Lawyers for the thousands of plaintiffs said it would be one of the biggest settlements ever in a class-action suit.[102]

On March 23, 1994, three major makers of implants, Dow Corning Corporation, the Bristol Myers-Squibb Company, and the Baxter Healthcare Corporation, agreed to finance a $3.7 billion fund. Although the companies continued to claim that the implants were not harmful, they said they wished to resolve the lawsuits in this manner.[103] It would clear the courts of some 12,000 cases involving more than 25,000 women. The women would have up to 30 years to collect from $200,000 to $2 million. U.S. District Judge Sam Pointer, in Birmingham, Alabama, gave preliminary approval to a $3.7 billion settlement on April 4. When Minnesota Mining and Manufacturing, General Electric, and two other silicone manufacturers joined the settlement about a week later, the amount went up to the original settlement proposal of $4.75 billion.[104]

A schedule and procedure for women to join the class-action suit was also set up. By April 11, manufacturers had to start notifying women in the United States of the settlement by spelling out in advertisements how they could join it. A June 16 deadline was set, at which time comments or objections to the settlement could be made. Also at that time, women could declare they were not joining the settlement but would sue on their own. A woman choosing to sue on her own had the possibility of a larger settlement as well as the possibility of losing the lawsuit and getting nothing. A fairness hearing was to be held in Birmingham, Alabama, on August 8 to determine whether the proposed settlement was fair, reasonable, and adequate and should get final approval. A deadline of September 16 was set for women who had certain diseases or medical conditions and wanted to seek damages under the settlement's Current Disease Compensation

Program to file claims. The settlement provided as well for women who had the implants but had had no physical problems. They had until December 1 to preserve their right to seek damages under the settlement's Ongoing Disease Compensation Program for women who develop defined diseases during the next 30 years.

On September 1, 1994, Judge Pointer gave final approval to a $4.25 billion breast implant liability settlement. At that point more than 90,500 women had agreed to the terms of the settlement. While some critics said the settlement was not large enough, Sandra Finestone, president of the Women's Implant Information Network, was pleased because, she said, "Now reason and calm can come to this issue."[105]

The settlement fell apart when Dow Corning filed for bankruptcy in May 1995. A new settlement was offered the following October by Baxter Healthcare, Bristol-Myers, and 3M. Women with implants manufactured by the three companies would be eligible. But the amount of money they would receive would be significantly lower than the original settlement. The total amount paid out by the three companies could reach $3 billion if all the women who are eligible make claims. About half of the 400,000 women in the original settlement are not affected because their implants were from Dow Corning.[106] They had to file a proof of claim form in Dow Corning's bankruptcy reorganization case by the end of 1995. For the latest information call the Breast Implant Litigation Settlement Agreement at (800) 887-6828.[107]

When the FDA ruled that silicone breast implants could only be used by women with breast cancer taking part in a clinical trial, saline implants were still available. In April 1992, the FDA made the saline implant a Class III medical device, which meant that it would call for safety data within a year. In January 1993, the FDA announced that to continue marketing saline implants, manufacturers would have to submit premarket approval applications demonstrating the safety and effectiveness of the devices. In October 1992, it was reported in the *Journal of the American Medical Association* that the presence of any implant, silicone or saline, impeded mammography by reducing the area that could be seen by 30 to 50 percent.[108] A study of 1,100 women who got saline implants between 1977 and 1991 was released in 1993. It found that 2 percent of the women had some discomfort from hardening of scar tissue around the implant and 1 percent had significant hardening. As for leakage of the implant, which is another problem, there was 20 percent leakage of the saline for a version used until the early 1980s, and 1 percent leakage for the new model. The findings in that study led Fort Worth, Texas, surgeon David Lavine, M.D., to say, "There's no question this is a viable and safe alternative to silicone gel implants."[109]

Not in agreement was Sybil Goldrich of Command Trust Network, an implant consumers group, who said, "We're hearing about a lot of ruptures with molds, fungus, and infection problems." She added that she questioned the objectivity of Lavine, "as these doctors have so much to gain from the success of this product."[110]

On June 2, 1994, the FDA held a hearing on saline implants. Sandra Finestone, president of the Women's Implant Information Network, said that breast reconstruction "should be available to me, to my daughter, and to the millions of women who may someday face the anguish of breast cancer."[111] And Cindy K. Wofford agreed, saying that "women should be allowed to make their own choices based on the information available." Wofford, who had had breast reconstruction, said, "My feelings of self-confidence in my body have been restored."[112]

Brenda Cannell testified against the saline implants because, she said, "They are not safe. The worst mistake I ever made was to trust the advice of a doctor who told me that saline implants were safe."[113] Cannell started getting back pain, mood swings, and repeated urinary, ear, mouth, gum, and throat infections shortly after she had the implants. Mary Spieker, who received saline implants for breast augmentation, said that the implants had disabled her, that she suffers from chronic fatigue, severe pain, memory loss, allergies to drugs, and other chronic problems. She attributed her health problems to a faulty valve in the implant, which resulted in a fungus that spread throughout her body.[114] Doctors' groups testified that there was no reason to ban saline implants immediately. William Riley, M.D., of the American Society for Plastic and Reconstructive Surgeons, said, "Right now the preliminary evidence shows no reason for alarm."[115]

Saline implants came under more attacks in August, when the Public Citizen Health Research Group called for a ban of the implants for most women until manufacturers prove they are safe. In a petition, the group urged the FDA to treat saline implants the same as silicone-gel implants are treated. Sidney Wolfe, founder of Public Citizen, cited FDA documents showing nearly 9,000 reports of serious injuries from saline implants from 1991 to March 1994.[116]

In August 1994, there was an annoucement that yet another kind of implant was being tested. The FDA gave approval to a Swiss company, LipoMatrix, to begin limited clinical trials of its natural soybean-oil implants on 50 American women. The company claims that it is the first implant through which a mammography can see. Some critics have charged that, like silicone and saline implants, the soybean-oil filling of the implant can grow bacteria while it is in its silicone shell and can cause harm if the shell leaks or ruptures, allowing the substance into the body. The chairman of the company, Terry Knapp, M.D., responded by saying that the filling is not capable of growing bacteria. "We found that those bacteria do not survive," adding that the shells were specially designed to stay intact longer than conventional implants. He did not claim that the implants would last a lifetime.[117]

There are other procedures that can be done to reconstruct the breast of a woman who has had a mastectomy. One method is abdominal advancement reconstruction, in which skin and fat from the chest and abdomen are moved to the breast area. In another method, after skin, fat, and muscle from other parts of the body are transplanted to the mastectomy site, an artery and vein are attached to existing blood vessels that had served the original breast. The surgery is far more invasive and extensive than an implant and can have unpleasant side effects as well.

Key questions remain. Why were silicone implants put into the bodies of so many women, as many as a million, before any real testing was done? If the FDA says the implants can only be used in clinical trials for breast reconstruction as women with breast cancer have "legitimate" reasons for it, why are they subjecting women who already have serious medical problems to the possibility of more down the road?

27

Multicultural Issues

Sometimes you think you're studying the psychological situation when you're really looking at a situation that could happen to anyone who doesn't have money.

— Harold Freeman, M.D.,
director of surgery at Harlem Hospital Center[1]

How do you get a woman to examine her breasts when she's grown up thinking that touching the breasts is masturbation?

— Karen Schmidt, R.N.[2]

The roles of the patient's partner and cultural background have also got to be examined.

— Julia Rowland, Ph.D.,
assistant professor of psychology at Georgetown University[3]

Different cultural beliefs and attitudes can have an impact on whether breast cancer is diagnosed and treated in a timely matter. For example, in the western world, the practice of health focuses largely on germ theory, the idea that diseases are caused by germs or physical dysfunction in the body. Treatment consists of destroying the germ or repairing the dysfunction.

Nonwestern nations frequently view health differently. It is not unusual for people in those countries to believe that there is a connection between the disease and an external force. Health is perceived as a result of physical and spiritual harmony with nature. When there is a state of disharmony, illness, disease, and disorder can result. Treatments such as prayer, religious ritual, herbs, home remedies, a witch doctor, a medicine man, voodoo, are designed to restore the harmony. When people emigrate to the United States, they bring their belief systems with them.

When Amy Langer, head of the National Alliance of Breast Cancer Organizations, attended an international conference on breast cancer, she came away with greater awareness of how breast cancer is viewed and treated in different parts of the world. "In Japan, daughters of breast cancer patients never discuss their mother's diagnosis because they would be considered unmarriageable. In Russia, a woman isn't told she has breast cancer, she's told she has an infection." Langer adds that in many countries "the woman's husband is addressed and consulted and not the woman herself."[4]

Within different minority groups, there can be variations of beliefs and adherence to them. The degree of assimilation into American society, how long people have lived in this country, can affect response to the traditional American way of treating disease and disorders. The extent to which traditional beliefs regarding health and disease prevail can have a significant impact on when and if a person goes to a medical doctor, and, if diagnosed, what treatment will be accepted.

One example of how cultural beliefs and attitudes can affect health in this country has been observed by Althea Smith, who is with the New York City Health and Hospitals Corporation, which serves many of the impoverished people in the city. A high percentage of minority women are among the impoverished. Smith says that they try to teach every woman how to do a breast self-exam, but "some women will say, 'My head is mine, my legs are mine, but my breasts belong to my husband.' We can't help those women do breast self-exam." Another problem is that "women in general, minority women in particular, always take care of others before they take care of themselves."[5]

Dr. Harold Freeman, director of surgery at Harlem Hospital Center in New York, says there really is very little known about psycho-social aspects of cancer in the minority population. "It's sort of confounded, in a way, by the people who don't have money, insurance, and access." Freeman says research related to social problems, such as poverty, has to be separated from the research related to the psychological and cultural, despite their interconnectedness. Unless a way is found to look at each factor individually, research in this area will not really be valid.[6]

In general, respect, authority, and family are highly valued in the Hispanic population. The premise of individualism in decision-making is foreign. Suffering is considered a part of life and an act of God. Hispanic women may be more concerned about how their disease is affecting family members than how it is affecting them. It is not uncommon for them to believe the disease is caused by an act of God to punish or test them, which can lead to passivity. They may not take the prescribed drugs because they feel since they cannot change their destiny, it is pointless to take medication. Those less inclined to take a passive role may seek out practitioners of folk medicine, as a substitute for, or in addition to, a medical doctor. The healer's remedies may provide a sense of hope and security, as well as reaffirm their self-worth and social integration.[7]

Jody Rogers, a cancer survivor in El Paso, Texas, says that plans are under way to build a breast care center at Texas Technical University but sponsors will face challenges in convincing women to use the facility. "El Paso is seventy percent Hispanic, so it is a very different situation there. . . . The reason Hispanic women don't go for mammography is embarrassment. They're shy about it, and they won't do it. It's their culture."[8]

In the first study of its kind in the United States, doctors at the University of San Francisco and Kaiser Permanente, a large health maintenance organization, looked at how the attitudes and beliefs of Hispanics affected their experience with cancer. They were trying to find out why Hispanics in general have lower rates of cancer than whites but are equally likely to die of the disease. Hispanics are also more likely to be diagnosed at a later stage. In 1992, they reported Hispanics are more likely than whites to have misconceptions about the causes and symptoms of cancer and that many have a sense of *fatalismo,* or fatalism, which can keep them from taking such steps as getting a mammography or getting the proper treatment when diagnosed. They found that 46 percent of the Hispanics in the study thought that cancer was a death sentence, whereas among whites 26 percent held that belief. In California, 42 percent of Hispanic women's breast cancer is diagnosed at a late stage compared to 32 percent of white women's.[9]

Fortunately for Ruth Mendoza, who lives in California, she did go for mammograms. She was 38 in 1989, when microcalcifications showed up on her mammogram.

> I didn't tell a soul. I didn't call anyone from church, which was different for me because I normally would have called some friends from church. . . . I went into the biopsy saying to myself, "This will be nothing, because these kinds of things don't happen to regular people." After the biopsy, the doctor came to the foot of the bed and he had that horrible look on his face. He said it was cancer and I remember thinking, "Oh, shit, get me out of here." I just wanted to go home and close my eyes. Then I became stoic again. I saw the doctor and told him I'd be having my breast off. I asked my husband, "Is this okay with you?" and my husband said, "Whatever's okay for you." I thought, now I have to go home and tell my family. I remember thinking, "These men are going to take good care of me." I was raised like that. I shouldn't ask for anything. They know what they're doing, I don't. . . . Our best friends who stood up for us at our wedding sent flowers and that was it. I never heard from them again. My family has been wonderful. My in-laws are trying to understand me. My brother and sister-in-law said to me in private, "How could you do this to our brother? How could you mutilate your body in that fashion for our brother?" This was late at night, very private, where no one else could hear. I didn't know how to answer them. They thought that I was ruining their brother's life and that I would not be a whole person anymore. My family was supportive; his family thinks that to cut off your breast is just the ultimate vulgarity and is a lack of respect for your body. It's been hard to try to educate them and share with them.[10]

Breast surgeon Alison Estabrook, chief of breast surgery at Columbia Presbyterian Hospital in New York, says that when Hispanic women are diagnosed with breast cancer, "They say their husbands will leave them if they have a mastectomy. Does it happen? It doesn't happen that often. Maybe husbands have girlfriends on the side but they don't leave them."[11] Social worker Roz Kleban, at Memorial Sloan-Kettering Cancer Center, says that Hispanic women seem to have a more difficult time with body integrity and the notion of being mutilated than do other ethnic groups.[12] And Karen Schmidt, R.N., who works with breast cancer screening at St. Luke's Hospital in Manhattan and is, herself, a member of the Hispanic community, says that more openness about sex is needed in her community. She adds, "People will listen about AIDS but not about breast cancer."[13]

Like Hispanics, African Americans frequently share in feelings of fatalism when confronted with breast cancer. In traditional African American culture, health and illness are believed to be related to and affected by religious beliefs. An illness may be seen to be caused by disobeying God, by witchcraft, or by the devil. Folk medicine can be as important as, or more important than, biomedicine. Supernatural phenomena, psychological support, the wearing of charms and other objects for protection from evil spirits, and home and herbal remedies are traditional healing practices.

A study published in 1993 confirmed earlier studies that found African American women at a more advanced stage of breast cancer when diagnosed than patients in higher income groups and those getting medical care through private physicians, private clinics, or HMOs. Access to health care, lifestyle, overweight and other anteced-ent medical experiences were shown to influence the stage of diagno-sis. However, white women from lower socioeconomic income strata also tended to have more advanced disease at diagnosis. The findings suggest that the advanced stage at diagnosis is related, in part, to poorer access to health care, which is common to socioeconomically disadvantaged populations, a point that is made by Harold Freeman, M.D., director of surgery at Harlem Hospital Center in New York City and head of the President's Cancer Panel, and is supported by many studies.[14] In 1995, it was reported that 37.5 percent of Amer-ican women diagnosed with breast cancer were stage 0 or 1 compared with 54.5 percent of white American women diagnosed with early-stage breast cancer.[15]

Janice Phillips, R.N., Ph.D., an assistant professor of nursing at the University of Maryland, is trying to come up with a "user-friendly" interview for African American women. In 1993, she surveyed 154

African American women teachers, service workers, and unemployed women to see how many did breast self-examination and got other breast cancer screening. She said that most of the interview surveys available were developed for white women. There was none specifically designed for African American women to measure factors that could give insight into their attitudes toward breast cancer screening. She has proposed development of just such a survey — an "African-American Woman's Breast Health Inventory."

When Phillips talked to African American women, she says, many women in their fifties and sixties said, "If I have breast cancer, it's God's will." Phillips heard other beliefs from women, such as that they couldn't get breast cancer because their breasts were too small or too large, and found an attitude expressed by the phrase "If you don't name it, you can't claim it," a form of denial.[16]

One of the best places for education and screening, according to Beverly Rhine, a breast cancer survivor, is African American churches. Rhine works with the Women of Color Breast Cancer Survivors Support Project in Compton, California. She is listed in the bulletin of her own congregation, which numbers between 3,000 and 4,000, as a breast cancer counseling contact. The support project reaches out not only to church members but to women at alcohol and drug facilities and public housing projects.[17]

For Chinese Americans, illness can be seen as a result of bad conduct by an individual or by a family member in this life or in a previous one. The ill person is expected to take responsibility for curing herself without complaint. Older women are particularly reluctant to seek medical help outside of the family unit. In a 1994 survey of about 775 Chinese women in San Francisco, nearly 40 percent believed that most diseases are caused by an imbalance of yin and yang. According to Confucian principles, health is maintained by a consistent balance of opposing forces of yin and yang, or hot and cold, light and heat, wetness and dryness, in the body. The balance can be disturbed by strong emotions and an improper diet.

Treatment for illness can include herbs, acupuncture, and meditation to help restore balance. Dr. Marion Lee, at the University of California in San Francisco, says that many Chinese will go to see a Western doctor only when Chinese medicine fails to help them.[18]

Traditional Vietnamese health beliefs can preclude the use of Western medical practices. According to Stephen McPhee, M.D., of the University of San Francisco, Vietnamese believe that disease is caused by an imbalance of the humoral forces in the body. They tend to accept illness as their destiny. Denial or tolerance of physical pain is considered a strong character trait. Vietnamese women tend to be modest and are frequently reluctant to undress for an examination, especially in front of a male doctor. Dr. McPhee says that in a survey he conducted, 59 percent of Vietnamese women preferred a female physician, while only 4 percent preferred a male.

When Vietnamese are ill, they may use Chinese herbal medicine to restore the balance or seek out an acupuncturist or other traditional healers. Dr. McPhee says that 18 percent of the Vietnamese who responded to his study felt that Western medicine was "too strong" and that Chinese medicine was better. While 9 percent agreed that Western medicine was better, 57 percent disagreed. However, he added that the use of traditional medical practices did not appear to prevent most Vietnamese women who found breast lumps from going to Western doctors.[19]

There is appallingly little data available on the impact cultural attitudes and behavioral practices have on minority women who get breast cancer. What is known is that too many nonwhite women are dying because their cancer is diagnosed in a late stage. Studies must be conducted to learn how to raise awareness among these women in ways that they can relate to in terms of their own beliefs and culture. Obviously, increased awareness is meaningless unless there is also access to breast cancer screening and timely, state-of-the-art-treatment available to all women.

28

Discrimination and Litigation

The gaps in insurance for breast cancer payments are inordinate.

— Barbara Balaban, *breast cancer advocate*[1]

One in four cancer patients report discrimination on the job.

— Kimberly Calder, *Cancer Care*[2]

I had to leave my job because I was not able to walk. My disability has run out and I have a month left of medical coverage. I don't know what I'm going to do.

— JoAnne S., *breast cancer survivor*[3]

Breast cancer survivors, like all cancer survivors, all too often face discrimination. While some legislation has been passed to eliminate the discrimination, it remains a major problem for many cancer patients, particularly women, who in general earn less than men. People with cancer lose jobs, can't new get jobs, earn less money, lose insurance, and can't get insurance. Frequently, one form of discrimination leads to a domino effect. A woman who is fired because she had breast cancer loses her medical benefits. Because she has a preexisting condition, she cannot get medical insurance. If she can, it is prohibitively expensive and frequently the policy is written so that benefits are limited. Although economics isn't the sole reason for the discrimination against patients, it plays a major role.

The importance of adequate health insurance cannot be overstated. It is difficult enough to get competent treatment with medical coverage. Without it, it is virtually impossible. Ellen Stovall, executive director of the National Coalition of Cancer Survivors, an organization created to address the issues facing many survivors, says, "We know a lot of people who are not getting state-of-the-art treatment because of insurance problems." She says that the exact numbers are hard to come by because of privacy issues and because many people are reluctant to reveal their current cancer status. Of the 37 million Americans without medical insurance, "we have no idea how many have had cancer," says Stovall.[4]

Women with insurance have their breast cancer detected earlier than women who do not have insurance or are on Medicaid. According to a study published in the *New England Journal of Medicine* in 1993, women with breast cancer who have private insurance are "better off."[5] John Z. Ayanian, M.D., of Brigham and Women's Hospital, who directed the study, believes that women with insurance may do better because they have easier access to mammography and breast exams.[6] Four to seven years after diagnosis, researchers found, uninsured women had a 49 percent higher risk of death and women on Medicaid a 40 percent higher risk of death than women with their own medical insurance. However, they do point out, it is possible that the longer survival of insured women may be a result of their being diagnosed earlier and thus living with the cancer for a longer period of time — and not necessarily surviving for a longer period of time.[7]

Insurance horror stories abound. Mary Katzke had to go to three different doctors before she was taken seriously and her breast cancer was diagnosed. A frightening and difficult situation soon became far worse.

In the middle of this, the insurance company dropped me retroactively. . . . I had graduated and just started a new alumni [medical insurance] policy. They have the right to look back five years. They asked for one year on the application but they went back five years. And that's when they found out I went to the doctor because I had menstrual cramps and ibuprofen was prescribed, and I hadn't reported that on my form under the heading of disorder of the urinary/genital tract. I said no because I thought that meant venereal disease . . . something serious, not menstrual cramps. I've gone to two lawyers now and they couldn't do anything. . . . Everything they did, as far as we can see, was legal. I had to scrimp around to find money. I'm now $40,000 in debt. . . . Insurance companies have the right to do these things, and even if I say I didn't understand the question that way, they can say that's too bad. The only thing I can do is keep going public and try to enrage people and somehow have it backfire on them.[8]

Cancer survivors constitute a disproportionate number of uninsured and underinsured Americans. Roughly one in four survivors cannot get adequate health insurance.[9] It is not uncommon for an insurance company to double the premium when it learns a subscriber has a cancer history. Zora Brown, a breast cancer survivor and the president of the Breast Cancer Resource Committee in Washington, D.C., can testify to that.

I'd worked for large companies, including the federal government, for over twenty years. When I turned forty, I went to work for a small venture capital company. There were only five people there. They were initially covered by Blue Cross/Blue Shield. When I signed up with the company, the rates went sky high, to the point where the company said, we can't afford this, and basically what they said was that it was since I had a preexisting condition. I was at the age where I was a likely candidate for having a recurrence. So my rates were much higher . . . twice as much as everybody else. I left the company because it was impossible for them to carry me and everyone else. We even shopped around for other forms of insurance. We finally found one, which said they would not cover me for any problems with my reproductive system (including cervical, breast, ovarian, endometrial). I just want my money back that I spent all those years paying. . . . It just makes me angry that for over twenty years I paid into a program where I got to use about five thousand dollars of my investment in that plan.[10]

Brown is worried about getting a recurrence of the breast cancer because she doesn't have adequate insurance coverage and is responsible for her own health care. She says, "I'm sure there are a lot more women than we know about who are affected."[11]

In June 1993, the Equal Employment Opportunity Commission (EEOC) declared that employers may not refuse to hire people with disabilities because of concern about their effect on health insurance costs. Under the directive, disabled workers must generally be given "equal access" to any health insurance provided to other employees. The EEOC adopted a broad policy statement based on the Americans with Disabilities Act, passed in 1990 to prevent discrimination by employers and insurers providing health benefits. Under the Americans with Disabilities Act (ADA) and the Federal Rehabilitation Act (FRA) it is illegal for a cancer patient/survivor to be treated differently from other employees. As of 1992, the ADA covered workers in companies with 25 employees. It took full effect, covering employers with 15 or more workers, in July 1994. Federal law and most state laws require a boss to provide a cancer survivor "reasonable accommodation" such as a change in work hours or duties, allowing flexible hours while the employee is undergoing treatment. The new policy does permit some types of discrimination to continue but stipulates that the employer will have the burden of proving that such practices are justified, for example, if the health insurance plan would no longer be solvent without them. It allows employers to make some "disability-based distinctions" in their health coverage. The policy applies to businesses that buy commercial health insurance and to companies that serve as their own health insurers. This means that an employer will be liable for any discrimination resulting from a contract or agreement with an insurance company, health maintenance organization, or other entity to provide or administer health insurance plans for its workers.

Irene Card, president of Medical Insurance Claims, says that job discrimination related to cancer is hard to prove. A company may be worried that its premiums will rise, that a worker with cancer will not be able to concentrate on her job, will need time off, will come in late and leave early. Card says that large companies are very savvy about the law and have whole departments which stay current so that they don't flagrantly abuse it. "But," she says, "they find a way to get rid of you."[12]

The ADA offers other protection as well. It is illegal to discriminate against an employee because a spouse or child has cancer. That means, for example, the employer cannot assume that a man will do a poor job or stay out more often because his wife has breast cancer. Every state but Idaho and Louisiana has a state agency that enforces the federal law. Every state has, to some extent, laws that ban employment discrimination against the disabled. Some states have laws that specifically mention cancer. (For information on the laws in your state, call the EEOC Public Information System at (800) 669-4000, which can help you find out the appropriate state agency to contact.)

One woman who might have benefited from the new regulations had they been in place in the late 1980s, when she was diagnosed with cancer, is Nancy Cardwell. She says she knew "the handwriting was on the wall" when she was told at the graphics firm where she had been working for five years that she would not be retrained to use the new equipment they were getting.

> I'd had seven operations in twenty-two months. I was working for a small company, so my employer was trying like hell to get rid of me. There was a woman who had lupus who was there before I came, and she was eventually no longer there. Any small company has to eventually do that, I guess. They have to get rid of those people who are racking up their insurance bills. After the first operation, it was, "How's everything, is everything okay? Can we do anything?" They send you flowers. After the second operation, it was, like, "Well, when do you think you'll be back?" By the third operation, they don't even bother to call you to wish you well. So you can imagine after seven, I was really on the hit list. I knew it was coming. But it was extremely unpleasant, because instead of just saying to me, "You're fired," or, "We just don't need you anymore," or, "We're downsizing," whatever, they waited until I was sick one day and they canceled my insurance and I received notification from Blue Cross that my insurance had been canceled. . . . I haven't found a job since then. I've been out of work two years and nobody would touch me, of course. When someone calls and asks, "Why did you let her go?" eventually it would come out and they'd say, "Well, she was too sick." They'd ask me, "Were you sick a lot?" and I'd say, "Well, no, I had some surgery."[13]

According to attorney Barbara Hoffman, studies indicate that at least one in four cancer survivors are treated differently from their coworkers because of their medical history.[14] Hoffman says that the problems survivors run into include dismissal, failure to be hired, denial of benefits, undesirable transfer, and hostility by coworkers, as well as the well-founded concern of the employer that the worker's illness will cause insurance premiums to increase. Some employers still believe long-standing cancer myths, including that cancer is an automatic death sentence, that it's contagious, and that survivors are unproductive workers.[15]

When Pam Onder was diagnosed with breast cancer in the late 1980s, she was a top executive with a staff of forty-five. She went to the human resources department where she worked and told officials that she'd be undergoing a mastectomy, chemotherapy, and radiation. After her first round of chemotherapy she was told that her job was "being put on hold" until she was cancer-free. She'd be kept on the payroll but would not have her rank, power, or staff. Onder was out three days every three weeks when she had the chemotherapy, which she says was "less than a lot of other people who were supposedly well." About seven months after her treatments started, the man who had taken over her responsibilities "brought me into his office, sat me down, and said to me, 'You will never manage again in this company. You are emotionally and physically incapable.' " The next morning she walked calmly into his office and said, "I finally realize what the problem is. You think I've had a lobotomy." She says she then whipped out her breast prosthesis, slapped it down on his desk, and said, "Not a lobotomy, a mastectomy." She left his office and called a lawyer.[16]

Joyce Salzburg also called a lawyer. She was diagnosed with breast cancer in 1989 on her forty-second birthday. In over nine months she missed 21 days of work, two days every other week for chemotherapy.

> I could have gone on disability, but felt I was more useful being there and doing my job. I'm a social worker. I feel there's mind-body connection and thought it would be better for me psychologically to go in and do work. . . . Near the end of my radiation treatment, my boss, who was the executive director, gave me a poor performance evaluation. He said he'd consulted with a lawyer to make sure he was doing the right thing. It was totally undeserved. I thought he was insensitive to give me this kind of evaluation at this low time in my life. A few

months earlier, the agency was having to get a new insurance carrier. One reason premiums were going up was that there were some high-risk people and I was one of them. It seemed clear to me that he was starting a paper trail to get rid of me. He was trying to make it look like I wasn't doing a good job. Then he backed off. I wrote a retaliatory response. When I requested vacation time, he asked how could I ask for vacation time when I'd taken so much sick leave. I spoke to my doctor, who wanted to do something. What she did was write a letter to my boss telling him that I should take vacation time, that I needed it. So he gave me the time and I took it. I had a very responsible position. I supervised many people and also held another title of program director of the early intervention program. Nineteen months later, I was told my position was being eliminated. I said I'd stay on at the early intervention program. They told me they'd hired someone for that job. It was someone who had been working under me. . . . At that moment it was crystal clear that they were getting rid of me because I had breast cancer, because I was a deficit to them. I felt my rights were being violated. I felt I had a duty to every other woman. How dare they treat someone with breast cancer like that![17]

About 80 percent of cancer survivors return to work after diagnosis.[18] Studies consistently show that cancer survivors are as productive as their coworkers.[19] However, in a survey done by Cerenex Pharmaceuticals of supervisors questioned about a worker with cancer, 66 percent said the cancer survivor might not perform his or her job adequately; 45 percent said the cancer survivor might not take the job seriously enough; 35 percent said the cancer survivor's job responsibilities would be changed; 13 percent said the cancer survivor would be pressured into early retirement; 8 percent said the cancer survivor would be denied a deserved promotion or raise; and 6 percent said it was likely that the cancer survivor would be fired because of the illness.[20] When coworkers were questioned, 13 percent said the survivor would probably not be able to do the job and 25 percent thought that other workers would be forced to work harder to compensate for the person who had survived cancer.[21]

Fighting an insurance company or an employer is what many cancer survivors, unfortunately, have to look forward to. Being well-informed about your rights, and you do have them, is essential.

Getting needed medical insurance after a diagnosis of cancer can be a nightmare. COBRA (Consolidated Omnibus Budget Reconciliation Act) is one option for people leaving a job. This national law, enacted in 1986, entitles you to pay for and continue your group health plan for a maximum of 18 months. In some situations that time may be extended.

About a dozen states have enacted a guarantee issue law which allows you, on a one-time basis, to sign up for medical insurance without listing preexisting conditions. As of 1996, New York, Pennsylvania, Idaho, Kentucky, Washington, Maine, New Hampshire, Connecticut, Vermont had such laws. Minnesota's law takes effect in July 1997. Check with your state commissioner of insurance to find out where your state stands on this issue and whether any other options are available to you under state law.

Before you start looking for insurance, you may want to check your status with the Medical Information Bureau, which keeps medical history data about you on file for insurance companies. For a fee of $8 they will send you the information they have so that you can check it for accuracy. The address is P.O. Box 105, Essex Station, Boston, MA 02112 or you can call (617) 426-3660.

If you are having a problem getting your insurer to reimburse you, fight! First read your policy carefully and make sure you are entitled to the specific coverage. Call and ask why you haven't been reimbursed or why the amount you have received is less than you think you should be getting. Ask to speak to a supervisor. Write down everything — the name of the person with whom you spoke, the date, the conversation, what he or she has promised to do. Follow up. When I had an MRI in the mid-1980s, my insurance company reimbursed me $400 for the MRI, which cost $1200. My doctor wrote a letter, I called radiologists in New York for comparison prices, and found articles on this new and costly procedure. I received my 80 percent reimbursement. Mary Thompson, who wrote *The Squeaky Wheel Gets the Grease: A Step by Step Guide to Health Insurance Reimbursement*, says that 90 percent of the people who put up a good fight against their carrier get results. Sometimes all it takes is a phone call from an attorney, as many women who have undergone a very expensive high-dose chemotherapy with bone marrow transplant have found out.

If you are looking for a job that will provide medical coverage, try to get into a large company with a payroll of at least 300. You also have rights when looking for new employment. In most cases it is illegal for a prospective employer to ask about your medical history, unless it affects your current ability to do that job. Under no circumstances should you lie on a job or insurance application. You will be giving your employer grounds to fire you and the insurance company may refuse to pay benefits or may cancel your coverage.

If you are being discriminated against on the job, let your employer know that you are aware of your legal rights and would rather work out a resolution informally within the company rather than file a lawsuit. If you belong to a union, talk with your representative. Keep complete written records of all job actions, both good and bad, such as an excellent evaluation or a conversation in which you are told of concern that you cannot do the job because of your illness. If you believe you are being treated differently from other workers because of your cancer and your employer is covered by the ADA, you must file a complaint with the Equal Employment Opportunity Commission (EEOC), which will attempt to settle the dispute. If you are filing a complaint with a federal agency, you have 180 days from the date of the discriminatory action. In most states the time frame is the same. Before you file a lawsuit, carefully consider all the positive and negative possibilities.

Surviving breast cancer, or any cancer, a feat in and of itself, is for many just the beginning of new obstacles to surmount.

Part VI

Fighting Back

29

Setting the Stage

I used to say, until you deliver the body bags to the steps of the Capitol, you won't get a response.

— Harvey Kushner, *Women's Breast Cancer Advisory Center*[1]

The answer is political action. . . . The time has really come when all women have to get obnoxious and we have to become so obnoxious about this issue that they do something just to shut us up.

— Susan Love, M.D., *director, UCLA Breast Center*[2]

The foundation for the breast cancer advocacy movement was laid in the 1960s. Feminists began urging women to understand their physiology and to take control of medical decisions previously reserved for physicians. In 1973, the book *Our Bodies, Ourselves,* by the Boston Women's Health Collective, was published. It challenged women to take responsibility for their health care and gave women the information they needed, and until then lacked, to understand their reproductive system. Another milestone was Rose Kushner's first book, "*Breast Cancer: A Personal History and Investigative Report,*" published in 1975. Kushner's unflagging efforts on behalf of herself and all the women of this country who faced the possibility of breast cancer continued from 1974, when she was diagnosed, until she finally lost her fight against breast cancer in 1990.

Many women I talked with cited the success of the AIDS movement as their inspiration to change from passive acceptance to angry words and actions. Amy Langer, executive director of the National Alliance of Breast Cancer Organizations (NABCO), says, "Women have traditionally played the role of private patient, private caretaker, discreet employee. But we have seen with AIDS that those who are able to speak out and transform the personal to the political have had some measurable effect."[3] Beverly Zakarian, president of CAN ACT, says, "We can speak of before-AIDS activism and after-AIDS as B.C. and A.D. I think [breast cancer activists] owe [AIDS activists] a great deal of gratitude."[4] Ellen Hobbs, with Save Ourselves (SOS), in California, knew exactly what she was doing and why when she took off her wig at a breast cancer rally to reveal her hairless head. "I was quite aware of the amount of money AIDS received. I figured if we did the same thing as the AIDS activists and got real noisy, we'd get the money too."[5]

Susan Claymon, cofounder of Breast Cancer Action (BCA) in San Francisco, says BCA tried to make contact with friends in the AIDS movement.

> I believe that we were the original advocacy group to say, "Hey, the AIDS movement has done some great stuff. It's changed the way the American medical system works. They've brought the patient into the process." And patients' intimate knowledge of this disease [AIDS] has become a very valuable commodity in the research world, in the legislative world. These were people who weren't trained scientists but who taught themselves well and kept educating themselves well. So we wanted to learn from them and do the same kind of thing for breast cancer. That idea was picked up by the media. The media thought it was a "hot story." And it started jumping from one to the other to the other — from *U.S. News* to "20/20" to the *New York Times* and so on because they kind of feed on each other.[6]

Eric Rofes, who was the executive director of an AIDS service organization in San Francisco, said, in a 1991 *New York Times* article, that the women's movement inspired the gay community. "Most people have no awareness that is where our roots are."[7]

In the late 1970s and early 1980s, support groups specifically for women with breast cancer were started. Before that time "breast" and "cancer" were two words you did not utter in polite company, either singly or together. But as support groups grew all over the United States, women with breast cancer began talking about breast cancer. They compared the different treatments they were getting and gave each other hints on what to do about side effects such as nausea and hair loss. They exchanged information on different doctors and encouraged each other to speak up and switch doctors if necessary. The support groups did a great deal to "demystify" the disease and empower women. The groups were a direct outgrowth of women's consciousness-raising groups of the 1970s that had enabled women to see their particular problems as part of a larger pattern of discrimination and inequality.

As these support groups cropped up around the country, it was not uncommon for doctors to be suspicious, even antagonistic. There were doctors who felt threatened and became defensive. They didn't want patients coming in and asking questions, and especially questioning the advice and treatment they advocated. They were worried that they would be undermined by these groups.

Diane Zarafonetis founded the breast cancer support organization Expressions in East Grand Rapids, Michigan, in 1988. She was 38 years old when she was diagnosed with breast cancer. "I thought a support group which did not give 'advice' but gave support would be helpful to women, to share experience and give state-of-the-art information. An important goal of the group was to empower women, to get them to understand it is up to them. If they're not happy with a doctor — for any reason — change! Ask questions and demand answers. We've seen over a thousand women since we started. We usually have forty to fifty women at our meetings." At first, however, "surgeons showed resistance. Some told me, 'I'm not turning my patients over to you.'" Zarafonetis says that today Expressions is supported by the entire medical community, including doctors.[8] As with Expressions, many groups are now supported by physicians and hospital staffs, even if that was not the case initially.

Today, it is not at all unusual for a woman who has been diagnosed with breast cancer immediately to call a breast cancer hotline and/or support group before making a decision about treatment. Many of the support groups have grown out of their original quarters, and expanded their mission as well. Although there were other factors, it was those grassroots support groups, sprouting up all over the country, that played the greatest role in the development of the breast cancer advocacy movement.

In 1970, the only formal support program available for a woman with breast cancer was the American Cancer Society's Reach to Recovery program, which was started in 1952 by Terese Lasser in New York. She had had a mastectomy and was well aware that there was virtually no emotional support for women who had gone through the devastating experience of having a breast removed. At that time breast cancer was a taboo subject.

The mission of the organization is simple. A Reach to Recovery volunteer, a woman who has been treated for breast cancer and undergone training from ACS, visits a breast cancer patient in the hospital. The volunteer gives the woman a soft, stretchy bra and a light temporary prosthesis that she can put in the bra so that she can leave the hospital looking as close as possible to the way she looked before she went in. At that time, as now, the Reach to Recovery visit had to be requested by the woman's doctor, not the woman herself.[9] In the early 1980s, Rose Kushner took exception to this practice, which she called an an anachronism. She said, "The letters M.D. no longer stand for Mystical Deity. It's ridiculous for the [American Cancer] Society to continue to act as if we are living in a vacuum surrounded only with information doctors dispense as they see fit. Newspapers, magazines, television, and radio have educated us about breast-cancer treatments and the unknown and controversies surrounding them."[10] Despite its legacy of paternalism, Reach to Recovery has helped thousands of women.

Helen is one of those women. She has been a Reach to Recovery volunteer more than 20 years. I asked her what kinds of changes she has seen during that time.

Women in general are much more informed, educated about the disease, their rights, their options. For example, most women will say their surgeon has talked about reconstruction. I don't think the fear of cancer has changed. . . . I never generalize when I get a call. I used to frame in my mind if it's an older woman, she wouldn't be so concerned about her appearance or sexuality, or a nun. You can't generalize on basis of age, marital status. . . . I visit women when they've just been diagnosed. Their biggest concern then is the extent of the disease. . . . I do strongly believe that the disease does not change the woman or the relationships [she has]. When I visit women, if there's some communication problem, it doesn't seem to be because of the cancer, but rather is longstanding. The disease may complicate or aggravate it.

Helen has been there for other women facing breast cancer but doesn't think the medical establishment has been equally supportive. "I still don't think enough is being done and I can't help but think if it had been a man's disease much more would have been done. I was on a panel with a plastic surgeon who said if breast cancer had been a man's disease, reconstruction would have been paid for by insurance companies many, many years before. It's definitely a bias and there's still a long way to go."[11]

In 1974, Betty Ford, the wife of the president, was diagnosed with breast cancer. At that time "cancer was a whisper, it was something people said behind closed doors, particularly breast cancer or anything that had a sexual connotation and that was taboo," said Ford. The extensive media coverage resulted in breast cancer's first small steps out of the closet. Ford got a lot of mail from people who had never been able to talk about it before, and now they "were so grateful that they could discuss it openly. Women were lining up to have mammograms — the thought was, well, if the First Lady of the United States could have breast cancer, maybe they could, too. It made an awareness for the whole public."[12]

A year later Kushner founded the Breast Cancer Advisory Center (BCAC), a hotline and mail service. Its goal was to make available help and information about breast cancer to women and men, many of whom would suddenly find themselves facing a disease about which they knew virtually nothing. From its start-up in 1975 through 1982, BCAC responded to over 20,000 callers. When I was diagnosed with a recurrence of breast cancer, Kushner was immensely helpful, suggesting questions to ask my doctor, advising me about the availability of NCI treatment, tamoxifen, and much more. In 1990, at a House subcommittee meeting, Samuel Broder, M.D., who was then director of NCI, described Rose Kushner as "one of the most persuasive and expressive advocates for women with breast cancer."[13]

In 1978, three years after Kushner started the BCAC and hotline, a small support group for breast cancer patients was begun by Ann Marcou and Mimi Kaplan in Chicago. That support group became Y-ME, which has grown into the largest and most comprehensive breast cancer support program in the country. Mimi Kaplan died of breast cancer in 1983. Ann Marcou was the director of counseling until she retired in 1994.

Ann Marcou was diagnosed with breast cancer in 1976 at the age of 44. She had had a history of fibrocystic disease and had already had three biopsies that were negative. Then she found another lump that she thought was suspicious. "I went to a doctor and he said, 'Well, you have benign problems, this is nothing, we'll just watch it.'" At that time, her sister was dying of breast cancer, which made her even more anxious. So she went for a second opinion and that doctor said the same thing: "We'll watch it." Ann says:

I insisted on a biopsy, and he very disgustedly said, "Yes, well all right, we'll do a biopsy." He kind of patted me on the head, and it turned out to be cancer. At that time I went through a one-step [biopsy and immediate surgery when biopsy was positive]. I wasn't given any options. I was so frightened I didn't look any further, didn't do any research. I just wanted to know what it was I had. Especially with a sister dying at the time, it was doubly frightening. I had a mastectomy. The doctors at that time told me I had to have the other breast removed because I had a very high likelihood of getting cancer in the second breast, so two months later I had a second mastectomy. When the doctors said I should have the other breast removed I was crushed, sad, and very scared for my life. My doctor said I could have the second mastectomy at any time in the next year. I opted to do it as soon as I could because I felt I was sitting on a time bomb. That was in the days before there were breast specialists. I had four children, all in their teens. They were pretty frightened. They knew about my sister, their aunt. I was working on my master's degree and met a gal [Mimi Kaplan] who'd also had a mastectomy. She was putting together a conference on breast cancer for the university. We got together and realized there was nobody out here to talk to; nowhere to get questions answered. She was on chemotherapy and had no one to talk to about side effects, where to get a wig, how to get a prosthesis, simple things. We decided to do something about it. We asked ten women who we knew had had breast cancer to come to a meeting. One even brought a friend. I thought we'd have some little group in the suburbs of Chicago. Before we knew it, it was spreading like wildfire. We never did anything to make it spread. The need was there. Our phones starting ringing off the wall. We were getting requests for meetings from all over. Then hospital requests were coming for lectures. It just kept burgeoning. I had a hotline in my home. We couldn't afford an office. We got tax-exempt status. Our original idea was to have a support and informational group. We were getting direct physician referrals in the Chicago area at that time. We made sure we were solid in Chicago and then branched out to make our local hotline national. We had established a good reputation before we even thought about a national hotline. We approached the National Cancer Institute and asked if they would do a pilot study with Y-ME and have its Cancer Information Service refer patients to us. NCI very readily accepted.[14]

At about the same time that Y-ME was taking off in Chicago, the first glimmerings of protest about breast cancer appeared on the East Coast. In March 1977, there was a relatively small article on page four of the Metro section of the *New York Times* with the headline, "Protestors Assail Refusal of Saks to Hire Woman After Mastectomy."

According to the story, about 20 women, many in fur coats, had demonstrated outside of the luxury department store during the lunch hour. The women were protesting on behalf of, and with, Jacqueline Bleibert of Bayside, Queens. She had been offered a job at Saks, but when she told the nurse at Saks she'd had a mastectomy, the job offer had been quickly rescinded.

The women chanted, "Don't shop at Saks, don't shop at Saks, this store discriminates against women." The protestors cut up their Saks credit cards.[15] Lee Miller, a breast cancer survivor and one of the organizers of the demonstration, went to some lengths to get there.

> I was working that day. I ran down, got a taxi, got on the picket line, borrowed a charge card to cut in half, because I did not own a Saks charge card, took a taxi back to work, and no one knew I was gone. That night some of [the demonstration] was on TV. At work the next day, one man said, "I could have sworn I saw you on TV last night, but there's no way you could have been at Saks at noon, was there?" and I said, "There sure was."[16]

Later in the day, Allan R. Johnson, the store's chairman and CEO, met with the women, including Bleibert. He apologized to Bleibert and said she could have the job selling pocketbooks whenever she wanted it. "It was a mistake," he said. "Our interviewer did not follow the procedure of asking the woman to get an opinion from her doctor on whether she can do the job." She told him she still felt too devastated to consider the offer.

Bleibert said later that she was thinking about taking legal action against the store. "I opened up a Pandora's box for other women, and I'm glad I did. How many other cases are there like mine that you don't hear about because the women are too embarrassed to come forward?"[17]

The women who demonstrated in front of Saks that day were from the National Organization for Women and from a group in Manhattan called the "Post Mastectomy Discussion Group," which had been in existence a year. The group had been organized by Eugene Thiessen, M.D., who specialized in breast cancer. Lee Miller was a cofounder of the group and says:

> The first meeting, held in August 1976, was led by [Thiessen]. Someone said we really should have a mental health person lead the group. So I volunteered to do it, because I was a counselor and did a lot of group counseling. I was the first facilitator. We had no money. The Strang Clinic [a clinic in Manhattan specializing in cancer screening] gave us a place where we could meet once a month. It was a real self-help group, real grassroots. We made some mistakes, we made some decisions. Our sole purpose was to help serve our members, to help ourselves. In the second year we had two groups and a hotline.[18]

Some years later the group changed its name to: Self Help Action Rap Experience (SHARE). Meanwhile, support groups were starting in places other than huge urban areas.

In Sidney, Montana, population 6,000, the breast cancer support group Bosom Buddies was started by Doris Erickson and another breast cancer patient in the early 1980s. Erickson says, "We had tried to get Reach to Recovery here for several years but weren't successful. So I visited women in the hospital on my own. One woman I visited said that it would be nice to have a support group. So we called some other women and started one."[19]

Terri Castagno is a nurse at a small community hospital in Delaware. She started the support group Looking Ahead in 1989.

We had five or six of our own nurses who had breast cancer. They felt they needed to get together. So we went to the administrator of the hospital and I said, "What about fulfilling the needs of people in the community?" The [administrator] said, "Go to it." I called Y-ME. They said there's nothing to starting a support group: find a date, time, and place. We had a core group of three nurses, myself, the director of nursing, and the social worker. Someone suggested getting marketing involved. . . . We made a mailing list of every doctor in the state of Delaware. We got a positive response and now have over 120 women [1993]. . . . When we first started, the women came for support. Now the women who were in that first group are the supporters. They do a lot of things together. There are a lot of things going on in the community. There's been a lot in the papers about breast cancer. Most of the women are now lobbyists and have branched out into legislation. We've written many letters, gone to insurance companies. In that sense we've become a more active part in the fight against cancer.[20]

Looking Ahead is just one of the many groups around the country that have switched, or are switching gears, from supporting the group members to taking action. For some groups, going from support to activism is a gradual transition, while others jump right in. Survivor Sandy Warshaw, one of the women who were involved in the formation of the group SHARE, says, "People who go to self-help groups don't necessarily turn into activists."[21] The Virginia Breast Cancer Foundation went through various stages of development. Mary Jo Kahn, who joined about a year after it started, says that different women are ready to take part in advocacy at different times:

Slowly this movement is getting to be nationwide. In my mother's time it was an embarrassment. We should have gotten concerned 20 years ago. It clearly is tied up in sexuality. [When my mother got breast cancer] she felt like she was no longer a woman. She was kidded by her friends. It was America's difficulty in dealing with sexuality on all issues.[22]

Women are used to being passive about things, which makes it hard to motivate them, says Y-ME cofounder Ann Marcou. "The older women are still pretty submissive to the doctors. We have to reeducate them in a big way. A lot of women are still intimidated by medical people." But she sees a change in younger women. "Today, women are being more outspoken. They're demanding more involved medical care, so that it's a partnership. They're demanding second and third opinions. Younger women are asking much more of the medical profession."[23] Mary Jo Kahn agrees, saying, "If there was one motivating factor in our group it was that we were all mothers of young girls. I don't know if women who are so used to being passive about their own needs would do it on their own, for themselves, but it was [for] our daughters."[24]

In 1987, Lee Miller, who was then president of SHARE, spoke at the Surgeon General's Conference on Self-Help about what she and others had learned during the 11 years of, as she put it, "groping pain, trial and error, sharing, and laughter" that had taken place as SHARE grew. One of the issues that the support group addressed was the feeling of helplessness and loss of control. She said, "We need to feel in control again, even if we know it is an illusion in the grand scheme of things. We need to feel we can take charge of our own bodies, be informed medical customers, and participate fully in decisions regarding our health. An uninformed choice is not a real choice."[25] The support groups formed by women to help themselves get through a terrifying and lonely time also served to educate and empower them. As women exchanged notes and stories, and became better informed, they started raising questions. Joanne Rathgeb was one of those women.

I met Joanne Rathgeb in May 1993 at a breast cancer rally in Washington, D.C. She was 63 years old and in a wheelchair because of the cancer that had spread to her bones. Her husband, Don, was beside her. She very quickly told me she was a "breast cancer survivor, not a victim, or patient!" I asked why she had traveled down from Vermont. It obviously had not been an easy ride. She answered without hesitation:

I never thought I'd ever become politically involved — it was just not my thing. Now I feel there's just no way I can't, and it's physically very hard right now. When I realized there was so little research available on this issue and that what was being focused on was chemicals or drugs. . . . It's a money issue and became a political issue and that's when I became involved. So I joined national organizations like NABCO [National Alliance of Breast Cancer Organizations] and NCCS [National Coalition of Cancer Survivors]. It was just at the time, in 1991, when this organization [National Breast Cancer Coalition, which sponsored the rally] was organizing. So I got embroiled in the Do The Right Thing [a letter-writing campaign to then President Bush and members of Congress]. From Vermont we were supposed to get 475 letters. We ended up getting over 13,000. I think that's what made Vermont sit up and take notice.

She told me that Vermont has officially recognized breast cancer as a national health emergency.

We've already done that, unanimously, last year. The governor declared Mother's Day a day of remembrance, recovery, and resolution for breast cancer patients. This year we collected 200 names of women who have died of breast cancer and had them read aloud and entered into the *Vermont State Journal*. As the names were read, someone would answer "mother," "wife," "daughter," "sister." . . . It was beautiful. We just need to keep this in front of the public. . . . There are a few states that are out there in terms of political action and getting it going. But Vermont, because we're small, we're able to get to things. For example, two years ago [1991] we had a law passed that insurance companies had to pay for mammograms. Some states don't even have that. Another woman active in the state [of Maine] brought her case to the newspaper when her insurance company wouldn't pay. She kind of embarrassed them into paying for it. So now Blue Cross/ Blue Shield in Maine pays for a lot of bone marrow transplants. . . . We found out there were a lot of small, little cells that are active [in Vermont]. We're trying to get ourselves to help each other. Certainly on legislative aspects we all work together toward the same goals. Congressman Bernard Sanders [I-Vermont] was given letters which caused him to go to find out more about [breast cancer]. He said he'd never realized it was such a problem. There was no real information and that's how they came up with the idea of the cancer registry bill [which would keep track of the women in Vermont who were diagnosed with breast cancer and those who died]. They also enlisted the aid of Senator Patrick Leahy [D-Vermont], who introduced the bill in the Senate. They got together and worked on the cancer registry bill, which was part of the women's health bill. . . . One of my issues has been trying to get everyone working toward the same goal.[26]

Joanne Rathgeb, who never thought she would be an activist, was instrumental in getting progressive legislation passed in Vermont and raised the awareness of many women and politicians. Still fighting, she died of the disease late in 1994.

In California, Breast Cancer Action (BCA) grew out of a support group made up of women with metastatic breast cancer. It was part of the Cancer Community Support Group in San Francisco. BCA co-founder Susan Claymon says that in her group,

> We talked a lot about our own situations and feelings and talked about our anger, and what [breast cancer] could do to our daughters, sisters, and what could we do. Finally a woman from New York, who has since died, said, "What's the matter with you guys? There are no activists here?" Elenor [Pred] was the catalyst, she picked up on that as a number of us did, but she wasn't working at the time. She was in treatment and kind of depressed and looking for something to focus on. We said, "Well, let's start an advocacy group, what the hell." So we set a date in July 1990. We met in someone's living room. We came up with the name Breast Cancer Action. Elenor said she'd be president. I said that I'd be vice president. There were certain things we thought were important right away. One was to have a newsletter so we could get the word out to people. We also wanted to get in touch with people we knew in the AIDS movement. The media thought that was a hot story. Elenor had a lot of charisma and a way of getting across her point and her anger without alienating people. So she became our media star. Our first emphasis was getting the word out and also starting to connect with other grassroots advocacy organizations which had begun popping up in different parts of the country. We started talking to each other on the phone. And tried to learn from each other, and we started making legislative contacts. There was a wonderful woman, Congresswoman Mary Rose Oakar, from Ohio, who was very helpful. She'd been working for about 20 years on women's health issues. So we started to learn about legislative stuff. We had monthly activist meetings. We felt that educating ourselves, one of the things we learned from the AIDS movement, was super

important. To keep up with as much as we could, we had monthly study groups where we would take topics and research them and then come back with the results of our research. . . . Medical journal articles seemed very foreign at first, all those big words, it's out of my league. But it's not. Once you start reading them, you get the gist of it. We learned a lot by doing that. Gradually we began to network around the country as well.[27]

Elenor Pred was influential in the formation of many groups. The Virginia Breast Cancer Foundation, which Mary Jo Kahn joined in 1989, is just one of those organizations. She discussed the impact Pred had:

In spring of 1991, someone in the hospital saw Elenor Pred on tele-vision and called her. They were going to have a Mother's Day rally. Elenor sent us material. We had a rally which was small but successful. It was spontaneous, we only had a month for planning. After the rally, Elenor asked if I'd come to see her. I ended up staying three days. Elenor's thrust was to support [Congresswoman] Mary Rose Oakar's bill, which called for additional funding for breast cancer. Once Elenor talked to her, Oakar decided to resubmit for $50 million instead of $25 million. After our Mother's Day rally we decided to do more, we had to do more. We had our first meeting in June and I called in people I thought would be supportive, like a lawyer who'd lost his wife. We had our first public meeting in July with about two dozen people. We now have five hundred and fifty members statewide. We're still in the process of pulling together interested groups throughout the state. The vast majority are women in the group who are living with breast cancer. One young woman said there was no woman in her family since her great-grandmother who'd lived past forty-two.[28]

Susan Shapiro saw her mother die of breast cancer after an eleven-year battle. When Shapiro was diagnosed with breast cancer, she was determined to do something to help other women. In 1989, several months before she died in 1990, she wrote the article "Cancer as a Feminist Issue," which appeared in the feminist newsletter *Sojourner*. In the article she explains that when she was first diagnosed, she didn't consider breast cancer a political issue. But then she started to ques-tion why there was so much silence in the feminist community when it came to the disease. She found there were many resources for other women's problems, such as incest, single parenting, stress, eating disorders, but nothing for women with cancer. It took some searching, but she eventually found ten women with breast cancer. She also started looking at the literature, organizations, legislation, and the food and drug industries to find out more about the politics of cancer. She found there was very little available.

Shapiro decided that an organization of women was needed that would treat cancer as a feminist issue and encompass political action, service, and education. She came up with an agenda for what she felt the organization should do:

- Question FDA decisions and press for longer testing periods, warning labels, bans, and consumer action when needed.
- Evaluate and change laws where necessary.
- Feminize the health care system, making room for our values of connectedness and emotional expression.
- Look at research and funding — how much was going for prevention and basic research and how much was going for finding a cure or slightly improved treatment.
- Pressure candidates and lawmakers to put cancer issues on their agendas.
- Promote widespread education about cancer prevention as well as treatment.

Shapiro noted a lack of any comprehensive understanding of the role that environment plays in cancer or what impact the combination of all that we're exposed to in the environment may have on us and the development of cancer. She cited the need for education about the environment and nutrition to start in elementary school and the need for a local volunteer network to help women with cancer in virtually all areas of their lives, from cooking to childcare to getting treatment. "Ideally," Shapiro said, "we would have a three-pronged approach to cancer activism: direct support, political action, and education." At the end of her article, she announced a meeting to be held on September 9, 1989, at the Cambridge, Massachusetts, YWCA to discuss plans for a Woman's Community Cancer Project (WCCP).[29] Susan Shapiro lived just long enough to see the group launched.

Rita Arditti was one of the founders of WCCP. Arditti was diagnosed with breast cancer at the age of 39 in 1974. She has survived recurrences in 1979 and 1983. She told me that about 25 women showed up at that first meeting in Cambridge. In 1993, the membership numbered upward of 400. Arditti says, "Our intention was to bring change in the social, political, and medical dimensions in the issue of women and cancer and offer free support groups." When they started looking at breast cancer, it didn't take them long to realize that the focus was on treatment. According to Arditti, it is obvious that treatment doesn't work because so many women still die of breast cancer. The group started realizing there was "no prevention, no one had any idea of the cause of breast cancer and that there was nothing that one could do not to get breast cancer. It didn't take us long to say 'What is going on?' "

The conclusions of Arditti and the WCCP about what was going on were that the cancer establishment, namely the National Cancer Institute, the American Cancer Society, and leading cancer centers, weren't open to new ideas. Nor were they being "challenged enough to think creatively." According to Arditti, those organizations had every reason to keep doing what they had been doing, that is, research into and the treatment of breast cancer with surgery, chemotherapy, and radiation. She charges that the drug industry and mammography industry are all tied in with the cancer establishment, so there is little if any impetus to find prevention.[30] This viewpoint was expressed by many of the people with whom I spoke, both women and men. The fact that such a small percentage of research has focused on prevention lends additional credence to that argument. Arditti also accuses the cancer establishment of ignoring alternative therapies and not giving them a fair chance.

In 1992, the Women's Community Cancer Project issued "A Woman's Cancer Agenda: Demands to the National Cancer Institute and US Government." The agenda, sent to Hillary Rodham Clinton, the chair of the Health Care Reform Task Force, was endorsed by numerous organizations and individuals. It called for, among other things, increased funding for research, with a focus on prevention, environmental causes, and nontoxic treatments; passage of the Women's Health Equity Act; and the input of women, minorities, and the poor into decisions being made that affect them.

On the West Coast, a local chapter of Y-ME called the Bay Area

Breast Cancer Network was formed in 1990. It was one of the first Y-ME chapters to call for radical activities. Sheila Swanson, one of the founders, was first diagnosed with breast cancer in 1979. When she had a second bout in 1990, she had a double mastectomy, quit her nursing job, and became a breast cancer activist. "I looked at my life and decided I have to make some sense out of getting breast cancer for a second time. I decided I had to be outspoken and not be one of the silent women." Her philosophy was very simple. "Fight the establishment, shock them, and then stay in their faces."[31]

In a letter to the *San Jose Mercury News* in September 1991, Swanson wrote about the much larger amount of money being spent on AIDS research projects compared to what was being spent for breast cancer research. She said, "I am not trying to minimize the crisis of AIDS, but we do know how to prevent this fatal disease. . . . We don't know how to prevent [breast cancer]!"[32] The following January, in a letter to *Coping* magazine, a magazine for cancer survivors, Swanson said the meaning was obvious — that as a group, women are expendable; that someone, some group, some elected officials with decision-making power are making it clear that breast cancer is a low priority.[33]

That January, the Bay Area Breast Cancer Network sent New Year's cards to every senator that said, "Welcome back, Senator. . . . Unfortunately, breast cancer never takes a vacation." At the bottom of the card was the line, "P.S. We will be monitoring your votes on the NIH Reauthorization Act of 1991, on behalf of the 96,000,000 women voters in America." They also sent Congress members a "before" and "after" poster of a 35-year-old woman nude from the waist up — on one side she looked normal and healthy, on the other side she was bald and bloated, with a missing breast. In June 1991, they sent letters to members of Congress threatening to publicize their votes against increased funding for breast cancer research. "I got a lot of flak for that," says Swanson. "I was told it doesn't work to be negative." Some members of Congress called Mary Rose Oakar, who was a big proponent of increased funding for breast cancer, and told her to get Swanson to back off. They vowed not to support the bill if she didn't. Swanson refused, saying, "We're not playing nice, but this is not a nice disease."[34] The additional funding was passed.

Another grassroots organization in California was Save Ourselves (SOS), founded by Ellen Hobbs in Sacramento in January 1991. This group was started specifically for the purpose of advocacy. Hobbs says,

I was diagnosed in October 1990. I had a lump in my armpit but nothing in my breast. Twenty-three of the twenty-four lymph nodes they removed were positive. I was told to get a bone marrow transplant at Stanford. I had to fight my insurance company. I also had to have a mastectomy to fit into the protocol even though I didn't need a mastectomy! At that same time articles came out in *Time* and *Newsweek* about the politics of breast cancer and I got really angry. I decided I wanted to do something and since I wasn't sure how long I'd be around, I decided to hold a demonstration at the state capital on Mother's Day. To do that I formed SOS to plan and organize the demonstration. I called a local newspaper columnist and told her I was starting a group for breast cancer, that we were planning a demonstration, and there would be ten thousand people. So she came out to interview me and people started calling me. The first meeting of SOS was at the end of January at my house. About forty people showed up. . . . We then met with Sheila Swanson and Elenor Pred, the founder of Breast Cancer Action. At that point we also formed the Northern California Breast Cancer Organization [which changed to CABCO later], again for the purpose of the rally. I called the gay community center, who were big supporters, and NOW. We met every Monday for the next two months, planning the demonstration.[35]

The rally received heavy media coverage, although 800 people, not 10,000, showed up. Hobbs was one of the speakers. Her speech was called "Look Good, Feel Better." (A program sponsored by ACS and the cosmetics industry called "Look Good, Feel Better" was founded to help cancer patients, primarily women, use makeup and wigs to improve they way they look, the idea being that when a woman looks better, she will feel better.) She waved her prosthesis in the air and pulled off her wig and said, "They gave me this and that didn't make me feel any better."[36]

The day after the rally, some members of SOS went to Washington, D.C., and met with Samuel Broder, the director of NCI at that time, and members of Congress. They also went to the first general National Breast Cancer Coalition (NBCC) meeting, where they met with grassroots breast cancer activists from all over the country.[37]

Barbara Balaban has been active with NBCC from its early days. She is the director of the Breast Cancer Support Program and hotline at Adelphi University, which was started in the early 1980s on Long

Island, New York. Its toll-free hotline number was expanded in 1991 in order to be accessible to women throughout New York State. The hotline offers support and information to women with breast cancer. However, Balaban also sees hotlines as another source of advocacy that is often overlooked. She says hotlines "have been there for years, women reaching out to each other. It's ongoing. They're doing a hell of a job."[38] The various breast cancer hotlines are an integral part of the advocacy movement, which would have gotten nowhere without women speaking to women — and being able, finally, to recognize, share, and express their anger.

Balaban has seen a lot of changes since 1991. She says, "Now we're getting calls about the environment and advocacy. The average age of women is younger than it was. There are more people getting involved. We have a men's group, a couples' group. We get a lot of calls when something is said on the media. We get a lot of calls about buying homes in safe areas. A lot of people call to give us information. They just found out, on their block, there were so many cases of breast cancer. They want it to be on record. And a lot of callers ask where to get low-cost screening mammography, find a doctor, a support group, are they doing the right thing?"[39]

When Francine Kritchek, a teacher and grandmother on Long Island, had a mastectomy, she discovered that a colleague also had had breast cancer. They sent a letter to everyone in their school about their disease. Then a study came out that showed a relationship between the high rate of breast cancer on Long Island and high income levels. The study virtually ruled out environmental factors.[40] The two women were outraged. They called Balaban at Adelphi University, put a small ad in a local paper, and wrote to hundreds of women asking them to come to a meeting. Fifty-seven women showed up, and that was the beginning of "1 in 9."

One-in-Nine, on Long Island, New York, was an advocacy group from the beginning. The women made local headlines when over 300 of them, some in wheelchairs, demonstrated in front of the courthouse in Nassau County. The demonstration prompted the Centers for Disease Control and Prevention (CDC) to hold a hearing on whether another study was warranted. The CDC heard testimony about environmental risks like auto emissions, polluted water, toxic wastes, pesticides, and electromagnetic fields (EMF). After six months, the CDC said the original study was sufficient.[41] The group said they would do their own study. Surgeon Susan Love and researcher Devra Lee Davis, with the International Organization for Breast Cancer Prevention, agreed to lead the study.

In its mission statement, 1 in 9 said, "We are not satisfied that the Department of Health reports have exhausted the field of inquiry as far as the high rate of breast cancer on Long Island is concerned. We are concerned about the difficulties in initiating and implementing research on breast cancer treatments." The statement then lists all the things the group found unacceptable, the first being that women get breast cancer. Others were:

- the existence of small geographic areas of [breast cancer] hot spots
- women who are healthy, exercise, and have no family history getting breast cancer
- increasing numbers of women under the age of 35 getting breast cancer
- the long time it takes for new medications to be available in the United States compared with other countries
- a greater focus on men, rather than women, in clinical trials of cancer treatments
- small percentage of research dollars going for breast cancer
- uncertified mammography equipment and radiology technicians
- inadequate insurance coverage for early detection and treatment
- the lack of research into the effects of environmental factors, including electromagnetic fields, on breast cancer

A hearing on breast cancer and the environment, sponsored by the New York City Commission on the Status of Women and the Women's Environment and Development Organization (WEDO), was held in March 1993. At the hearing, Balaban said, "As we are in contact with people around the state [New York], it becomes obvious that the grassroots movement is growing. It's there. It's a vital force." Balaban urged all the different groups in the state to join forces, share ideas and information, rather than "reinventing the wheel over and over."[42]

In May 1992, SHARE, which started out as a support group, held an advocacy meeting that was attended by some 500 people, mostly women. There were women there from other groups, like 1-in-9. *New*

York Newsday columnist Jimmy Breslin also attended. The headline on his article read "Women in the Fight of Their Lives." Although he had praise for how well organized the meeting was, he also had many reservations, saying that the meeting "showed how far women have to go. Many women were worried about their daughters. Only some seemed angry. The rest were living proof that women don't know how to fight over anything more important than a label or an expression. . . . With 50,000 [sic] women a year dying of breast cancer, women who don't organize like ACT UP [the activist AIDS organization] are ridiculous." Breslin said that there was one woman there who really knew what was going on. That woman spoke about taking action — she told the women that they should get a huge crowd and picnic on the runways at Kennedy Airport, O'Hare, and L.A.X. Then, the woman said, the "balding, gray-haired old men in Washington, most of whose emotions remain in high school, might understand that a woman's breasts, which so many politicians still think of as belonging on magazine covers, can be changed."[43]

In 1995, SHARE was running support groups for women newly diagnosed with breast cancer, women with recurrent breast cancer, single women, family members, husbands, and Chinese, Hispanic, and African American women. (It had also expanded to include ovarian cancer.) SHARE has a breast-cancer advocacy committee of 8 to 12 women who meet regularly and is a member of the NBCC board.

Y-ME has also gotten involved in advocacy. It's using its newsletter to alert members to upcoming legislation and has set up a nationwide phone network to call lawmakers when necessary. Ann Marcou says, "We've always been pretty outspoken but never lobbied in Washington. I hope we're going to do something as good as the AIDS people did. I think women can have the power and force that the AIDS people have. There are lots of little splinter groups, a lot of little factions. We're trying to get all those people together — that's what it's all about."[44]

The grassroots movement — breast cancer patients in support groups and in advocacy groups — has had some noteworthy accomplishments, and continues to do so. In May 1979, the Massachusetts state legislature passed a bill making it illegal for women to be railroaded through a breast cancer surgical procedure without being informed, beforehand, of all the alternatives. What this means, in effect, is that a two-step procedure is required. If the biopsy proves to be positive, the woman can then research her treatment options and make a decision. The exception is the woman who signs a consent form allowing the doctor to perform whatever surgery he or she feels is indicated after getting preliminary results of the biopsy. Even if a doctor tells the woman all the possible options before the biopsy is performed, the options may change as a result of what is found in the biopsy. Informed consent cannot be obtained from a woman who is unconscious or on an operating table. Massachusetts was the first state to pass such a law.

In Springfield, women marched demanding that breast reconstruction be included in their medical coverage. The state's Blue Cross and Blue Shield plans had refused to cover it, calling it cosmetic. The women said that the breast reconstruction was "rehabilitation" and should be covered just the way penile and testicular implants in men had *always* been covered.[45] The women won.

On May 20, 1992, Massachusetts became the first state to declare breast cancer an epidemic and to launch a campaign to fight the disease. The state announced a three-part plan:

1. pilot education programs to reach poor, uninsured women who don't get regular medical checkups and often find the disease too late
2. a bill that would require state licensing of mammography facilities
3. improved surveillance, by the state, of the incidence of breast cancer

The stage at which breast cancer was diagnosed in various parts of the state was of particular interest. For example, if it were found that inner-city women were being diagnosed at a later stage of the disease, when the cancer is not as likely to respond to treatment, that would give a good indication of where intervention programs were needed.

Ann Maguire, president of the Massachusetts Breast Cancer Coalition, says, "The realization of the epidemic proportions of this disease . . . is the kind of public awareness that is going to help us find what causes it, how you can treat it, and ultimately how you can cure it. . . . We are drawing the line at one in nine. We want to change that to one in none."[46]

In 1987, the Susan G. Komen Foundation for the Advancement of Breast Cancer Research, Education and Training, a national breast cancer advocacy group based in Texas, had volunteers lobbying members of the Texas state legislature to pass a bill mandating insurance coverage for a baseline (first) mammogram for any woman over 35. Then "people nearly laughed us out of Austin, but we got it through in one session," says foundation president Linda Cadigan.[47] Since then many states have passed similar legislation.

It took California two years to pass its breast cancer informed-consent law, which became effective January 2, 1981, and made California the second state in the nation with such legislation. California's law can be credited to the efforts of Juliet Ristom, a breast cancer patient. Before she was even definitively diagnosed with breast cancer, her doctor had reserved an operating room for the mastectomy she would be getting. When she asked about alternatives, he refused to give her any other information. She did her own research and ended up getting a lumpectomy and keeping her breast. In a letter to members of the California Assembly, she said that she had taken control of her treatment and always would, but that many women wouldn't — and that all women should have the opportunity to be well informed of all the possible treatments before making a decision.

CABCO (California Breast Cancer Organizations) was instrumental in getting a special "breast cancer check-off" on the state income tax for breast cancer research. When filing a return, you can indicate a certain amount of money to be used for breast cancer research. A special research fund was set up with patient advocates on its board. In its first year the check-off raised about $300,000. Another, and potentially far richer, source of income is the two-cent-a-pack cigarette tax enacted by the California Assembly. The money generated by that levy will fund breast cancer research, awareness, and education.

The gains made by grassroots groups at the state level are impressive and the women behind them deserve a lot of credit. They show what can be done locally by working together and persevering. Although at times it may appear that they are overshadowed by groups on a national level, that must never become a deterrent and distract from the grassroots movement that started the ball rolling. The ultimate victory will be a result of winning one battle at a time.

30

A National Movement

You found billions of dollars for the war in the Persian Gulf — you've gotta find money for us. You've found billions of dollars to bail out the savings and loans when the white men in suits destroyed that system — you better find billions of dollars for us.

— Fran Visco, *president, NBCC*[1]

One B-1 bomber is about equal to the breast cancer research budget. Instead of trying to defend the Kuwaitis, we need more money to defend women in this country.

— Susan Love, M.D., *director, UCLA Breast Center*[2]

It doesn't only make a difference who's in the White House. It makes a difference when we elect women to Congress.

— Donna E. Shalala, *Secretary of Health and Human Services*[3]

As grassroots support and advocacy groups were burgeoning, various national groups were developing as well. The Susan G. Komen Foundation was one of the first and most successful nonprofit volunteer organizations. Its primary mission was to raise money specifically to fight breast cancer. It was founded by Nancy Brinker in 1982 in Dallas, Texas, after the breast cancer death of her sister Suzy Komen at the age of 36. Suzy's last request had been for her sister Nancy to make it better for other women. To raise money, the foundation sponsors a yearly Race for the Cure. The first race, held in Washington, D.C., in 1990, raised half a million dollars. As of 1995, there were 56 cities holding a Race for the Cure and 26 chapters of the Komen Foundation throughout the United States. Over $27.5 million has been raised. That money has been used for more than 200 grants for research and for providing care to the underserved.[4]

The Komen Foundation has also played a major role in calling attention to breast cancer. When Rae Evans, a Hallmark executive, met Brinker at a luncheon in Washington, she called her close friend Marilyn Quayle, whose mother had died of breast cancer. After meeting Brinker, the wife of then vice president Dan Quayle told her own story several months later at a Komen Foundation fund-raiser. "We hit it off from the very beginning," Quayle says. "She's just got so much drive. And — let's face it — because of her husband she has the wherewithal to have mounted a campaign."[5] (Brinker's husband, Norman Brinker, is the founder of Bennigans, Steak and Ale, and Chili's restaurants.)

Another national organization is the National Alliance of Breast Cancer Organizations (NABCO). According to Harvey Kushner, NABCO was originally the idea of his late wife, Rose, and several others. Rose Kushner wanted breast cancer organizations to band together and take political action. She left the project when it didn't seem to be taking the political direction she'd been striving for and decided she'd take on Congress on her own. (Early in 1988 she created "Breastpak," a political action committee. Breastpak disolved after Kushner died.)[6] Other women who played a role in the formation of NABCO include Ruth Spear, Nancy Brinker, and Diane Blum, head of Cancer Care.

Amy Langer has been the executive director of NABCO since October 1990. She can be credited with making it a nationally known and respected organization. Langer, who was diagnosed with breast cancer in 1984, became a volunteer in 1987.

I saw NABCO mentioned in *Ms.* magazine and called Diane Blum. I told her I was a businesswoman and I was interested in helping. She said, "I'm not sure how we could use you," and I said, "Great, I'll be there tomorrow." It had just started and had, I think, forty member organizations. At that time I had my own consulting business. I spent time here [at the NABCO office] mostly getting them organized, computerized, and then got very seduced by the potential of a national organization that would be an alliance of members and be able to supply information. The more I did this, the less I did my consulting. And then I decided to make this my career. . . . When I became executive director, I think it was really still the era when breast cancer carried a big stigma. People still talked about cancer like the "big C." There was very little media coverage of breast cancer. It wasn't talked about openly except in a support group context. Most people associated breast cancer with mutilation and death. So it was a very uncomfortable subject to a lot of people.[7]

NABCO, which began by providing information to cancer patients, is now lobbying for legislation for patients' and survivors' rights and concerns.

NABCO and Amy Langer played a key role in the formation of the biggest and most effective political organization for breast cancer, the National Breast Cancer Coalition. In December 1990, Langer met with breast surgeon Susan Love, at that time director of the Faulkner Breast Centre in Boston, and Susan Hester of the Mary-Helen Mautner Project for Lesbians with Cancer in Washington, D.C. They discussed the possibility of starting a coordinated effort to fight breast cancer. The idea was to have breast cancer patients lobbying on their own behalf for such things as research, legislation, and regulations. The coalition was to be comprised of grassroots organizations from all over the United States.

Langer contacted Diane Blum of Cancer Care, Nancy Brinker and Linda Cadigan of the Susan G. Komen Foundation, and Sharon Green of Y-ME, and suggested they all meet sometime in late January as a "first step in organizing a joint effort." In her December 17 memo, Langer wrote, "Although each of our organizations has been active in some aspects of patient advocacy, I feel we can accomplish more, faster, if we work together."[8]

Two months later, on February 28, there was an announcement that a national breast cancer advocacy coalition was being formed. The planning group was NABCO, Y-ME, Cancer Care, CAN ACT, the

Faulkner Breast Centre, the Mautner Project, and the Women's Community Cancer Project (WCCP). The press release listed three major goals:

- To promote **research** into the cause of, cure for, and optimal treatments for breast cancer through increased funding, recruitment, and training of scientists and improved coordination of funds distribution
- To improve **access** to high-quality breast cancer screening, diagnosis, treatment, and care for all women, particularly the underserved and uninsured, through legislation and beneficial changes in the regulation and delivery of breast health care
- To increase the involvement and **influence** of those living with breast cancer in the areas of legislation, regulatory process, and all aspects of clinical trial design, including access to trials

The announcement concluded by saying, "Breast cancer patients and their supporters will be invited to participate in national and local grass roots advocacy efforts on behalf of American women, all of whom are at risk for developing breast cancer."[9]

On May 1st, the NBCC released its Action Agenda. At the end of May, NBCC sent a letter to Congressman William Natcher (D-Kentucky), chair of the Labor, Health, Human Services, and Education Appropriations Subcommittee, which addressed the need for more funding, a major concern. It read in part:

The Breast Cancer Coalition, a national network of breast cancer advocates representing tens of thousands of women, their families and supporters, strongly supports an increase in funding for breast cancer research. We request that an additional $25 million be appropriated for basic breast research, as well as $25 million for clinical trials and treatment.

By the time it takes to read this statement, another woman will be diagnosed with breast cancer — the most common form of cancer among the women in the U.S. Every 12 minutes, another death will occur. The incidence of breast cancer — currently one in nine women — is escalating annually for reasons which remain unclear. The Breast Cancer Coalition believes these facts should make all women fear for their lives, should mobilize individuals and groups across the

country into demanding progress, and should compel all elected officials into immediate action. Elected officials must make breast cancer
research a national priority by enabling more breast cancer research
through meaningful increases in funds.... We demand a new and
appropriate level of attention to the need for progress against the
epidemic of breast cancer, and strongly urge these appropriations.[10]

The first major undertaking of NBCC was "Do the Right Thing,"
a letter-writing campaign. Its goal was to generate 175,000 letters that
would go to members of Congress and President Bush, asking them
to show their support of breast cancer–related legislation and regulation. The goal of 175,000 letters represented the number of new
breast cancer cases projected for 1991. Each state was asked to collect
the number of letters that represented the number of new cases
in their state for that year. The first campaign was coordinated by
Y-ME, which found the state captains. The second campaign, a
year later, was coordinated by Mary Jo Kahn, of the Virginia Breast
Cancer Foundation. "At times I was working sixteen- or eighteen-
hour days. I can remember many all-nighters. Board members did
everything. We made our own flyers, got them printed, and distrib-
uted them."[11]

Women all over the country heard the call. Some states collected
many more letters than needed. Thirty-three-year-old Kathy Welsh of
Ellisville, a small town in Missouri, was newly diagnosed with breast
cancer. Welsh wrote her own letters and spread the word at the church
where she works. Instead of the 4,000 letters requested, Missouri
came up with over 14,000 letters, thanks to Welsh and many other
women and men.

In the end, some 600,000 letters were collected. Fran Visco, president of NBCC, says the 600,000 letters "told us it would be a success, that there was a real movement out there, waiting to happen."
The letters were sorted by state and most were delivered to senators
and representatives from that state. The rest, 140,000, were brought
to the White House. Visco told me that they were led to a side door.
"The person who opened it gave the impression that our letters were
going on a conveyor belt, straight into trash cans. President Bush
never answered one of the letters. He never acknowledged that he
received them." They did get a response from some members of

Congress. "We felt we made our mark [on the Hill] and they now knew we existed and we expected them to be responsive."[12]

In February 1992, NBCC held hearings in Washington that were open to both the public and the media. Fifteen scientists from around the United States were chosen to participate in the hearings. Their specialties covered all areas of breast cancer research. The hearings were organized into three sessions: Prevention and Epidemiology, Basic Science, and Clinical Science. The purpose of the hearings was to get an overview of breast cancer research in progress and, more important, to determine the direction future research should take. NBCC intended to use the information from the hearings to compute the amount of funding needed to achieve near and long-term goals. Rather than just asking for some arbitrary amount of additional funding, NBCC members were determined to justify every cent being requested. The following summary conclusions were reached:

- *Prevention and epidemiology:* Prevention efforts are hampered by the lack of understanding of how breast cancer is caused. Research is needed on susceptibility, environmental exposures, and hormone manipulation. New risk and epidemiology studies are needed, in particular on exogenous hormones (those derived from outside the body).
- *Basic science:* The knowledge and tools necessary to examine and potentially reverse the genetic effects of carcinogens are available. Identification of the early hereditary changes in both hereditary and nonhereditary breast cancer are close to being made. Studies of cytology (structure and function of cells) and growth factors (materials that stimulate the production of blood cells) have developed hypotheses which are ready for clinical trials. The use of suppressor genes which can be used to switch off the malignant process is being studied.
- *Clinical science:* Research has made the most progress in the treatment of breast cancer. Clinical trials studying various surgical approaches, drug combinations and treatments, adjuvant therapy, have made important contributions. There are many clinical issues still unresolved, such as treatment for carcinoma in situ, mammography, the role of immune-directed therapies, and the development of quality-of-life measurements, and interventions of clinical protocols. These issues are crucial.

The general conclusions cited the need for more money across the board for breast cancer research. The additional funding was especially appropriate at that time because of the financially impoverished state of basic research. The researchers and NBCC felt that with sufficient funding a powerful impact could be made on the prevention, treatment, and cure of breast cancer.[13] As a result of the hearings, the NBCC said that in addition to the $133 million for fiscal year 1992, an additional $300 million in funding would be needed for fiscal year 1993, which would bring the funding to $433 million.

At the 1992 Democratic convention, then candidate Bill Clinton (whose mother had breast cancer, which caused her death in 1994) promised $400 million for breast cancer research. Congress appropriated an additional $64 million for breast cancer research at NCI for a total of $197 million. In addition, Senator Tom Harkin (D-Iowa) and Congressman John P. Murtha (D-Pennsylvania) found funding in an unconventional source, the Pentagon budget. The Army budget already had $25 million in place for breast cancer research. They worked out a plan to get an additional $185 million in that budget. The additional $210 million added to the $197 million resulted in a total of $407 million. When the Senate voted on the funding from the Department of Defense (DOD), the vote was a whopping 89 to 4. (When it became evident that the measure was going to pass, 30 senators suddenly developed sensitivity to women's issues and switched their votes to be on the winning side.) NCI ended up spending $211.5 million for breast cancer research in fiscal year 1993.

Mary Rose Oakar, who at that time was a Democratic congresswoman from Ohio, was pleased about the additional funding. She was not at all pleased when the money was not transferred out of the DOD, as had been promised. "They're buying that baloney that the military will take a fresh approach. They don't have the capacity to do those kinds of research, nor experience in giving grants out. We did studies on how the military deals with health care and women, and it's terrible."[14]

Oakar's concerns about the Army having control of so much money for breast cancer research was echoed by many. To deal with the issue, the Institute of Medicine (IOM), a private, nonprofit corporation set up by the National Academy of Sciences, assembled a ten-member panel to advise DOD on how to best manage the $210 million appropriation. The IOM committee took into account the views of and information from over 250 individuals. Kay Dickersin, Ph.D., assistant professor of epidemiology and preventive medicine at the University of Maryland Medical School, was part of the group. "There were twelve people sitting on a panel and nine of them were women. That was a wonderful feeling. Not only were there mostly women, most were not breast cancer research specialists. They were all top-notch researchers. They didn't bring to the table a set notion of how things should go."[15] The IOM issued its report "Strategies for Managing the Breast Cancer Research Command" in 1993. It recommended that most of the money be for research, with money allocated also for recruiting and training researchers and for enhancing the infrastructure of research such as tumor registries, banks of tumor samples, breast tissue banks, information systems, and so on.[16]

Oakar had wanted a special department set up for breast cancer research, like the one for AIDS. She says, "Two hundred million bucks isn't a lot when you compare it to AIDS research or the military budget. The fact is, it could be dramatic money for those researchers who get turned down every year."[17]

In October 1994, the Army finished a year-long evaluation of 2,700 grant applications and announced 433 winning proposals. The guidelines set up by the IOM were basically met, with 78 percent of the money going for investigator-initiated research. Another 12 percent was to be used for training grants to support graduate students, postdoctoral researchers, and midcareer scientists who want to switch to breast cancer studies. Kay Dickersin, an NBCC board member, said the Army was "excellent to work with" and that the NBCC's expectations of where the money should go had been met. She added that the Coalition would encourage more psychosocial and epidemiologic proposals in the future.[18] And while many thought the Army money was a "one-shot" deal, Congress allocated an additional $25 million for fiscal year 1994 and in October 1994 allocated $115 million in the Army's 1995 budget for breast cancer.[19]

In October 1994, it was reported that 18 NCI-designated cancer centers had been granted a total of about $5 million to set up or expand breast cancer research programs. The funding was a joint effort of NCI, the National Institute of Environmental Sciences, and the National Institute on Aging. Margaret Holmes, Ph.D., chief of NCI's Cancer Center Branch, said, "We expect it to improve the quality of breast cancer research and increase the number of investigators studying breast cancer in NCI-designated centers. . . . The initiative will stimulate research on the important but understudied question of the role of environmental factors in breast cancer. The grants will primarily help institutions in staff recruitment and in the conduct of exploratory research projects."[20]

In 1993, NBCC launched another letter-writing campaign. This one was kicked off at a rally in May in Washington, D.C. At that rally, Dr. Susan Love called for an overall national strategy to address the problem of breast cancer. This time the call was for 2.6 million signatures — one representing every woman in the United States with breast cancer.

The day after the rally, NBCC sponsored a conference on the skills needed for advocacy. At the conference, women were given the latest information on breast cancer research and legislation; they took part in workshops to hone advocacy skills, met and networked with NBCC members and other breast cancer advocates, and collected materials that could be used to motivate and teach breast cancer advocacy to those who were not at the conference.

Also in May, Fran Visco was appointed to the President's Cancer Panel, replacing Nancy Brinker, whose term had expired. The appointment was further recognition and validation of NBCC and marked the beginning of a new era of cancer patient activism.

I attended a march and rally for breast cancer in Washington the following October. In five months, women around the country had collected over 2.6 million signatures from people in every part of the United States, from every state in the Union. I walked down Independence Avenue with thousands of women — young and old, white, black, Hispanic, Asian, with friends, husbands, children in tow, women wearing brightly colored T-shirts with slogans from the polite to the abrasive, women chanting and screaming and yelling for a cure, for a way to prevent cancer, for life. People leaned out of office building windows and cheered. We walked 12 abreast behind a flat-bed truck piled high with boxes of petitions and letters for the president.

Later, at the rally on the Ellipse, the usual people spoke — some members of Congress, an actress, various celebrities and breast cancer activists. But what I found most moving were the letters written by women around the country and read aloud by several of the women at the rally.

From Adele in New York: President Clinton, I had a lumpectomy and then lymph node surgery; I had 33 treatments of radiation and eight months of chemotherapy. In my school of 30 teachers 7 women have faced breast cancer. Please help us to solve this problem forever.

From Linda in Maine: My mother died at the age of 46 of breast cancer. Then it struck me at the age of 34. It struck me three more times since then. I lost my job because of this disease. My worst nightmare is thinking how breast cancer might strike my daughter. Please, please, please help.

The reaction from the Clinton administration to NBCC and its letters was quite different from that of the Bush administration. In addition to having a mother with breast cancer, Clinton was pressing for health care reform, and with over two and a half million signatures urging him on, he had nothing to lose and everything to gain by supporting a movement that was fighting to save lives. So the president and First Lady Hillary Rodham Clinton, who was the chief architect of the health care reform plan, welcomed some 200 women into the White House East Room, where the president accepted some of the petitions.

Besides signing a proclamation declaring October 19 National Mammography Day, the president called on state governments, insurance companies, medical facilities, and businesses to adopt policies that would make mammography more accessible and affordable. Declaring it time for the health care system to stop treating women as second-class citizens, Clinton said that his reform agenda would put women on equal footing with men for the first time. He also pledged additional money for research, saying that spending on breast cancer research would increase by 44 percent in his budget, from $208 million to almost $300 million.[21]

Congress appropriated $2.082 billion to NCI for fiscal year 1994, an increase of 103 million. However, there was no earmarking of funds for breast cancer research as there had been in the previous budget. It was estimated that funding for breast cancer research would be $262.9 million.

The Clinton budget for fiscal year 1995 had a 4.7 percent increase for NIH, which came out to an additional $118 million for NCI, with breast cancer research getting a proportionally bigger share of the increase. It was estimated that breast cancer would get $323.7 million. Ten million dollars was included in the budget for breast cancer "outreach activities" to be supported by NCI and the Centers for Disease Control and Prevention (CDC).

The additional money that NBCC managed to wrangle did not win cheers from everyone. Marc Lippman, M.D., director of the Vincent T. Lombardi Cancer Center at Georgetown University in Washington, whose main focus is breast cancer research, says he doesn't want to appear ungrateful, but "I am worried about advocacy going overboard. It worries me deeply to see monies removed from other viable programs because of that kind of advocacy." It is obvious that advocacy works, he says. "Squeaky wheels do get funded."[22]

Former *New York Times* columnist Anna Quindlen says that there are people who believe that the increase in funding has "little to do with smart science and everything to do with political attempts to look sensitive to women's issues." She adds that, with a finite amount of money available at the National Cancer Institute, choices do have to be made. "Today," she says, "those choices have as much to do with petitions and demonstrations as with medicine."[23]

There are, however, many who question whether the pie cannot be made larger, and if the finite amount of money cannot be increased. Susan Love points out that one B-1 bomber is about equal to the breast cancer research budget. "Instead of trying to defend the Kuwaitis, we need more money to defend women in this country."[24] Congressman Jerry Nadler (D-New York) says that while $33 billion was spent on the Star Wars program between 1985 and 1992, during the same time the United States spent a little over one billion dollars for breast cancer. He called it "a travesty of priorities, shameful in the extreme."[25]

Another point of contention is whether funds should be earmarked for research for one particular disease such as breast cancer. Congresswoman Barbara Vucanovich believes that money should be earmarked for breast cancer research.[26] Margaret Foti, executive director of the American Association for Cancer Research, urged rejection of the practice of earmarking funds. Testifying at the 1994 House subcommittee hearing, she said, "We understand that the entire increase provided to NCI in fiscal year 1994 will be devoted to breast cancer."

She made the objection, frequently heard, that increases in other areas will have to be cut, leading to a reduction in other critical research. She said there should be a balanced cancer research program that should also address the needs of the underserved, those people who do not have access to cancer screening and state-of-the-art treatment.[27]

How the available money is spent is of major concern to the women who strove so hard to get it. When breast cancer advocate Rose Kushner was appointed to the National Cancer Advisory Board (NCAB) by then president Jimmy Carter, she felt that to solve the problem of breast cancer there must be more basic research. In the past, the major research focus had been on treatment. As a board member she started lobbying against the emphasis on research into treatment. She believed if the appropriate investment into basic research was made to find out more about causes and biologic interventions, that chemotherapy would become obsolete.[28]

More than a decade after Kushner lobbied for increased basic research, NBCC president Fran Visco was calling for at least half of the money for research to be spent investigating prevention and environmental issues, with less money going for treatment research. Breast surgeon Susan Love says that too great a share of the available money for research has been spent on studying different variations of the same treatment for breast cancer, and that advancements in treatment have done little to decrease the mortality rate. Love is calling for more research into the prevention of breast cancer, identifying possible promoters of breast cancer, as well as genetic research to identify women who are predisposed to develop the disease.[29]

"Do we let NCI decide what research to do?" asks Kay Dickersin. "What's their record so far?" Answering her own question, she says their record is poor. So far, she says, "We haven't gotten anywhere." As for Congress, Dickersin contends that "their interest is in saving money, not saving lives. . . . We, the women, need to be part of that decision-making, too, and how that money is spent."[30] Kimberly Calder, director of public policy at Cancer Care, agrees, saying, "In the future I think we'll see an increase in the number of advocates who have a seat at the table. We're not going to go silently into the night. . . . Patient advocates have to be much more involved in the decision-making rooms."[31] Susan Love cites the fact that it is the breast cancer activists who have "increased research funding for the first time and now we're demanding a seat at the table and a say in how that research money is spent." Love wants NBCC to monitor how that money is spent and to be included in the decision-making process for spending the money at every level.[32]

That raises the question of just how much input breast cancer advocates like members of NBCC and interested consumers in general should have in clinical studies. Larry Norton, M.D., chief of the breast and gynecologic medical service at Memorial Sloan-Kettering Cancer Center, fears that bad research may be supported because it's politically correct. "People have to know how to use experts and how to gather expert opinions and make decisions on the basis of them. There's a danger sometimes in discounting opinions of experts because they've been in the field for a while." Happy that more money is being allocated for breast cancer research, he's also concerned about the money being used in the best way possible, and that the people involved really understand research. "Bad research on an important topic is not as good as doing good research on a topic that may not seem directly related."[33]

Frederick Becker, chief of research at M. D. Anderson Cancer Research Center in Houston, expresses some reservations. "The tidal wave of advocacy . . . may wash away certain bulwarks of basic science that have been the greatest contributors towards the potential for cancer prevention and cure." At a National Cancer Advisory Board meeting in December 1993, he gave an impassioned speech, stressing the importance of nontargeted research. His concern was that the trend toward targeted research will make it harder to support speculative research that has resulted in some discoveries crucial to understanding breast cancer, such as information on oncogenes (defective genes that can cause cancer) and tumor suppressor genes.[34]

The bigger piece of the pie finally allocated for breast cancer was viewed as a victory by many of the women in the movement and at the same time just the beginning. There are breast cancer advocates who say the additional money is still not sufficient, adding that it has come much later than it should have. One of those advocates is former Congresswoman Mary Rose Oakar, who says, "I wish this had happened sooner, because we'd be about ten years closer to finding a cure." Oakar also worries that some women may now become complacent.[35] Susan Love says, "The next step is making sure that the money is maintained."[36] Most breast cancer advocates do not want to take money from AIDS or any other cancer, but if that is the only way to get more money, so be it.

Besides the additional funding, NBCC wanted formulation of a national plan to fight breast cancer. At the October 1993 meeting with 200 breast cancer activists at the White House, President Clinton responded by promising a major planning conference in December. He designated Health and Human Services secretary Donna Shalala to take charge.

The "Conference to Establish a National Action Plan on Breast Cancer (NAPBC)," called by Shalala, took place on December 14 and 15, 1993, at the National Institutes of Health in Bethesda, Maryland. More than 125 people — including experts and leaders in education, access, screening, research, and treatment as well as journalists, breast cancer activists, and breast cancer survivors from all over the country — were asked to be active participants at the conference and charged with coming up with a national strategy for breast cancer. Also attending were close to 200 observers from different government agencies, legislative aides, military officials, breast cancer organizations, and other organizations. Altogether, there were over 300 people, which did not go unnoticed by Shalala. When she got up to speak, she said, "As I was walking in, someone said there aren't enough chairs, and I said, 'It's about time that there aren't enough chairs when we're discussing women's health.' "

Shalala said that the purpose of the conference was to produce an operational action plan that would give direction to the president, the policy-makers, and the decision-makers. She added, "We don't want this conference to produce another study. I specifically told those putting this together that we don't need another long-term commission report. . . . We need to build this action plan on the wealth of knowledge we already have and the recommendations we already have, and over the next two days [are] asking you to come up with a plan of what more needs to be done to find out why the incidence of breast cancer is rising in the United States and what action we have to take in the private and public sector to detect breast cancer earlier when there's a better chance of saving lives." Shalala then defined what she called the biggest challenges we face:

1. What other screening tests can we develop so that we can detect breast cancer early, especially in younger women?
2. How can we promote incorporation of research findings into daily practice so that women can benefit immediately from the advances in our knowledge; how can we do something about what just happened in the reports on mammography, in which we tripped over ourselves and probably confused a whole generation of women on what the messages were?
3. How can we improve our education efforts so that women, especially older women and minority women, make use of preventive services that are available to them?[37]

To brainstorm and come up with recommendations for a final plan, the designated participants were organized into ten different work groups looking at different aspects of research, information dissemination, and access to health care.

The document "Proceedings of the Secretary's Conference to Establish a National Action Plan on Breast Cancer," issued in March 1994, outlined the plan's three major components: health care, research, and policy.[38]

The health care component included improved access to breast health services, increased participation of underserved women and those at risk in programs related to risk factors, early detection, diagnosis, and treatment, coordination of doctors, patients, scientists, and the media in disseminating information, and establishment of public and private partnerships to enhance breast health education.

The research component included expanding biomedical and behavioral research activities related to breast cancer, making clinical trials more widely available, supporting research on prevention, cause, quality of life, and psychosocial issues.

The policy component addressed issues such as inclusion of advocacy groups in health policy decision-making, development of new, stable sources of funding for research and public health activities, and making breast health management, diagnosis, treatment, and follow-up care comprehensive, compassionate, widely available, and of high quality.

On December 14, 1994, a year after the initial meeting, cochairs of the NAPBC, Susan Blumenthal, M.D., M.P.A., deputy assistant secretary for women's health, and Fran Visco, president of NBCC, summarized what they described as the "substantial progress [that] has been made in implementing the action plan." The following six priority actions were identified:

- *Information superhighway:* Identify strategies to disseminate information about breast cancer and breast health to scientists, consumers, and doctors.
- *National patient data registry:* Establish biologic resource banks and comprehensive patient data registries to ensure a national resource of information for multiple areas of breast cancer research.
- *Consumer involvement:* Ensure consumer input at all levels in the development of public health and service delivery programs, research studies, and educational efforts by involving advocacy groups and women with breast cancer in setting research priorities and in patient education.
- *Breast cancer etiology:* Expand the scope and breadth of biomedical and behavioral research activities related to the etiology of breast cancer.
- *Clinical trials:* Make clinical trials more widely available to women with breast cancer and women who are at risk for breast cancer using consumer/clinician dialogue, reduction of economic barriers, and other strategies.
- *Breast cancer susceptibility gene:* Implement a comprehensive plan to address the needs of individuals carrying breast-cancer susceptibility genes and recommend educational interventions for consumers, health care providers, and at-risk patient groups.

Implementation strategies were to be developed along with timelines early in 1995. The fiscal year 1995 budget to fund NAPBC activities was $10 million.[39]

In April 1995, the first Request for Applications (RFA) was announced for grants using money appropriated to fund initiatives developed by NAPBC. Three million in total costs per year for two years would fund about 40 small grants in breast cancer research and outreach activities. The RFAs will be reviewed jointly by NCI and members of NAPBC. Suzanne Haynes, at the Office of Women's Health (OWH), which released the request, said, "It is very exciting because consumers are intimately involved for the first time in making recommendations for how money is being spent." She added that later that month OWH would announce a $2 million program in administrative supplements to current federal grants to address the priority areas of NAPBC. Fran Visco said she was pleased with the pace at which the NAPBC was progressing.[40]

It has taken a long time for breast cancer advocacy groups and women in general to get their message to legislators in Washington. With few women in Congress, either in the House or Senate, there were not many members of Congress with a large interest in issues predominantly affecting women. In 1977, the Congressional Caucus for Women's Issues was founded by Pat Schroeder. The caucus and Schroeder went on to become major advocates for breast cancer legislation.

Mary Rose Oakar was another one of the pioneer women in the House of Representatives who fought staunchly for women's health issues. She became involved when she saw, firsthand, what was happening to women. Her mother had died of breast cancer. "My sister had gotten breast cancer, her next-door neighbor had gotten breast cancer. I thought, this is an epidemic and nobody seems to be paying attention to it. So I was motivated on a personal basis. It seemed that everywhere I went, some member of the family had this terrible disease."[41]

In 1984, Congressman Claude Pepper, who was chair of the House Subcommittee on Health and Long-Term Care, held a long-overdue hearing on breast cancer. In his opening statement, Pepper said the hearing "may be one of the most meaningful hearings we shall have." Of the seven medical doctors who testified, there was one woman.[42]

Over a decade later, a similar proportion of male to female doctors is still frequently seen at breast cancer meetings. Sharon Green, who was at an American Cancer Society Conference on breast cancer in Boston in August 1993, said, "The focus of the group was very male oriented and there was a lot of discussion about it. Of the eight or nine plenary speakers, only one was a woman and she was from Reach to Recovery. There was a lot of grumbling about that. . . . It was an absolutely stupid move on behalf of the ACS. They should have known it was politically wrong to do."[43] About two dozen women from the Women's Community Cancer Project of Cambridge were outside the Sheraton Hotel in Boston carrying signs and demanding that the ACS pay more attention to the cause of breast cancer, particularly environmental toxins. In contrast, the Y-ME conference on breast cancer, held in July of that year, managed to find ten female physicians who could report on breast cancer, along with 11 male doctors. Of all those speaking at that conference, there were about twice the number of women speakers as men.

In October 1993, the report *Breast Cancer: A National Strategy, A Report To The Nation* was released. The report was the culmination of 11 hearings held by the President's Cancer Panel's Special Commission on Breast Cancer, which was convened in April 1992 at the request of then vice president Dan Quayle. It focused on breast cancer's causes and prevention; the development of new and more accurate technologies for detection and diagnosis; improvement in the effect of treatment on the quality of life; education; patient advocacy; and special issues for minority and underserved women.

The commission's overall findings were that "modest improvements" had been made in the detection and treatment of breast cancer, but they said there is a "widespread sense of urgency that more can and should be done to address the problem of breast cancer in this country." It estimated that in the 1990s, two million women would be diagnosed with breast cancer and 460,000 would die of it. It called for improvements in detection and treatment and noted that they were not uniformly applied throughout the population. The report acknowledged that there was no period of time after being treated for breast cancer that a woman could be assured that the breast cancer would not recur. Citing the advocacy movement, the report said, "There is a growing public demand for even greater levels of funding of a national breast program and an outcry for the development of cure and prevention." It also said that a minimum of $500 million a year would be needed to meet its goals, which were "to make substantial progress in developing effective methods to cure and to prevent breast cancer and to make current and future proven methods of early detection, treatment, and prevention universally available." The recommendations were outlined in eight specific sections: causes and prevention, earlier detection and diagnosis, treatment strategies, psychosocial effects, access, public policy, partnership of breast cancer advocates and breast cancer scientists, and information and empowerment. Its recommendations were similar to those made two months

later at the Conference to Establish a National Action Plan on Breast
Cancer called by Donna Shalala.[44]

Besides its major accomplishments of getting breast cancer funding
substantially increased and gaining a greater voice in federal hallways,
NBCC can take credit for raising the awareness of hundreds of thousands of women and motivating many other local activities around the
country. For example, as part of its 1992 "Stop Breast Cancer: A
Mother's Day Challenge" there was a run, marathon, and rally in New
York, as well as rallies in Burlington, Philadelphia, Sacramento, Chicago, Fayetteville, and Seattle. There was a march in Richmond, a
picnic in New Orleans, a candlelight ceremony in Phoenix, and in
Pennsylvania the state senate declared breast cancer a national emergency. And those are only some of the events.

Though NBCC has had stunning success in terms of raising the
funding for breast cancer research, there are some women who express
concerns about the future of the organization. Some of the questions
I've heard are: Will there be infighting in the organization? Will
NBCC, which started out as a grassroots movement, become another
bureaucracy with little input from the groups all over the country that
contributed so much in the beginning? Will NBCC keep up the momentum, keep up the fight? Following are comments from some of
the women involved in the movement:

Sharon Green, executive director, Y-ME:

> The National Breast Cancer Coalition movement probably hasn't
> reached the plateau yet. We're going to have a rude awakening. I don't
> think we're going to get support for individual disease issues. As hard
> to sell as it was in the past, I think it's going to be even harder to sell.
> I think it's going to be increasingly difficult.[45]

Ellen Hobbs, founder of Save Ourselves:

> The NBCC is doing fairly well, they've made some inroads, they've
> gotten some attention, they have some powerful people involved with
> them. However, those of us who started out on a grassroots basis were
> totally committed on a much more personal and creative angle; I think
> the NBCC has become another big bureaucracy. Anytime your success
> is tied to how much money you can get, you have to make a lot of
> compromises. Though they are a little bit more outspoken than ACS,

I really think they've become another of those organizations and then you're more limited with how aggressive you can be. For example, on evidence you have about cutting out dairy and meat, you could tell people that. A lot of cancer has been linked to pesticides and environmental toxins. They're reluctant to bring that out because of how powerful those industries are. . . . A lot of breast cancer stuff, it wears me out — even my own organization has become more bureaucratic. If I was coming into it now, I wouldn't get involved in these organizations, because they are too mainstream. I think what happened with the breast cancer movement and NBCC is that you had a lot of women who were very ambitious and were using this for a vehicle. . . . A lot of that grassroots element was lost.[46]

Virginia Soffa, cofounder of Breast Cancer Action Group (BCAG):

The NBCC leadership was starting to act more like a bureaucracy than a grassroots organization. The decision-making process was no longer one of consensus but of majority rule which was greatly affected by the power and money of those who considered themselves to be the powers that be. . . . The most profound thing was that it was not any longer a melding of the grassroots voices — but a power struggle that has resulted in a single, solitary voice that didn't necessarily represent our point of view at all. In a general sense, our point of view is that breast cancer is an incredibly diverse disease — and that the more diversity contained in any position, the more accurate the perspective is that you're portraying. We've been dealing with a medical establishment that has distilled down what breast cancer is about for years. It has never represented the patient.[47]

Although the Breast Cancer Action Group in Vermont, one of the original board members of the NBCC, left the organization in October 1993, saying it could "no longer support some of the major policy decisions of the National Breast Cancer Coalition . . . [nor] endorse some of the recent actions of the NBCC,"[48] its defection has had no apparent impact on the coalition.

As with any movement, there are different opinions within the breast cancer movement as to what should be done, how it should be done, and who should do it. Opinions run the gamut — from holding that women should quietly and politely write letters and hold bake sales to proposing that women should be demonstrating at major airports by sitting on runways. Many women who started out baking cookies have thrown out the flour and shortening and instead attend rallies, write letters to, and call members of Congress, and in general take part in much more aggressive activities.

The advocacy movement must continue on both the state and national level. With greater cuts anticipated in health appropriations, vigilance is mandatory. Women must be elected to state governments and to Congress to protect women's interests and make sure that there is maximum funding for research and access for the underserved. While it may be too late for many of us to benefit from our efforts, the benefit will be for our daughters and granddaughters, who deserve no less.

Epilogue

When I started working on this book, the breast cancer advocacy movement was just gearing up. Funding for breast cancer research was low. Stories about breast cancer were few and far between and appeared exclusively in women's magazines. And although today, in the 1990s, women are much more prone to talk about their breast cancer, there are still many who are reluctant or unwilling to reveal that they had breast cancer, for various reasons. They feel embarrassed or stigmatized. They also worry that it could affect their employment and insurance — a valid concern. Women celebrities have hidden the fact that they have breast cancer. One well-known news personality, Linda Ellerbee, revealed it only when warned that a newspaper was about to publish a story about it.

Now funding for breast cancer research has increased substantially and stories in newspapers, magazines, radio, and television are plentiful, including those that we wish did not have to be written, such as the manipulation of data in some large and significant breast cancer studies, the possible dangers of the silicone implants used for breast reconstruction, the lack of access to screening and competent care for so many women.

It is heartening to see women organizing, working together, and having an impact. On Long Island, before the November 1994 election, the breast cancer advocacy group 1 in 9 sponsored a meet-the-candidates night.

At the meet-the-candidates night before the 1994 election, members of 1 in 9 were stunned when 36 Democrats and Republicans seeking congressional seats and state offices showed up. Gerri Barish, cochair of the group, said, "It was just unbelievable. And every single one of them spoke." Obviously the candidates and their staffs were well aware of the media coverage the breast cancer groups had been successful in getting and the importance of showing their support to what could be a large group of voters. Each candidate spoke of his or her commitment to finding out why Long Island women are being diagnosed with breast cancer in such great numbers. The influence and power of 1-in-9 was recognized by the politicians and was ultimately productive in getting funding to study the high rate of breast cancer in the area.[1]

Years ago, if you were diagnosed with breast cancer, it could be difficult getting information about it. That is no longer the case. There are hotlines, support groups, and advocacy groups available to offer information and assistance. There are books in libraries and bookstores. And there have even been television shows on breast cancer. Information is out there and accessible.

If you are diagnosed with breast cancer, it is crucial to make sure you know all you have to know to make the best treatment decisions for yourself. You cannot rely on anyone else. Ask questions. Get answers you can understand. Many women have told me that their doctor "wouldn't answer my questions." I say, find one who will. It is true that doctors are frequently busy and working under time demands and constraints. You may be lucky and have a doctor who takes plenty of time to explain everything to you and repeat explanations if necessary. If you don't, it is up to you to ask the questions for which you need answers and make sure you get an answer that you understand. If you are not satisfied that a mechanic who is working on your car is doing a good job, you are going to find another mechanic. If you are not satisfied that your doctor is doing a good job, you must find one whom you trust and believe in.

I don't mean to make this sound simple. It's not. When you're under a lot of stress because of a life-threatening illness, it is frequently hard to be assertive and to question the doctor. Many of us have been brought up not to challenge authority, but this is a matter of life and death. So whatever it takes — bringing your spouse or a good friend in with you for moral support or just for an extra set of ears (which is very helpful, and recommended), writing a letter, sending a fax to a doctor whom you feel too uncomfortable to confront — do it! And if you have to find a different doctor, do it!

Although the information is out there, not every woman knows how to get it or even that it exists. As I was doing research for this book and talking with women all over the country, my biggest concern became the disenfranchised women in our society. These are the women who are poor, the greatest percentage of whom are minority women. There are too many women dying unnecessarily because their breast cancer is at a late stage when diagnosed. There are too many women dying unnecessarily because they don't have access to competent care when they are diagnosed, or they don't know how to get it. Dr. Harold Freeman, head of the President's Cancer Panel and chief of surgery at Harlem Hospital in New York, says, "One of the most critical issues in breast cancer is access to getting mammograms, physical exams and treatment. . . . that's just reality, the need to solve the problem of access."[2]

We desperately need and must fight for funding to provide mammograms for women who don't have medical insurance and can't afford to get them, as well as funding for competent treatment for women who are diagnosed with breast cancer. Money is also needed for things as basic as transportation to the mammography or treatment site, child care for the young children of a mother getting a mammogram or undergoing debilitating treatment, and, last but not least, education. Besides the money needed for access, the other thing affecting poor women, says Joyce Ford, "is not necessarily having the wherewithall to get into the system in the first place, how to access it to get the kind of care that they need. . . . So there are barriers that they themselves can't even penetrate to start dealing with the problem of breast cancer."[3] Every woman in this country, regardless of her economic class, race, or age, deserves state-of-the-art competent medical treatment. It is an issue that *all of us* must confront and fight for. Despite the fact that there is no "sure cure" for breast cancer, the high breast cancer mortality rate should not be as high as it is.

Education is important for every woman. Some women know virtually nothing about breast cancer, while many others have misconceptions about it. It is not uncommon for a woman whose mother has had breast cancer to be sure that she too will get it. That woman may live in a state of anxiety, obsessed with checking her breasts and check-ing with doctors, while another woman with a family history of breast cancer may decide not to do anything because she thinks she's doomed anyway.

Too many women do not get a mammogram for inappropriate reasons. Many think they'd never get breast cancer because nobody in their family has had it and they eat well and do the right things. So why should they bother with a time-consuming and frequently costly procedure? They are shocked beyond belief when they are diagnosed with breast cancer. Many women don't get a mammogram because they've had one and it was painful. There are women who are afraid that something will be found and they don't want to know. And there are women who think that they will die of breast cancer if they have it, so why find out. And then there are the women who say, "Well, I got a mammogram and it was fine." When you ask how long ago, they say five or six or ten years. Some women don't examine their own breasts because they've been taught it's a sin to touch themselves, or they think their breasts belong to their husbands, or they're afraid they will find something, or they do examine their breasts but ineffectively because they've never been shown how to do it.

We need education on every level, from high schools to senior centers, to make sure all women are aware of breast cancer and what they can do to reduce their risk or make sure it is detected as early as possible. And we have to make sure that the information they are getting is understandable and accurate. We must educate doctors as well, and not just gynecologists. Many physicians are not skilled at examining breasts and so are unable to teach a woman how to do it or what to look for. Postmenopausal women frequently stop seeing gy-necologists and go instead to internists, who just as frequently do not tell a woman to get a mammogram. We must devise strategies to raise the awareness of all women as well as the predominantly male medical establishment.

We must educate ourselves on our rights as patients and as survi-vors and work to make changes where they are needed. It took years to get legislation mandating Medicare reimbursement for mammo-grams, but with pressure and lobbying from breast cancer advocates, and a few dedicated members of Congress, it eventually passed. There are many ways to find out what your rights are and to what you are entitled. There are phone numbers in the appendix of this book for organizations that can provide you with information and answers to your questions. National organizations can inform you about your rights under federal legislation, laws that you can use to fight discrimination on the job or for your insurance. Local organizations are best for laws in your state.

Virtually every woman I met talked about the need for research. Research is needed to discover why only 20 to 30 percent of women diagnosed with breast cancer have one of the known risks. Is breast cancer caused by something in the environment that wasn't there years ago? Is it a combination of things in the environment? Research on new and more effective ways of treating breast cancer is needed. Research is also needed for prevention, which ideally would solve the problem.

The increase in funding for breast cancer research holds much promise. The participation of breast cancer advocates and consumers in the development and monitoring of new studies holds promise as well. As a result of the advocacy movement, more environmental studies are being done and developed. The effects of environmental factors such as pesticides, chemical wastes released into the air and water, electromagnetic fields, and radiation are hard to measure and have in the past more often than not been ignored. The fact that the environmental role in cancer is finally being taken seriously and will be subjected to scientific study is an optimistic sign not only for breast cancer but for all cancers.

Psychosocial issues is another area that is finally getting more attention and interest. More studies are being done and developed to examine psychosocial issues in the treatment and development of breast cancer. Data such as that published by David Spiegel,[4] in which a counseling group for women with metastatic breast cancer not only improved the quality of their lives but increased the length of survival as well, is exciting and promising for the future.

There have been some recent encouraging developments. How beneficial they will be remains to be seen. In 1994, the location of the BRCA1 breast cancer gene was found. It is a major scientific discovery that was hailed throughout the world. Its direct impact on breast cancer could be relatively small, however, since the gene is thought to be responsible for, at the most, 5 percent of the breast cancer cases.

One hopes that its discovery will lead the way to more information on the development and prevention of cancer.

How this new information on the BRCA1 gene will be used to help women with breast cancer is still a question. Although it is possible to test someone for the gene, a screening test is not readily available. And when one is developed, how will it be used? What options will be available to a young woman with a family history of breast cancer who tests positive for the gene? The present alternatives are far from pleasant and can have a great impact on her quality of life. She can choose to have a prophylactic double mastectomy that will give her a much greater chance of not getting breast cancer but is not foolproof. Or she can be followed closely with anxiety-provoking mammograms and biopsies for a longer period of time than the average woman. Another possible problem is safeguarding the information that she tested positive. If the information is readily accessible to insurance companies, and there's no reason to believe that it wouldn't be, does it mean that she faces denial of medical insurance because she has a "preexisting condition"?

We are making progress in finding new ways of detecting breast cancer earlier than can be done with mammography. There is the possibility of a blood test, which is certainly less cumbersome and uncomfortable than a mammogram and very possibly less expensive. If microscopic breast cancer can be found using new techniques long before it can be detected by mammography, how could that be regarded as anything but great progress and good news? But what do we do about it once we find it at such an early stage? Is it possible that many women walk around with microscopic breast cancer cells their entire lives that never develop into breast cancer? Even today, with our current screening, there are questions about how and when to treat in-situ breast cancer that can now be detected much more frequently by mammography than in past years.

Within a few years the first data from the breast cancer prevention trial should be in and we should know if tamoxifen can prevent breast cancer in women at risk. The trial itself has been a major source of controversy. No doubt its findings will be, too. If tamoxifen proves to prevent breast cancer in some women but not others, how will we know which women at risk will benefit from a treatment that is not only financially costly but possibly physically costly as well? Tamoxifen does have some side effects and puts a woman at an increased risk of endometrial cancer. Another question that the study will not answer is how long can a woman take tamoxifen and what will happen when she stops taking it.

High-dose chemotherapy with the support of peripheral stem cells is a treatment being investigated in three NCI-sponsored clinical trials. Originally there were four, but one was stopped because too few women were taking part. What role this treatment will play in the treatment of breast cancer in the future has yet to be determined. That may be hard to do since so many women who see high-dose therapy with peripheral stem cell support as their only possibility for life are demanding the treatment and getting it outside of a clinical trial. One woman told me that she understood the need for participation in clinical trials but said that if it meant giving up a promising treatment she would not be willing to take that chance with her life. If we are demanding research for new treatments for breast cancer, we must be willing to take part in a clinical trial testing the efficacy of a new treatment.

There are things each of us can do, whether we are breast cancer survivors or at risk of being diagnosed one day with breast cancer. There are breast cancer support groups all over the country. Many of those groups have become political to one degree or another. Find a group to join or support, or start a group. Both inside and outside of a group setting, you can keep an eye on local politicians and national politicians from your state. If there is a bill regarding breast cancer on the table, call and/or write the politician and express your view. Get friends to write and call as well. If there's an issue for which legislation is needed, call your local politician. If the politician has a person on staff to handle medical issues, talk to that person. Always have facts and figures to back up your proposal. If you're concerned about what appears to be a cluster of cancer cases, call the local health department, the newspaper, politicians. You may have to do what women on Long Island, New York, did when they became frightened and angry about the above-average levels of breast cancer cases. First they got a local paper to print, on its front page, a survey on breast cancer. They followed that up with a mass mailing of the survey. After that, they went door to door. They succeeded in getting facts and figures to support their demands while at the same time raising the awareness of many women.

If your local newspaper writes a story or a television station does a program that is inaccurate, call or write and get as many others as you can to do the same. Those in charge of newspapers and radio and television stations pay attention to the calls and letters that come in. Write and call to ask for more stories on breast cancer. When a good job has been done by a television station or newspaper, acknowledge it.

Organize a rally or demonstration. Offer to talk to girls at the local high school. Give a talk at a woman's organization. Pass out flyers. Donate some books on breast cancer to the library or talk the librarian into purchasing some. Hold a bake party with the proceeds going to a breast cancer support group or for breast cancer research. Your goal should be twofold: to raise the awareness of every woman and to encourage more and more women to join the movement.

We have made some progress. But we cannot afford to take even one backward step. We are waking up. We are fighting back. And now we must continue to fight until we win.

Appendix A

Organizations/Resources

American Association of Retired Persons (AARP). 601 E Street NW, Washington, DC. 20049 (202) 434-2560; (800) 424-3410. Legislative advocacy for programs like Medicare, breast cancer, mammography; provides insurance supplemental to Medicare.

American Cancer Society (ACS). 1599 Clifton Road NE, Atlanta, GA 30329. (404) 320-3333; the toll-free cancer response line is (800) ACS-2345 and is in operation from 8:30 A.M. to 4:30 P.M. ACS is a nationwide voluntary health organization. It supports and funds research; provides education on cancer prevention, early detection, and treatment; provides services for cancer patients and their families and provides free literature. There are 57 chartered divisions and about 3,000 local units. Following are the chartered divisions by state:

Alabama: 505 Brookwood Blvd., Homewood, AL 35209; (205) 879-2242

Alaska: 406 W. Fireweed Lane, Anchorage, AK 99503; (907) 277-8696

Arizona: 2929 E. Thomas Rd., Phoenix, AZ 85016; (602) 224-0524

Arkansas: 901 N. University, Little Rock, AR 72207; (501) 664-3480

California: 1710 Webster St., Oakland, CA 94612; (415) 893-7900

Colorado: 2255 S. Oneida, P.O. Box 24669, Denver, CO 80224; (303) 758-2030

Connecticut: Barnes Park S., 14 Villate Lane, Wallingford, CT 06492; (203) 265-7161

Delaware: 92 Read's Way, New Castle, DE 19720; (302) 324-4227

District of Columbia: 1875 Connecticut Ave., Washington, DC 20009; (202) 483-2600

Florida: 3709 W. Jetton Avenue, Tampa, FL 33629-5146; (813) 253-0541

Georgia: 2200 Lake Blvd., Atlanta, GA 30319; (404) 816-7800

Hawaii: Community Services Center Bldg., 200 N. Vineyard Blvd., Honolulu, HI 96817; (808) 531-1662

Idaho: 2676 Vista Ave., Boise, ID 83705-0836; (208) 343-4609

Illinois: 77 E. Monroe, Chicago, IL 60603-5797; (312) 641-6150

Indiana: 8730 Commerce Park Place, Indianapolis, IN 46268; (317) 872-4432

Iowa: 8364 Hickman Rd., Suite D, Des Moines, IA 50325; (515) 253-0147

Kansas: 1315 S.W. Arrowhead Rd., Topeka, KS 66604; (913) 273-4114

Kentucky: 701 W. Muhammad Ali Blvd., Louisville, KY 40203-1909; (502) 584-6782

Louisiana: Fidelity Homestead Bldg., 837 Gravier St., Suite 700, New Orleans, LA 70112-1509; (504) 523-4188

Maine: 52 Federal St., Brunswick, ME 04011; (207) 729-2339

Maryland: 8219 Town Center Dr., White Marsh, MD 21162-0082; (301) 931-6868

Massachusetts: 247 Commonwealth Ave., Boston, MA 02116; (617) 267-2650

Michigan: 1205 E. Saginaw St., Lansing, MI 48906; (517) 371-2920

Minnesota: 3316 W. 66th St., Minneapolis, MN 55435; (612) 925-2772

Mississippi: 1380 Livingston Lane, Lakeover Office Park, Jackson, MS 39213; (601) 362-8874

Missouri: 3322 American Ave., Jefferson City, MO 65102; (314) 893-4800

Montana: 313 N. 32nd St., Suite #1, Billings, MT 59101; (406) 252-7111

Nebraska: 8502 W. Center Rd., Omaha, NE 68124-5255; (402) 393-5800

Nevada: 1325 E. Harmon, Las Vegas, NV 89119; (702) 798-6857

New Hampshire: 360 Route 101, Unit 501, Bedford, NH 03110-5032; (603) 472-8899

New Jersey: 2600 Route 1, CN 2201, North Brunswick, NJ 08902; (201) 297-8000

New Mexico: 5800 Lomas Blvd. NE, Albuquerque, NM 87110; (505) 260-2105

New York: 6725 Lyons St., P.O. Box 7, East Syracuse, NY 13057; (315) 437-7025

   Long Island: 75 Davids Drive, Hauppauge, NY 11788; (516) 436-7070

   New York City: 19 W. 56th St., New York, NY 10019; (212) 586-8700

   Queens: 112-25 Queens Blvd., Forest Hills, NY 11375; (718) 263-2224

   Westchester: 30 Glenn St., White Plains, NY 10603; (914) 949-4800

North Carolina: 11 S. Boylan Ave., Raleigh, NC 27603; (919) 834-8463

North Dakota: 123 Roberts St., P.O. Box 426, Fargo, ND 58107; (701) 232-1385

Ohio: 5555 Frantz Rd., Dublin, OH 43017; (614) 889-9565

Oklahoma: 4323 63rd St., Suite 110, Oklahoma City, OK 73116; (405) 843-9888

Oregon: 0330 S.W. Curry, Portland, OR 97201; (503) 295-6422

Pennsylvania: P.O. Box 897, Route 442 & Sipe Ave., Hershey, PA 17033-0897; (717) 533-6144

   Philadelphia: 1422 Chestnut St., Philadelphia, PA 19102; (215) 665-2900

Puerto Rico: Calle Alverio #577, Esquina Sargento Medina, Hato Rey, PR 00918; (809) 764-2295

Rhode Island: 400 Main St., Pawtucket, RI 02860; (401) 722-8480

South Carolina: 128 Stonemark Lane, Columbia, SC 29210; (803) 750-1693

South Dakota: 4101 Carnegie Place, Sioux Falls, SD 57106-2322; (605) 361-8277

Tennessee: 1315 Eighth Ave. South, Nashville, TN 37203; (615) 255-1227

Texas: 2433 Ridgepoint Dr., Austin, TX 78754; (512) 928-2262

Utah: 941 E. 3300 S. Salt Lake City, UT 84106; (801) 483-1500

Vermont: 13 Loomis St., P.O. Box 1452, Montpelier, VT 05601-1452; (802) 223-2348

Virginia: P.O. Box 6359, Glen Allen, VA 23058-6359; (804) 527-3400

Washington: 2120 First Ave. North, Seattle, WA 98109-1140; (206) 283-1152

West Virginia: 2428 Kanawha Blvd. East, Charleston, WV 25311; (304) 344-3611

Wisconsin: P.O. Box 902, Pewaukee, WI 53072-0902; (414) 523-5500

Wyoming: 2222 House Avenue, Cheyenne, WY 82001; (307) 638-3331

American Civil Liberties Union (ACLU): 132 W. 42nd Street, New York, NY 10036. (212) 944-9800 (or call local listing) for legal assistance on discrimination.

American College of Radiology: 1891 Preston White Drive, Reston, VA 22091. (800)-227-5463.

American College of Surgeons (ACOS). 55 E. Erie Street, Chicago, IL 60611. (312) 664-4050. Will provide list of ACOS-approved cancer programs in all states and will copy names of member surgeons by area.

American Medical Association (AMA). 515 North State Street, Chicago, IL 60610. (312) 464-5000. Can provide information on a doctor — when he/she was licensed, his/her speciality, if he/she is board certified. (The *Directory of Medical Specialists* lists the qualifications of medical doctors and should be available in medical libraries and the public library.)

American Society of Clinical Oncology (ASCO). 435 N. Michigan Avenue, Suite 1717, Chicago, IL 60611. (312) 664-0828.

American Society of Plastic and Reconstructive Surgeons. 444 E. Algonquin Road, Arlington Heights, IL 60005. (312) 228-9900; (800)-635-0635. Has written information on reconstruction and can provide list of certified reconstructive surgeons by geographic area.

Blue Cross and Blue Shield Association. 676 N. St. Claire Street, Chicago, IL 60601. (312) 352-6533. Provides information on Blue Cross/Blue Shield coverage offered by every state, including availability of annual open enrollment periods.

Board Certification. (800) 776-2378. Can provide information on whether a doctor is board certified. (The *Directory of Medical Specialists* lists the qualifications of medical doctors and should be available in medical libraries and the public library.)

BMT Newsletter. 1985 Spruce Ave., Highland Park, IL 60035. (708) 831-1913. Publishes free, bimonthly newsletter; also publishes book *Bone Marrow Transplants: A Book of Basics for Patients,* which is available for $5.00.

Breast Implant Information Network. (800) 887-6828. Provides assistance and information to women with implants or who are considering getting them; material packets, newsletters available.

CAN ACT (Cancer Patients Action Alliance). 26 College Place, Brooklyn, NY 11201. (718) 522-2400.

Cancer Care. 1180 Avenue of the Americas, New York, NY 10036. (212) 221-3300. A nonprofit social service agency, it helps patients and family members cope with the emotional and financial consequences of cancer; generally serves the New York metropolitan area but responds to phone calls and letters from all over the United States, providing information and referrals whenever possible.

Cancer Information Service (CIS). The nationwide toll-free (800) 4-CANCER number is available 9:00 A.M. to 7:00 P.M. weekdays; funded largely by the National Cancer Institute. Information specialists can tell callers the latest state-of-the-art treatment for a particular cancer and where clinical trials are taking place, as well as provide information about detection, prevention, diagnosis, and support groups. Free NCI booklets are available.

Disability Rights Center. 1346 Connecticut Avenue NW, Washington DC 20036. (202) 223-3304.

Greenpeace. 1017 W. Jackson, Chicago, IL 60607. (312) 666-3305. Organization investigating the role of various environmental hazards in the development of cancer.

Health Insurance Association of America (HIAA). 555 13th Street NW, Suite 600 East, Washington, DC 20004-1109. (202) 824-1600. Trade association; has free publications for consumers, including *The Consumers Guide to Health Insurance* and *The Consumers Guide to Disability Insurance*.

Hereditary Cancer Institute. Henry Lynch, M.D., Creighton University School of Medicine, California at 24th, Omaha, NE 68178. (402) 280-2942. Provides free cancer-risk information and other forms of genetic counseling.

Job Accommodation Network. (800) 526-7234. A project of the President's Committee on the Employment of People with Disabilities, in which a hotline provides information for employers, employees, job applicants, and job placement specialists about reasonable accomodation strategies.

Look Good . . . Feel Better. (800) 395-LOOK or (800) ACS-2345. Helps women recovering from cancer handle changes in appearance as a result of treatment; print and videotape materials available.

Medical Information Bureau, Incorporated (MIB). P.O. Box 105, Essex Station, Boston, MA 02112. (617) 426-3660. Provides your medical records so that you can verify the information in them and correct any inaccuracies.

National Action Plan on Breast Cancer (NAPBC). Office on Women's Health, Hubert H. Humphrey Building, Room 730-B, 200 Independence Avenue SW, Washington DC 20201. For comments, suggestions, and progress.

National Alliance of Breast Cancer Organizations (NABCO). 9 East 37th Street, 10th floor, New York, NY 10016. (212) 889-0606.

National Bone Marrow Transplant Link. 29209 Northwestern Highway, #624, Southfield, MI 48034. (313) 932-8483. Information; can link patients or family members with former patients or family members.

National Breast Cancer Coalition (NBCC). 1707 L Street NW, Suite 1060, Washington DC 20036. (202) 296-7477; fax (202) 265-6854. National advocacy group for breast cancer.

National Coalition for Cancer Survivorship (NCCS). 1010 Wayne Avenue, 5th floor, Silver Spring, MD 20910. (301) 650-8868. A network of independent groups and individuals offering support to cancer survivors, family members, and friends; provides information and resources on support and life after a cancer diagnosis, with special attention to job and insurance discrimination; advocates for rights of survivors.

National Rehabilitation Information Center (NARIC). 8455 Colesville Road, Suite 935, Silver Spring, MD 20910. (800) 34-NARIC. Information on resources, adaptive equipment, and services for disabled people.

National Institute of Environmental Health Services (NIEHS). 100 Capitola Drive, Suite 108, Durham, NC 27713. (800) 643-4794; fax (919) 361-9408. Sponsors ENVIRO-HEALTH Clearinghouse.

National Insurance Consumer Helpline. (800) 942-4242. Joint project of the American Council on Life Insurance, the Health Insurance Association of America, and the Insurance Information Institute; provides information on all types of insurance.

National Lymphedema Network. 2211 Post Street, Suite 404, San Francisco, CA 94115. (800) 541-3259. Provides counseling, support, and information.

National Women's Health Network. 1325 G Street NW, Washington, DC 20005. (202) 347-1140. Advocacy organization for women's health.

Office of Alternative Medicine. OAM/NIH, 6120 Executive Blvd., Suite 450, Rockville, MD 20892-9904. (301) 402-2466; fax (301) 402-4741. Has various fact sheets on alternative treatments.

Older Women's League (OWL). P.O. Box 1242, Ansonia Station, New York, NY 10023-1409.

Pesticide Action Network. 116 New Montgomery Street, Suite 810, San Francisco, CA 94105. (415) 541-9140.

Susan G. Komen Breast Cancer Foundation. 3005 LBJ Freeway, Suite 370, Dallas, TX 75244. (214) 980-8841; (800) I'M AWARE. Funds breast cancer research, education, screening, and treatment; has publications available.

U.S. Consumer Product Safety Commission (CPSC). Washington, DC 20207. (800) 638-CPSC. Free publications.

U.S. Department of Health and Human Services. Social Security Administration, Baltimore, MD 21235. (800) 772-1213. Consumer information on Medicare.

U.S. Department of Health and Human Services. 200 Independence Avenue SW, Washington, DC 20201. (202) 619-0257. Handles complaints under Section 504 of the Federal Rehabilitation Act.

U.S. Department of Labor. Office of Federal Contract Compliance Programs, 200 Constitution Avenue NW, Room C-3325, Washington, DC 20210. (202) 523-9410.

U.S. Department of Labor. Pension and Welfare Benefits Administration, Room N-5669, 200 Constitution Avenue NW, Washington, DC 20210. (202) 523-8521. Enforces individuals' rights under COBRA (insurance) and ERISA (employment).

U.S. Environmental Protection Agency (EPA). 4001 M Street, Washington, DC 20460. (202) 829-3535. Provides information on hazards in the environment.

U.S. Equal Employment Opportunity Commission (EEOC). (800) 669-EEOC for the publications that explain your rights under the Americans with Disabilities Act and how to enforce your rights; (800) 669-4000 for the location of your local EEOC office.

U.S. Food and Drug Administration (FDA). (HFE-88), 5600 Fishers Lane, Rockville, MD 20857. (301) 245-8012; (800) 532-4400. Information on breast implants and mammography.

Women's Environment and Development Organization (WEDO). 845 Third Avenue, 15th floor, New York, NY 10022. (212) 759-7892.

Y-ME. 212 West Van Buren, 4th floor, Chicago, IL 60607. (312) 986-8338; hotline (800) 221-2141. Offers information, advocacy, and support; has a prosthesis and wig bank for women with financial need.

Appendix B

Comprehensive Cancer Centers
(designated by the National Cancer Institute as of 1995)

ALABAMA: University of Alabama Comprehensive Cancer Center, 1918 University Blvd., Basic Health Sciences Building, room 108, Birmingham, AL 35233. (205) 934-5077.

ARIZONA: University of Arizona Cancer Center, 1501 North Campbell Avenue, Tucson, AZ 85724. (602) 626-6372.

CALIFORNIA: The Kenneth Norris Jr. Comprehensive Cancer Center, University of Southern California, 1441 Eastlake Avenue, Los Angeles, CA 90033-0804. (213) 226-2370.

Jonsson Comprehensive Cancer Center, University of California at Los Angeles, 100 UCLA Medical Plaza, Suite 255, Los Angeles, CA 90027. (213) 206-0278.

CONNECTICUT: Yale University Comprehensive Cancer Center, 333 Cedar Street, New Haven, CT 06510. (203) 785-4095.

DISTRICT OF COLUMBIA: Vincent T. Lombardi Cancer Research Center, Georgetown University Medical Center, 3800 Reservoir Road NW, Washington, DC 20007. (202) 687-2192.

FLORIDA: Sylvester Comprehensive Cancer Center, University of Miami Medical School, 1475 Northwest 12th Avenue, Miami, FL 33136. (305) 545-1000.

MARYLAND: The Johns Hopkins Oncology Center, 600 North Wolfe Street, Baltimore, MD 21205. (301) 955-8964.

MASSACHUSETTS: Dana-Farber Cancer Institute, 44 Binney Street, Boston, MA 02115. (617) 632-3476.

MICHIGAN: Meyer L. Prentis Comprehensive Cancer Center of Metropolitan Detroit, 110 East Warren Avenue, Detroit, MI 48201. (313) 745-4329.

University of Michigan Cancer Center, 101 Simpson Drive, Ann Arbor, MI 48109-0752. (313) 936-9583.

MINNESOTA: Mayo Comprehensive Cancer Center, 200 First Street SW, Rochester, MN 55905. (507) 284-3413.

NEW HAMPSHIRE: Norris Cotton Cancer Center, Dartmouth-Hitchcock Medical Center, 2 Maynard Street, Hanover, NH 03756. (603) 646-5505.

NEW YORK: Memorial Sloan-Kettering Cancer Center. 1275 York Avenue, New York, NY 10021. (800) 525-2225.

Kaplan Cancer Center. New York University Medical Center, 550 First Avenue, New York, NY 10016. (212) 263-6485.

Roswell Park Cancer Institute. Elm and Carlton Streets, Buffalo, NY 14263. (800) 761-9355.

NORTH CAROLINA: Duke Comprehensive Cancer Center, P.O. Box 3814, Durham, NC 27710. (919) 684-2748.

Lineberger Comprehensive Cancer Center, University of North Carolina School of Medicine, Chapel Hill, NC 27599. (919) 966-4431.

Cancer Center of Wake Forest University at the Bowman Gray School of Medicine, 300 South Hawthorne Road, Winston-Salem, NC 27103. (919) 748-4354.

OHIO: Ohio State University Comprehensive Cancer Center, 410 West 10th Avenue, Columbus, OH 43210. (800) 638-6996.

PENNSYLVANIA: Fox Chase Cancer Center, 7701 Burholme Avenue, Philadelphia, PA 19111. (215) 728-2570.

University of Pennsylvania Cancer Center, 3400 Spruce Street, Philadelphia, PA 19104. (215) 662-6364.

Pittsburgh Cancer Institute, 200 Meyran Avenue, Pittsburgh, PA 15213-2592. (800) 537-4063.

TEXAS: The University of Texas M. D. Anderson Cancer Center, 1515 Holcombe Boulevard, Houston, TX 77030. (713) 792-3245.

VERMONT: Vermont Cancer Center, University of Vermont, 1 South Prospect Street, Burlington, VT 05401. (804) 656-4580.

WASHINGTON: Fred Hutchinson Cancer Research Center, 1124 Columbia Street, Seattle, WA 98104. (206) 667-5000.

WISCONSIN: Wisconsin Clinical Cancer Center, University of Wisconsin, 600 Highland Avenue, Madison, WI 53792. (608) 263-8090.

Appendix C

Grassroots Organizations by State

ALASKA

The Anchorage Women's
  Breast Cancer
  Support Group
3340 Providence Drive
Anchorage, AK 99508
(907) 261-3151

ALABAMA

Woman to Woman
Gadsden, AL 35901
(205) 494-HOPE

UPFRONT Support Group
809 University Blvd.
Tuscaloosa, AL 35401
(205) 759-7000

ARIZONA

Phillips Cancer Support
  House
2510 Datson Avenue
Fort Smith, AZ 72901
(602) 782-6302

Maryvale Samaritan Hospital/
  New Beginnings
5102 West Campbell
Phoenix, AZ 85031
(602) 848-5588

Y-ME Breast Cancer Net-
  work of Arizona
P.O. Box 1652
Scottsdale, AZ 85252
(602) 952-9793

Cerelle Center for Women's
  Health
Breast Cancer Resource
  Center
3100 North Campbell, Suite
  103
Tucson, AZ 85719
(602) 325-3000

Arizona Cancer Center
1515 West Campbell
Tucson, AZ 85724
(602) 626-6044

ARKANSAS

CARTI Cancer Answers
P.O. Box 5210
Little Rock, AR 72215
(501) 660-7614

CALIFORNIA

Breast Care For Life
  Program
Anaheim Memorial Hospital
1111 West La Palma Ave-
  nue
Anaheim, CA 92804
(714) 999-3880

Woman's Cancer Resource
  Center
3023 Shattuck Avenue
Berkeley, CA 94705
(510) 548-9272

Beyond Breast Cancer Sup-
  port Group
Enlow Breast Screening
  Outpatient Center
888 Calgeswe Village Com-
  mons
Chico, CA 95928-3979
(916) 891-7445

Breast Cancer Recovery Plus
Culver City, CA
(310) 391-0068

The Health Concern
Pallmar Pomerado Health
  System
1260 Auto Park Way,
  Suite B
Escondido, CA 92029
(619) 737-3960

St. Agnes Medical Center/
  Breast Cancer
  Support Group
P.O. Box 27500
Fresno, CA 93720
(209) 449-5222

Family Service Center
3030 W. Fresno St.,
  Suite 106
Fresno, CA 93703
(209) 227-3576

Bloomers
Y-ME of Orange County
921B W. Las Lomas
La Habra, CA 90631
(714) 447-6975

Steven's Cancer Center
Scripps Memorial Hospital
9888 Genesee Avenue
La Jolla, CA 92037
(619) 457-6756

Ladies of Courage/Y-ME
P.O. Box 2413
Lancaster, CA 93539-2413
(805) 266-4811

Y-ME South Bay/Long
Beach
P.O. Box 8546
Long Beach, CA 90808
(310) 984-8456

Long Beach Memorial
Breast Center
701 E. 28th Street,
Suite 200
Long Beach, CA 90806
(310) 933-7821

Breast Self-Help Group
100 Barnet Segal Lane
Monterey, CA 93940
(408) 649-1772

Breast Center
Queen of the Valley Hospital
1000 Tramcas
Napa, CA 94558
(707) 257-4047

The Breast Care Center
1140 West Lavet, #460
Orange, CA 92668
(714) 541-0101

Breast Cancer Support Group
UC Irvine Medical Center
101 City Drive
Orange, CA 92688
(714) 456-6968

Desert Comprehensive
Breast Center
1695 N. Sunrise
Palm Springs, CA 92262
(619) 323-6676

Discovery Breast Cancer
Support Group
Mid-Peninsula YWCA
4161 Almast
Palo Alto, CA 94306
(415) 494-0972

Breast Cancer Networking
Group
200 East Del Mar Boule-
vard, Suite 118
Pasadena, CA 91105
(818) 796-1083

Save Ourselves/Y-ME Sacramento
1832 Tribute Road, #219
Sacramento, CA 95815
(916) 921-9747

Orange County Chapter
Susan G. Komen Founda-
tion
380 Caminode Estrella,
Suite 137
San Clemente, CA 92672
(714) 496-5624

Women's Cancer Task
Force/Y-ME
San Diego Chapter
555 W. Beech, Suite 452
San Diego, CA 92101
(619) 239-9283

Breast Cancer Peer Support
Group
University of California San
Diego Cancer Center
9500 Gilman Drive
La Jolla, CA 92093
(619) 543-7397

The Cancer Support Com-
munity
185 Lundys Lane
San Francisco, CA 94110
(415) 648-9400

Aurora Medical
2211 Post Street, Suite 404
San Francisco, CA 94115
(415) 921-2911

Breast Cancer Action
55 New Montgomery Street,
#624
San Francisco, CA 94105
(415) 922-8279

The Resource Center/Mt.
Zion Cancer Center
P.O. Box 7921
San Francisco, CA 94120
(415) 885-3693

Bay Area Breast Cancer Network
4010 Moor Park Avenue,
Suite 105
San Jose, CA 95117
(408) 261-1425

Wellness Community
2716 Ocean Park Boulevard,
1040
Santa Monica, CA 90405
(310) 314-2555

Center for Attitudinal Healing
333 Buchanan Street
Sausalito, CA 94965
(415) 331-6161

The Breast Center
14624 Sherman Way, Suite
600
Van Nuys, CA 91405
(818) 787-9911

John Muir Medical Center
Breast Cancer Resource
Center
1601 Ygnacio Valley Road
Walnut Creek, CA 94596
(510) 947-3322

Queen of the Valley Breast
Cancer Support Group
1115 South Summit Drive
West Covina, CA 91790
(818) 962-4011

CANADA

Burlington Breast Cancer
Support Services
777 Guelen Line
Burlington, Ont. CAN
L7R4K3
(905) 634-2333

Breast Cancer Research and
Education Fund
8 Pearl Ann Drive
St. Catharine's, Ont. CAN
L2T3B3
(905) 687-3333

COLORADO

Daryleen Emmons Breast
Cancer Support Group
Penrose Cancer Center
P.O. Box 7021
Colorado Springs, CO
80933
(719) 630-5273

AMC Cancer Research Center
1600 Pierce Street
Denver, CO 80214
(303) 239-3393 / (800)
321-9526

Rose Breast Cancer Center
4500 E. 9th Avenue, Suite
1305
Denver, CO 80220
(303) 320-7142

CONNECTICUT

Y-ME of New England
1169 Main Street, Suite B3
Branford, CT 06405
(203) 483-8200 / (800)
933-4963.

I Can
16 Hospital Drive, Suite 201
Danbury, CT 06810
(203) 830-4621

St. Francis Hospital and
Medical Center
1161 Woodland Street
Hartford, CT 06105
(203) 548-4000

Cancer Care, Inc
120 East Avenue
Norwalk, CT 06851
(203) 854-9911

Ridgefield Breast Cancer
Support Group
The Revivers
90 East Ridge
Ridgefield, CT 06877
(203) 438-5555

DELAWARE

Looking Ahead Support
Group
St. Francis Hospital
Seventh and Clayton Street
Wilmington, DE 19805
(302) 421-4180

DISTRICT OF COLUMBIA

Lombardi Breast Cancer
Support Group
Georgetown University
3800 Reservoir Road NW
Washington, DC 20007
(202) 784-4000

The Mary-Helen Mautner
Project for Lesbians with
Cancer
1707 L Street, NW, Suite
1060
Washington, DC 20036
(202) 332-5536

George Washington Hospi-
tal Breast Care Center
2150 Pennsylvania Avenue
NW
Washington, DC 20037-
2396
(202) 994-4589

Betty Ford Comprehensive
Cancer Center
2440 M Street, NW, Suite
224
Washington, DC 20037
(202) 293-6654

FLORIDA

Halifax Medical Center
Women's Services
303 West Clyde Morris
Blvd.
Daytona Beach, FL 32114
(904) 254-4211

Bosom Buddies
Florida Community
College
Women's Center
101 West State Street
Jacksonville, FL 32202
(904) 633-8246

South Florida Comprehen-
sive Cancer Center
1750 Bird Road
Miami, FL 33175
(305) 227-5582

Center for Women's
Medicine
Florida Hospital
2501 North Orange Avenue,
Suite 340
Orlando, FL 32804
(407) 897-1617

Bosom Buddies
Women's Center
7727 Lake Underhill Drive
Orlando, FL 32822
(407) 281-8663

Ann L. Baroco Center for
Women's Health
5147 N. Ninth Avenue
Pensacola, FL 32504
(904) 474-7878

Woman to Woman
Sarasota Memorial Hospital
1900 South Tamiami Trail
Sarasota, FL 34239
(813) 917-1375

Woman to Woman
Woman's Resource Center
Tallahassee Memorial
Regional Medical Center
1300 Magnolia
Tallahassee, FL 32308
(904) 681-2255

FACTORS / H. Lee Moffit
Cancer Center
12902 Magnolia Drive
Tampa, FL 33612-9497
(813) 972-8407

GEORGIA

Northside Hospital
100 Johnson Ferry Road
Atlanta, GA 30342
(404) 851-8052

Bosom Buddies of GA
Men's Bereavement Support
Group
P.O. Box 874
Tucker, GA 30085
(404) 493-7517

HAWAII

Queens Medical Center
1329 Lusitana Street,
Suite B5
Honolulu, HI 96813
(808) 537-7555

IDAHO

Mountain States Tumor In-
stitute
151 East Bannock
Boise, ID 83712
(208) 386-2764

North Idaho Cancer Center
700 Ironwood Drive
Coeur d'Alene, ID 83814
(208) 666-3800

The Wellness Group /
  Hospice of the Wood
  River Valley
P.O. Box 4320
Ketchum, ID 83340
(208) 726-8464

ILLINOIS

CARE
Alton Memorial Hospital
One Memorial Drive
Alton, IL 62002
(618) 463-7311

A Time to Heal
Wellspring Women's Health
  Center
Good Shepherd Hospital
450 W. Highway 22
Barrington, IL 60010
(708) 381-9600

Mastectomy Club
St. Elizabeth Hospital
211 South Third
Belleville, IL 62222
(618) 234-2120

Breast Cancer Support
  Group
Elmhurst Memorial Center
200 Berteau Avenue
Elmhurst, IL 60126
(708) 833-1400

Positive People
Sister Theresa Cancer Care
  Center, St. Joseph Medical Center
333 North Madison
Joliet, IL 60435
(815) 741-7560

Women's Health Resource
  Center
McDonough District
  Hospital
525 East Grant Street
Macomb, IL 61455
(309) 833-4101, ext. 3198

Quad City Mastectomy Sup-
  port Group
435 17th Street
Moline, IL 61265
(309) 764-2888

Mastectomy Support Group
Pekin Hospital
600 S. 13th Street
Pekin, IL 61554
(309) 353-0807

Susan G. Komen Breast
  Center
4911 Executive Drive
Peoria, IL 61614
(309) 689-6622

Breast Cancer Support
  Group for
  Younger Women
2350 Rockton Avenue,
  Suite 108
Rockford, IL 61103
(815) 961-6215

Sangamon Breast Cancer
  Support Group
Springfield, IL
(217) 787-7187

INDIANA

Women's Cancer Support
  Group
223 West Washington
Bluffton, IN 46714
(219) 824-6493

Yes, We Can, Methodist
  Hospital
Northlake Campus
600 North Grant Street
Gary, IN 46402
(219) 886-4328 / (800)
  952-7337

Uplifters Breast Cancer Support Group
1500 North Ritter
Indianapolis, IN 46219
(317) 355-1411

Y-ME of Central Indiana
11651 Capistrano Drive
Indianapolis, IN 40236
(317) 823-7292

Y-ME of Wabash Valley
Union Hospital
c/o Hux Cancer Center
1606 N. Seventh
Terre Haute, IN 47804-
  2780
(812) 877-3025 / 877-
  3266

Women Winning Against
  Cancer
2267 Dubois Drive
Warsaw, IN 46580
(219) 269-9911

IOWA

"Especially for You" After
  Breast Cancer
701 Tenth Street SE
Cedar Rapids, IA 52403
(800) 642-6329 / (319)
  365-HOPE

Marshalltown Cancer
  Support Group
1401 Fairway Drive
Marshalltown, IA 50158
(515) 752-8775

ABC-After Breast Cancer
  Support Group
Marion Health Center
P.O. Box 3168
Sioux City, IA 51102
(712) 279-2989

KANSAS

Breast Cancer Care Group
  Victory in the Valley
P.O. Box 2210
971 N. Market
Wichita, KS 67214
(316) 262-7559 / (800)
  657-7202

KENTUCKY

Breast Cancer Support
  Group
Cancer Care Office
2201 Lexington Avenue
Ashland, KY 41101
(606) 327-4535

St. Elizabeth Women's
  Center
20 Medical Village Drive
Doctor's Building, Suite 209
Edgewood, KY 41017
(606) 344-3939

The Thursday Group
119 Desha Road
Lexington, KY 40502
(606) 269-4836 / 233-
  3601

Breast Center / Breast Cancer Support Group
Box 668
Prestonburg, KY 41653
(606) 886-8511, ext. 160

LOUISIANA

Bosom Buddies
West Jefferson Medical
Center
1101 Medical Center Boulevard
Marrero, LA 70072
(504) 349-1640

Center for Living with Cancer
4200 Nouma Boulevard
Metairie, LA 70006
(504) 454-5071

Breast Cancer Support
Group
4429 Blara, Suite 340
New Orleans, LA 70115
(504) 897-5860

Lakeland Medical Center
6000 Ballard Avenue
New Orleans, LA 70128
(504) 245-4855

Patricia Trost Friedler
Cancer Counseling
1430 Tulane Avenue, SL68
New Orleans, LA 70112
(504) 587-2120

Bosom Buddies
NorthShore Regional
Medical Center
100 Medical Center Drive
Slidell, LA 70461
(504) 646-5014

MARYLAND

Y-ME of the Cumberland
Valley
1035 Haven Road
Hagerstown, MD 21742
(301) 791-5843

Arm In Arm
302 Pressway Road
Timonium, MD 20193
(410) 561-1650 / (410)
494-0083

MASSACHUSETTS

1 In Eight
Massachusetts Breast Cancer
Coalition
10 Post Office Square
Boston, MA 02109
(617) 423-6222 / (800)
649-6222

Margaret Gosselin Counseling Center
664 Main Street
Amherst, MA 01002-2418
(413) 256-4600

Cross Roads
Dana Farber Cancer
Institute
44 Binney Street
Boston, MA 02115
(617) 632-3459

Evening Exchange / Life
After Breast Cancer /
Living with Recurrent
Breast Cancer
New England Medical
Center
750 Washington Street
Boston, MA 02111
(617) 956-5757 / (617)
956-5261

Lahey Clinic Breast Cancer
Treatment Center
611 Mall Road
Burlington, MA 01805
(617) 273-8989

Harvard University Faculty
Mid & Staff Assistance Program
46 Brattle Street
Cambridge, MA 02138
(617) 495-4357

Cancer Care Center
Metro West Medical Center
99 Lincoln Street
Framingham, MA 01701
(508) 383-1240

Faulkner Breast Centre Cancer Support Group
1153 Centre Street
Jamaica Plain, MA 02130
(617) 983-7777

Y-ME of the Berkshires
42 Wendell Avenue
Pittsfield, MA 01201
(413) 243-4822 / (800)
439-4821

Strength for Tomorrow
P.O. Box 137
Marion, MA 02738
(508) 748-1611

University of Massachusetts
Breast Cancer Education
Awareness Group
7 Oak Street
Worcester, MA 01609
(508) 752-2210

MICHIGAN

Breast Cancer Support
Group
1500 E. Medical Center
Drive
Ann Arbor, MI 48109
(313) 936-6000

Comprehensive Breast
Center
Harper Hospital
4160 John Street, Suite 615
Detroit, MI 48201
(313) 745-2754

St. John Hospital
Breast Cancer Support
Group
22101 Moross Road
Detroit, MI 48736
(313) 343-3684

Breast Cancer Detection
Center
Michigan Cancer Foundation
110 East Warren Avenue
Detroit, MI 40201
(313) 833-0710

"EXPRESSIONS" for
Women
1427 Breton Road, SE
East Grand Rapids, MI
49506
(616) 957-3223

Cancer Counselling Program / Sinai Hospital
Department of Medicine
6767 West Outer Drive
Detroit, MI 48235
(313) 493-6507

McLaren Mastectomy Support Group
401 South Ballenger
Flint, MI 48532
(810) 762-2375

Woman to Woman / St.
Mary's Breast Center
260 Jefferson SE
Grand Rapids, MI 49503
(616) 774-6756

WINS Support Group
Sparrow Hospital
1215 East Michigan Avenue
Lansing, MI 48912
(517) 483-2689

Marquette General Hospital
420 West Magnetic
Marquette, MI 49855
(906) 228-9440

Midland Community Cancer
    Services
220 West Main
Midland, MI 48640
(517) 835-4841 / (800)
    999-3199

Just For Us
888 Grand Avenue
Petoskey, MI 49770
(616) 347-8443

"Unique" Breast Cancer
    Support Group
Michigan Cancer Founda-
tion
110 East Warren
Detroit, MI 48201
(313) 833-0710, ext. 770

MINNESOTA

Breast Diagnostic Center
Duluth Clinic
400 East Third Street
Duluth, MN 55805
(218) 725-3195

Mercy Hospital Oncology
    Program
4050 N.W. Coon Rapids
    Boulevard
Coon Rapids, MN
(612) 422-4524

Cancer Center
Methodist Hospital
6500 Excelsior Boulevard
St. Louis Park, MN 55440
(612) 932-6086

MISSISSIPPI

Biloxi Regional Medical
    Center
150 Reynoir Street
Biloxi, MS 39533
(601) 432-1571

MISSOURI

FOCUS
St. Luke's Hospital
232 South Woods Mill
    Road
Chesterfield, MO 63017
(314) 851-6090

TOUCH Breast Cancer
    Program,
Menorah Medical Center
4949 Rockhill Road
Kansas City, MO 64110
(816) 276-8848

Cancer Hotline
4410 Main
Kansas City, 64111
(816) 932-8453

The Cancer Institute of
    Health Midwest
P.O. Box 413035
Kansas City, MO 64111
(816) 751-2929

Reach Together
Women's Center
Breast Care Clinic
1000 East Primrose, Suite
    170
Springfield, MO 65807
(417) 886-LADY

Breast Cancer Network
Mid American Cancer
    Center
St. John's Hospital
1235 East Cherokee
Springfield, MO 65804
(800) 432-CARE / (800)
    364-6120

St. Joseph Health Center
300 First Capital Drive
St. Charles, MO 63301
(314) 947-5614 / (800)
    835-1212

"We Can" Missouri Baptist
    Medical Center
3015 North Ballad Road
St. Louis, MO 63131
(314) 569-5263

St. John's Mercy Cancer
    Center
615 South New Ballad Road
St. Louis, MO 63141
(314) 569-6400

SHARE Breast Cancer
    Education and Support
    Program
9378 Olive Boulevard
St. Louis, MO 63132
(314) 991-4424

Reflections and Can Survive
Barnes Jewish Hospital
    Breast Cancer Support
    Groups
1 Barnes Hospital Plaza
St. Louis, MO 63110
(314) 362-5574

Jewish Hospital
216 South Kings Highway
St. Louis, MO 63110
(314) 454-7000

MONTANA

Bosom Buddies
401 North Central
Sidney, MT 59270
(406) 482-2423

NEBRASKA

St. Elizabeth Community
    Health Center
555 S. 70th Street
Lincoln, NE 68510
(402) 489-7181

NEVADA

On With Life
St. Mary's Women's Center
235 W. Sixth Street
Reno, NV 89520
(702) 789-3282

NEW HAMPSHIRE

Concord Hospital
250 Pleasant Street
Concord, NH 03301
(603) 225-2711, ext. 3872

Catholic Medical Center
100 McGregor Street
Manchester, NH 03102
(603) 626-2049

Elliot Hospital
1 Elliot Way
Manchester, NH 03103
(603) 628-2338

NEW JERSEY

Breast Disease and Surgery
Center
1541 Sjak Highway 88 West
Bricktown, NJ 08724
(908) 458-4600

Comprehensive Breast Care
Center
Cooper Hospital University
Medical Center
3 Cooper Plaza, Suite 411
Camden, NJ 08103
(609) 342-2474

Dover General Hospital and
Medical Center/
Oncology
24 Jardine Street
Dover, NJ 07801
(201) 989-3106

Mid-Monmouth County
Recurrence Support
Group
Fair Haven, NJ 07704
(908) 229-9535

Hackensack Medical Center
5 Summit Avenue
Hackensack, NJ 07601
(201) 996-5800

St. Barnabas Medical Center
94 Old Short Hills Road
Livingston, NJ 07039
(201) 533-5633

Cancer Center at Mon-
mouth Medical Center
300 Second Avenue
Long Branch, NJ 07740
(908) 870-5429

Elm Lifelines Center for
Cancer Counseling and
Support
23 South Main Street, Suite 1
Medford, NJ 08055
(609) 654-4044

Cancer Care, Inc.
241 Millburn Avenue
Millburn, NJ 07041
(201) 379-7500

Woman to Woman
Jersey Shore Medical Center
1945 State, Route 33
Neptune, NJ 07754-0397
(908) 776-4240

Cancer Institute of New
Jersey
303 George Street, Suite
501
New Brunswick, NJ 08901
(908) 235-6790

Brick Hospital
2121 Edgewater Place
Point Pleasant, NJ 08742
(908) 295-6424

Atlantic City Medical
Center
RNS Regional Cancer
Center
Simmie Leeds Road
Pomona, NJ 08240
(609) 652-3500

B.E.S.T. Care
Ruth Newman Shapiro
Medical Center
Simmie Leeds Road
Pomona, NJ 08240
(609) 652-3500

Breast Cancer Resource
Center
Princeton YWCA
Paul Robeson Place
Princeton, NJ 08540
(609) 497-2126 / (609)
252-2003

Beyond Cancer
4570 Provine Line Road
Princeton, NJ 08540
(609) 683-0692

Women at Risk / Breast
Cancer Coalition
500 B Oberline Pines
Lakeview, NJ 08701
(800) 82-BREAST

Riverview Regional Cancer
Center
1 Riverview Plaza
Red Bank, NJ 07701
(908) 530-2382 / (800)
564-3551

Cancer Care
141 Dayton Street
Ridgewood, NJ 07450
(201) 444-6630

Talking It Over
Valley Hospital
223 N. Van Bien Avenue
Ridgewood, NJ 07450
(201) 447-8656

After Breast Cancer Support
Group
Somerset Medical Center
110 Rehill Avenue
Somerville, NJ 08876-2598
(908) 704-3740

WISE (Women's Interna-
tional Support Environ-
ment)
510 Old Bridge Turnpike
South River, NJ 08882
(908) 257-6611 / (800)
870-6616

Community Medical Center
99 Route 37 West
Toms River, NJ 08755
(908) 240-8076

After Breast-Cancer Surgery
605 Pascack Road
Washington Township, NJ
07675
(201) 666-6610

NEW MEXICO

People Living Through
Cancer
323 Eighth Street SW
Albuquerque, NM 87102
(505) 242-3263

NEW YORK

1 in 9
Nassau County Medical
Center
2201 Hempstead Turnpike
East Meadow, NY 11554
(516) 357-9622

Breast Cancer Support
Group
Box 718
Binghamton, NY 13902
(607) 693-1759 / (607)
797-4222

Othmer Cancer Center at
Long Island
College Hospital
340 Henry Street
Brooklyn, NY 11209
(718) 780-1135

Cancer Institute of Brooklyn
927 49th Street
Brooklyn, NY 11219
(718) 972-5816

St. John's Queens Hospital
9002 Queens Boulevard
Elmhurst, NY 11373
(718) 457-1300, ext. 2250

Flushing Hospital Medical
 Center
40 Fifth Avenue and Parsons
 Boulevard
Flushing, NY 11355
(718) 670-5640

Adelphi Breast Cancer
 HOTLINE and Support
 Program
Support Group for Women
 under 40
Adelphi University School of
 Social Work
Garden City, NY 11530
(516) 877-4444

After Breast Cancer
Glens Falls Hospital
100 Clark Street
Glens Falls, NY 12801
(518) 761-2204

Huntington Hospital
270 Park Avenue
Huntington, NY 11743
(516) 351-2568

Tompkins Community
 Hospital
Oncology Department
101 Dates Drive
Ithaca, NY 14850
(607) 274-4101

Womens Health Connection
United Health Services
33-57 Harrison Street
Johnson City, NY 13790
(607) 763-6546

Oncology Support Program
 for Cancer Patients and
 Their Families
North Shore University
 Hospital
300 Community Drive
Manhasset, NY 11030
(516) 926-HELP

Side by Side
UNIT #5
154 Martling Avenue
Tarrytown, NJ 10591
(914) 347-2649

Post Lumpectomy Support
 Group
Long Island Jewish Medical
 Center
Radiation Oncology Depart-
 ment
270-05 76th Avenue
New Hyde Park, NY 11040
(718) 470-7188

SHARE: Support Services
 for Women with Breast
 or Ovarian Cancer
19 W. 44th Street,
 Suite 415
New York, NY 10036
(212) 719-0364

Post-Treatment Resource
 Program
Memorial Sloan-Kettering
 Cancer Center
1275 York Avenue
New York, NY 10021
(212) 639-3292

New Beginnings
Beth Israel Medical Center,
 North Division
170 East End Avenue
New York, NY 10128
(212) 870-9502

Breast Friends
Mount Sinai Medical Center
100th Street & Fifth Avenue
New York, NY 10029
(212) 241-7748

Breast Examination Center
 of Harlem
163 W. 125th Street
New York, NY 10027
(212) 864-0600

Live, Love, and Laugh
 Again
John T. Mather Memorial
 Hospital
North Country Road
Port Jefferson, NY 11777
(516) 476-2707

Breast Cancer Support
 Group
19 Butterfly Lane
Putnam Valley, NY 10579
(914) 528-8213

Cancer Action, Inc.
255 Alexander Street
Rochester, NY 14607
(716) 423-9700

University of Rochester
 Cancer Center
601 Elmwood Avenue
Rochester, NY 14620
(716) 275-5908

Cancer Support Team, Inc.
18 Rye Ridge Plaza
Port Chester, NY 10573
(914) 253-5334

Franklin General Hospital
 Mastectomy
 Discussion Group
900 Franklin Avenue
Valley Stream, NY 11580
(516) 825-8800, ext. 2205

NORTH CAROLINA

Life After Cancer/Pathways,
 Inc.
121 Sherwood Road
Asheville, NC 28803
(704) 252-4106

Chapel Hill Support
1030 Torrey Pines Place
Chapel Hill, NC 27514
(919) 929-7022

Charlotte Organization for
 Breast Cancer Education
9809 Four Mile Creek Road
Charlotte, NC 28277-9038
(704) 846-2190

Presbyterian Hospital
200 Hawthorne Lane
Charlotte, NC 28204
(704) 384-4750

Women Living with Cancer
100 Blythe Boulevard
 Medical Center
Charlotte, NC 28203
(704) 355-3789

Duke Cancer Patient Sup-
 port Program
Duke Comprehensive Can-
 cer Center
Erwin Road
Durham, NC 27710
(919) 684-4497

Living with Cancer
Moses Cone Memorial
Hospital
1200 N. Elm St.
Greensboro, NC 27401
(910) 574-7000

Breast Cancer Coalition of
North Carolina
P.O. Box 988
Mebane, NC 27302
(800) 419-5481

Triangle Breast Cancer
Support Group
621 West Morgan Street
Raleigh, NC 27603
(919) 881-9754 / (919)
781-7070

Rocky Mount Area Breast
Cancer Alliance
Nash Day Hospital
2450 Curtis Ellis Drive
Rocky Mount, NC 27803
(919) 443-8607

Boice Willis Clinic
901 N. Winston Avenue
Rocky Mount, NC 27803
(919) 937-0202

Kathy Farris Memorial
Breast Cancer Group
1505 Kenan
Wilson, NC 27893
(919) 243-4098

Pink Broomstick / Cancer
Services, Inc.
107 Westdale Avenue
Winston-Salem, NC 27101
(910) 725-7421 / (800)
228-7421

NORTH DAKOTA

Mastectomy Support Group
Great Plains Rehabilitation
Services
1120 E. Main
Bismarck, ND 58502
(701) 224-7988

OHIO

Cancer Family Care
7162 Redding Road
Cincinnati, OH 45237
(513) 731-3346

Bethesda Oak Hospital
Breast Center
619 Oak
Cincinnati, OH 45206
(513) 569-5152

University of Cincinnati
Hospital
234 Goodman Street
Cincinnati, OH 45267
(513) 558-3465

Support Groups for Women
Arthur G. James Cancer
Hospital
300 West Tenth Avenue,
Rm. 775
Columbus, OH 43210-
1228
(614) 293-3237

Post-Mastectomy Support
Group
Elizabeth Blackwell Center
3635 Olentangy River Road
Columbus, OH 43214
(614) 566-5153

Riverside Cancer Institute
3535 Olentangy River Road
Columbus, OH 43214
(614) 566-4321 / (800)
752-9119

St. Elizabeth Breast Center
601 Edwin Moses Boulevard
Dayton, OH 45408
(513) 229-7474

Y-ME of the Greater Day-
ton Area
311 Trailwoods Drive
Dayton, OH 45415
(513) 274-9151

Fort Hamilton Hughes
Hospital
630 Eaton Drive
Dayton, OH 45013
(513) 867-2700

SOAR / Strength, Opti-
mism & Recovery
Kettering Medical Center
3535 Southern Boulevard
Kettering, OH 45429-
1298
(513) 296-7231

Evening Exchange
Marietta Memorial Hospital
401 Matthew Street
Marietta, OH 45750
(614) 374-1450

HERS-Breast Cancer Sup-
port Network
Mercy Medical Center
1343 N. Fountain Boule-
vard
Springfield, OH 45501
(513) 390-5030

Cancer Care
Southside Medical Center
345 Oak Hill Avenue
Youngstown, OH 44501
(216) 740-4176 / (216)
788-5048

OKLAHOMA

Central Oklahoma Cancer
Center
SW Medical Center
1001 Southwest 44
Oklahoma City, OK 73109-
3607
(405) 636-7104

Oklahoma Breast Care Cen-
ter
13509 North Meridian,
Suite 6
Oklahoma City, OK 73120
(405) 755-2273 / (800)
422-4626

OREGON

Breast Specialty Center
9155 Southwest Barnes
Road, Suite 934
Portland, OR 97225
(503) 291-4673

McKenzie-Willamette Hos-
pital
1460 G Street
Springfield, OR 97477
(503) 726-4452

Meridian Park Hospital
19300 S.W. 65th
Tualatin, OR 97062
(503) 692-2113

PENNSYLVANIA

John and Dorothy Morgan
Cancer Center
Cedarcrest and J-78
P.O. Box 689
Allentown, PA 18105-1556
(215) 402-0500

Bryn Mawr Hospital
Office of Cancer Programs
130 Bryn Mawr Avenue
Bryn Mawr, PA 19010
(215) 526-3073

WomanCare Resource Center
989 East Park Drive
Harrisburg, PA 17111
(717) 558-2125

Brandywine Breast Center
201 Repleville Road
Coatesville, PA 19320
(215) 383-8549

"A New Beginning" Self
Help Group
Abington Memorial
Hospital
1200 Old York Road
Abington, PA 19001
(215) 646-4954

Advanced Care Associates
575 Virginia Drive, Suite D
Ft. Washington, PA 19034
(800) 289-8001

Penn State University
Milton S. Hershey Medical
Center, Suite 3135
P.O. Box 850
Hershey, PA 17033
(717) 531-5867

Wyoming Valley Health
Care System
61 Poplar Street
Kingston, PA 18704
(717) 283-7851

Lancaster Breast Cancer
Network
208 Willow Valley Dr.
Lancaster, PA 17602
(717) 393-7477

Montgomery Breast Cancer
Support Program
1330 Powell Street
Norristown, PA 19401
(610) 270-2703

Fox Chase Cancer Center
7701 Burholme Avenue
Philadelphia, PA 19111
(215) 728-2668

Linda Creed Breast Cancer
Foundation
Bodine Center, Room
1-310
111 S. 11th Street
Philadelphia, PA 19107
(215) 955-4354

Thomas Jefferson University
Hospital
Bodine Center for Cancer
Treatment
11th and Sansom
Philadelphia, PA 19107
(215) 955-8227

Cancer Support Network
Essex House, Suite L10
Baum Boulevard at S. Negley Avenue
Pittsburgh, PA 15206
(412) 361-8600

Magee-Women's Hospital
300 Halket Street
Pittsburgh, PA 15213
(412) 641-1178

Berger King Cancer Caring
Center
4117 Liberty Avenue
Pittsburgh, PA 15224
(412) 622-1212

Magee-Women's Hospital
Peer Counseling
Program
300 Halket Street
Pittsburgh, PA 15213
(412) 641-4253

Taylor Hospital
Caring and Sharing
East Chester Pike
Ridley Park, PA 19078
(610) 595-6000

York Hospital Outpatient
Cancer Center
25 Moument Road,
Suite 194
York, PA 17403
(717) 741-8100

RHODE ISLAND

Focus on Us
8 Juniper Hill Drive
Coventry, RI 02816-6434
(401) 822-0095

Roger Williams Medical
Center
825 Chalkstone Avenue
Providence, RI 02908
(401) 456-2284

Hope Center for Life
Enhancement
297 Wickenden Street
Providence, RI 02903-4422
(401) 454-0404

Breast Health
528 N. Main Street
Providence, RI 02904-5721
(401) 751-6890

Breast Cancer Coalition
8 Juniper Hill Drive
Coventry, RI 02816-6434
(800) 216-1040

SOUTH CAROLINA

Breast Cancer Support
Group
Center for Cancer Treatment & Research
Richland Memorial Hospital
7 Richland Medical Park
Columbia, SC 29203
(803) 434-3378

Bosom Buddies and Man to
Man
Baptist Medical Center
Taylor at Marron Street
Columbia, SC 29220
(803) 771-5244

Mcleod Resource Center
Caring Friends Support
Group
555 E. Cheves Street
Florence, SC 29501
(803) 667-2888

Supporting Sisters
481 Frye Branch Road
Lexington, SC 29072
(803) 796-6009

SOUTH DAKOTA

Volunteer & Information
Center
1321 W. 22nd Street
Sioux Falls, SD 57105
(605) 339-HELP

Friends Against Breast
Cancer
1000 E. 21st Street
Sioux Falls, SD 57105
(605) 339-7808

Sioux Valley Hospital
1100 S. Euclid Avenue
Sioux Falls, SD 57117
(605) 333-5244

Dakota Midwest Cancer In-
stitute
1000 E. 21st Street
Sioux Falls, SD 57105
(605) 331-1111

TENNESSEE

Y-ME of Chattanooga
P.O. Box 51
Chattanooga, TN 37401
(615) 886-4171

Knoxville Breast Center
6307 Lonas Drive
Knoxville, TN 37909
(615) 584-0291

Wellness Community
1844 Terrale Avenue
Knoxville, TN 37916
(615) 546-4661

TEXAS

Images by MM
1020 N. Daud Drive
Arlington, TX 76012
(817) 277-7434

Virginia R. Cetko Patient
Education
Baylor-Charles A. Sammons
Cancer Center
3500 Gaston Avenue
Dallas, TX 75246
(214) 820-2608

Between Us
Breast Treatment Associates
3404 Worth Street
Dallas, TX 75246
(214) 521-5225

Patient to Patient
Breast Treatment Associates
3409 Worth Street
Dallas, TX 75246
(214) 821-2962

Woman to Woman
Presbyterian Hospital of
Dallas
8200 Walnut Hill Lane
Dallas, TX 75231
(214) 345-2600

Breast Reconstruction
Educational Support
Group
800 8th Avenue
Ft. Worth, TX 76104
(817) 332-4311

Doris Kupferle Breast Center
1301 Pennsylvania Avenue
Ft. Worth, TX 76104
(817) 882-3650

The Rose Garden
(Pasadena)
12700 N. Featherwood,
Suite 260
Houston, TX 77034
(713) 484-4708

The Rosebuds (Southwest)
9121-C Stellalink
Houston, TX 77025
(713) 665-2729

Women's Information
Network
Medical City Hospital,
Dallas
2404 Hosan Hill
McKinney, TX 75070
(214) 562-7717

Texas Oncology
3320 Line Oakcs
Dallas, TX 75204
(214) 824-4639

Bosom Buddies / Women's
Center
Richardson, TX 75080
(214) 238-9516

UTAH

Holy Cross Hospital Breast
Care Services
1050 E. South Temple
Salt Lake City, UT 84102
(801) 350-4973

Ashley Valley Medical Center
151 W. 200 North
Vernal, UT 84078
(801) 789-3342

VERMONT

Breast Center
1 South Prospect Street
Burlington, VT 05401
(802) 656-2262

Woman to Woman
Rutland Regional Medical
Center
160 Allen Street
Rutland, VT 05701
(802) 747-3713

VIRGINIA

My Image After Breast
Cancer
6000 Stevenson Avenue,
Suite 203
Alexandria, VA 22304
(703) 461-9616 / (800)
970-4411

Cardwell Cancer Center
Martha Jefferson Hospital
459 Locust Avenue
Charlottesville, VA 22902
(804) 982-8407

Fairfax Hospital
3300 Gallows Road
Falls Church, VA 22042-
3300
(703) 698-3731

Women's Health Focus
Rockingham Memorial Hos-
pital
235 Cantrell Avenue
Harrisonburg, VA 22801-
3293
(703) 433-4641

Santara Leigh Hospital
6015 Poplar Hall Drive,
Suite 103
Norfolk, VA 23502
(804) 466-6837

M.C.V. Hospital
401 N. 12th Street
Richmond, VA 23219
(804) 828-9000

Virginia Breast Cancer
  Foundation
P.O. Box 17884
Richmond, VA 23226
(804) 285-1200

Lewis-Gale Regional Cancer
  Center
1900 Electric Road
Salem, VA 24153
(800) 543-5660

WASHINGTON

Overlake Hospital Medical
  Center
1035 116th NE
Bellevue, WA 98004
(206) 688-5261

Breast Cancer Support
  Group of Kitsap County
718 Lebo Boulevard
Bremerton, WA 98310
(206) 373-1057

Puget Sound Tumor Insti-
  tute
21605 76th Avenue West
Edmonds, WA 98026
(206) 640-4300

Providence Hospital
916 Pace Fox Avenue
Everett, WA 98201
(206) 258-7255

Evergreen Hospital
12040 NE 128
Kirkland, WA 98034
(206) 899-2264

A Touch of Strength
St. Peter Hospital Regional
  Cancer Center
413 Lilly Road, NE
Olympia, WA 98506
(206) 493-7510

Operation Uplift
P.O. Box 547
Port Angeles, WA 98362
(206) 457-5141

Seattle Breast Center/
  Northwest Hospital
1560 N. 115th Street
Seattle, WA 98133
(206) 368-1457

Providence/Breast Cancer
  Support Group
500 17th Avenue
Box 34008
Seattle, WA 98124
(206) 320-2100

Highline Community
  Hospital Cancer Care
  Program
16251 Sylvester Road SW,
  Burien
Seattle, WA 98166
(206) 439-5577

Cancer Lifeline
1191 Second Avenue,
  Suite 680
Seattle, WA 98101-2938
(206) 461-4542

Swedish Hospital Tumor
  Institute
1221 Madison
Seattle, WA 98104
(206) 386-2323

WEST VIRGINIA

CAMC Family Resource
  Center
Women & Children's
  Hospital
800 Pennsylvania Avenue
Charleston, WV 25302
(304) 348-2545

WISCONSIN

Meriter Hospital Women's
  Center
After Breast Surgery
309 West Washington
Madison, WI 53703
(608) 258-3750

Lifestream Women's Health
  Center
Sheboygan Memorial Medi-
  cal Center
2624 N. Seventh
Sheboygan, WI 53083
(414) 459-5536

WYOMING

United Medical Center
300 E. 23rd
Cheyenne, WY 82001
(307) 633-7895

Appendix D

Abbreviations

AARP American Association of Retired Persons

ACR American College of Radiologists

ACS American Cancer Society

ADA Americans with Disabilities Act

AMA American Medical Association

ASPRS American Society of Plastic and Reconstructive Surgeons

BCA Breast Cancer Action

BCAC Breast Cancer Advisory Center

BCDDP Breast Cancer Detection Demonstration Project

BCPT Breast Cancer Prevention Trial

BCT Breast Conservation Therapy

BENT Breast Exposure Nationwide Trends

BRH United States Bureau of Radiologic Health

BSE Breast Self-Exam

CABCO California Breast Cancer Organizations

CDC Centers for Disease Control and Prevention

DCIS Ductal Carcinoma in Situ

DOD Department of Defense

DCPC Division of Cancer Prevention and Control

EEOC Equal Employment Opportunity Commission

EMF Electromagnetic Fields

EPA Environmental Protection Agency

ER Estrogen Receptor

ERT Estrogen Replacement Therapy

EUSOMA European Society of Mastology

FDA Federal Drug Administration

FRA Federal Rehabilitation Act

GAO General Accounting Office

HDC/ABMT High Dose Chemotherapy/Autologous Bone Marrow Transplant

HIP Health Insurance Plan

IOM Institute of Medicine

LCIS Lobular Carcinoma in Situ

LIBCSP Long Island Breast Cancer Study Project

MQSA Mammography Quality Standards Act

MRI Magnetic Resonance Imaging

NABCO National Alliance of Breast Cancer Organizations

NAPBC National Action Plan on Breast Cancer

NBCC National Breast Cancer Coalition

NBSS [Canadian] National Breast Screening Study

NCAB National Cancer Advisory Board

NCCR National Coalition for Cancer Research

NCCS National Coalition for Cancer Survivors

NCI National Cancer Institute

NEXT Nationwide Evaluation of X-ray Trends

NIEHS National Institute of Environmental Health Sciences

NIH National Institutes of Health

NHIS National Health Interview Survey

NSABP National Surgical Adjuvant Breast and Bowel Project

OAM Office of Alternative Medicine

OTA Office of Technology Assessment

ORI Office of Research Integrity (replaced OSI)

ORWH Office of Research on Women's Health

OSI Office of Scientific Integrity

OWH Office of Women's Health

OWL Older Women's League

RFA Request for Application

SES Socioeconomic Status

SOS Save Ourselves

WEDO Women's Environmental and Development Organization (called WEDO 10/20/94)

WHEA Women's Health Equity Act

WHT Women's Health Trial

WINS Women's Intervention and Nutrition Study

WHO World Health Organization

WCCP Woman's Community Cancer Project

Notes

PART I. WAKING UP

CHAPTER 1. HEALTH CARE ON THE BACK BURNER

1. Paul Cotton. "Women's Health Initiative Leads Way as Research Begins to Fill Gender Gaps" [News]. *Journal of the American Medical Association.* 1/22, 29/1992.
2. Senator Barbara Mikulski at the Conference to Establish a National Action Plan on Breast Cancer, 12/16/93.
3. K. J. Armitage, L. J. Schneiderman, and R. A. Bass. "Response of Physicians to Medical Complaints in Men and Women." *Journal of the American Medical Association.* 5/18/79.
4. Lewis Harris and Associates. *The Commonwealth Fund Survey of Women's Health.* 7/14/93.
5. Carol Stevens. "How Women Get Bad Medicine." *Washingtonian.* June 1992.
6. Ruth B. Merkatz, Grant Bagley, and E. Jane McCarthy. "A Qualitative Analysis of Self-Reported Experiences Among Women Encountering Difficulties with Silicone Breast Implants." *Journal of Women's Health.* Volume 2, Number 2, 1993.
7. Personal interview with Mary Rose Oakar.
8. C. H. Hennekens and J. E. Buring. "Methodologic Considerations in the Design and Conduct of Randomized Trials: The Physicians' Health Study." *Controlled Clinical Trials.* 12/10/89.
9. Shari Roan. "Working on a Cure for Unequal Medicine." *Los Angeles Times.* 6/9/92.
10. Rebecca Dresser. *The Hastings Center Report.* January/February 1992.
11. Bernadine Healy. "Rx for Women's Better Health." *USA Today.* 8/16/92.
12. James S. Todd, M.D. "Better Late Than Never." *Good Housekeeping.* March 1993.
13. "Women's Health Report of the Public Health Service Task Force on Women's Health Issues." *Public Health Report*, volume I, pp. 74–106. 1985.
14. *NIH Guide to Grants and Contracts.* November 1986.

15. Linda Roach Monroe. "Let Us Heal Ourselves, Women Scientists Say." *Miami Herald.* 7/18/93.
16. "National Institutes of Health: Problems in Implementing Policy on Women in Study Populations." General Accounting Office. 6/18/90.
17. *NIH Guide to Grants and Contracts.* August 1993.
18. Ruth L. Kirschstein, M.D. "Public Health Policy Forum: Research on Women's Health." *American Journal of Public Health.* March 1991.
19. Kirschstein, March 1991.
20. Hearing before the House Committee on Government Operations Subcommittee on Human Resources and Intergovernmental Relations. 12/11/91.
21. Hearing before House Subcommittee, 12/11/91.
22. Warren Leary. "Study of Women's Health Criticized by Review Panel." *New York Times.* 11/2/93.
23. Sam Ward. "Goals Aren't at Issue; Cost and Focus Are." *USA Today.* 11/2/93.
24. President's Cancer Panel Special Commission on Breast Cancer, October 1993.
25. Conference to Establish a National Action Plan on Breast Cancer, 12/16/93.

CHAPTER 2. DOLLARS AND SENSE

1. Rose Kushner. *Alternatives: New Developments in the War on Breast Cancer.* Cambridge, Mass.: Kensington Press, 1984.
2. Louise Slaughter. "Women Deserve Parity in Medical Research." *USA Today.* 10/30/91.
3. National Cancer Institute Act, P. L. 244, 8/5/37.
4. Robert Pear. "Report Finds Pills Cost More in U.S. Than Great Britain." *New York Times.* 2/3/94.
5. Francis X. Mahaney, Jr. "Retail Drug Prices Found Higher in U.S. Than Abroad." *Journal of the National Cancer Institute.* 9/21/94.
6. Mahaney, 9/21/94.
7. Women's Environment and Development Organization (WEDO) Public Hearing of the Commission on the Status of Women. City Hall, New York City, 3/2/93.
8. Personal interview with Mary Katzke.
9. Personal interview with Jeff Soper.
10. Martin Brown and Lou Fintor. "The Economic Burden of Cancer." In *Cancer Prevention and Control.* Peter Greenwald, Barrett S. Kramer, and Douglas L. Weed, eds. Marcel Dekker, 1995.
11. "Cancer Facts & Figures: 1995." The American Cancer Society. 1995.
12. Lauren Chambliss. "The Cost of Breast Cancer." *Working Woman.* October 1994.
13. WEDO, 3/2/93.
14. Congressional Research Report for Congress. Library of Congress. 3/10/94.
15. Melinda Beck, Emily Yoffe, Ginny Carroll, et al. "The Politics of Breast Cancer." *Newsweek.* 12/10/90.
16. Hearing before the House Committee on Government Operations Subcommittee on Human Resources and Intergovernmental Relations, 12/11/91.

PART II. RISK FACTORS, CAUSE, AND PREVENTION

CHAPTER 3. STARTLING STATISTICS

1. "Progress in Controlling Breast Cancer." Hearing before the House Select Committee on Aging Subcommittee on Health and Long-Term Care. Chaired by Claude Pepper. 98th Congress. 6/28/84.
2. Personal interview with Loretta Steen.
3. Russell Harris, M.D. "Breast Cancer Among Women in Their Forties: Toward a Reasonable Research Agenda" [Editorial]. *Journal of the National Cancer Institute.* 3/16/94.
4. Jill Walden. "Studies Link Familial Breast, Prostate Cancers." *Journal of the National Cancer Association.* 5/19/93.
5. Nancy Axelrad Comer. "Early Warning." *Mirabella.* February 1993.
6. Centers for Disease Control and Prevention (CDC), 1994.
7. CDC, 1994.
8. CDC, 1994.
9. CDC, 1994.
10. Sandra G. Boodman. "Fear of Breast Cancer." *Washington Post.* 1/5/93.
11. CDC, 1994.
12. "Cancer Facts and Figures: 1994." American Cancer Society. 1994.
13. Philip J. Hilts. "U.S. Breast Cancer Deaths Fell Nearly 5 Percent in Three Years." *New York Times.* 1/12/95.
14. "Executive Summary of the President's Cancer Panel Special Commission on Breast Cancer." In "Cancer at a Crossroads: A Report to Congress for the Nation." National Cancer Advisory Board. September 1994.
15. Hearing before the House Committee on Government Operations Subcommittee on Human Resources and Intergovernmental Relations, 12/11/91.

CHAPTER 4. POVERTY

1. Personal interview with Joyce Ford.
2. Personal interview with Harold Freeman.
3. Joycelyn Elders speaking at the "Secretary's Conference to Establish a National Action Plan on Breast Cancer." Bethesda, Maryland. 1993.
4. M. V. Graham, L. M. Geitz, R. Byhardt, et al. "Comparison of Prognostic Factors and Survival Among Black Patients and White Patients Treated with Irradiation for Non-small Cell Lung Cancer." *Journal of the National Cancer Institute.* 11/18/92.
5. Don Colburn. "Disadvantaged Blacks More Prone to Cancer." *Washington Post.* 6/14/94.
6. Arlene Draper in speech at breast cancer rally in Washington, D.C., 1993.
7. Louis Harris and Associates. *The Commonwealth Fund Survey of Women's Health.* 7/14/93.
8. Cynthia Costello and Anne J. Stone, eds. *The American Woman, 1994–1995: Where We Stand.* New York: W. W. Norton, 1994.
9. National Cancer Institute.
10. "Breast Cancer Twice as Deadly in Blacks." *New York Times.* 9/28/94.

11. President's Cancer Panel, Special Division on Breast Cancer, October 1993.
12. U. K. Henschke, L. D. Leffall, Jr., C. H. Mason, et al. "Alarming Increase of Cancer Mortality in the U.S. Black Population (1950–1967)." *Cancer.* April 1973.
13. Harold Freeman. "Cancer in the Economically Disadvantaged." *Cancer.* 7/1/89.
14. Personal interview with Joyce Ford.
15. "Update: National Breast and Cervical Cancer Early Detection Program, 1992–1993." *Journal of the National Cancer Institute.* 10/20/93.
16. Kolata, Gina. "Deadliness of Breast Cancer in Blacks Defies Easy Answers." *New York Times.* 8/3/94.
17. Kolata, 8/3/94.
18. Kolata, 8/3/94.
19. Harold Freeman, M.D. "Subcommittee on Cancer in the Economically Disadvantaged." American Cancer Society. 1986.
20. Centers for Disease Control and Prevention, 1991.
21. The United States Bureau of the Census, 1990.
22. Harold Freeman. "Race, Poverty, and Cancer." *Journal of the National Cancer Institute.* 4/17/91.
23. Personal interview with Sandy Warshaw.
24. Personal interview with Harold Freeman.
25. Personal interview with Joyce Ford.
26. C. P. Hunter, C. K. Redmond, Vivien Chen, et al. "Breast Cancer: Factors Associated with Stage at Diagnosis in Black and White Women." *Journal of the National Cancer Institute.* 7/21/93.
27. Bernadine Healy at the hearing before the Subcommittee on Human Resources and Intergovernmental Relations of the House Committee on Government Operations. 12/11/91.

CHAPTER 5. HEREDITY

1. Personal interview with Joan D'Argo.
2. Personal interview with Zora Brown.
3. Rick Weiss. "Breast Cancer Gene's Impact Limited." *Washington Post.* 9/20/94.
4. Personal interview with Susan Love.
5. Eliot Marshall. "The Politics of Breast Cancer." *Science.* 1/29/93.
6. Personal interview with Alison Estabrook.
7. D. E. Anderson and M. D. Badzioch. "Breast Cancer Risks in Relatives of Male Breast Cancer Patients." *Journal of the National Cancer Institute.* 7/15/92.
8. Jill Walden. "Studies Link Familial Breast, Prostate Cancers." *Journal of the National Cancer Institute.* 5/19/93.
9. H. Tulinius, H. Sigvaldison, G. Olafsdottir, et al. "Epidemiology of Breast Cancer in Families in Iceland." *Journal of Medical Genetics.* 3/29/92.
10. Graham A. Colditz. "Family History, Age, and Risk of Breast Cancer." *Journal of the American Medical Association.* 7/21/93.
11. Geoffrey Cowley. "Family Matters." *Newsweek.* 12/6/93.

12. Natalie Angier. "Scientists Identify a Mutant Gene Tied to Hereditary Breast Cancer." *New York Times.* 9/15/94.
13. Kenneth Offit. "Hostage to Our Genes?" *New York Times.* 9/22/94.

CHAPTER 6. THE FAT FACTOR

1. Gina Kolata. "Big New Study Finds No Link Between Fat and Breast Cancer." *New York Times.* 10/21/92.
2. W. C. Willett, D. J. Hunter, M. J. Stampfer, et al. "Dietary Fat and Fiber in Relation to Risk of Breast Cancer: An 8-Year Follow-Up." *Journal of the American Medical Association.* 10/21/92.
3. Claudia Wallis. "A Puzzling Plague." *Time.* 1/14/91.
4. L. A. Cohen, D. P. Rose, and E. L. Wynder. "A Rationale for Dietary Intervention in Postmenopausal Breast Cancer Patients: An Update." *Nutrition and Cancer.* 1993.
5. Susan Rennie. "Breast Cancer Prevention: Diet vs. Drugs." *Ms.* May/June 1993.
6. Eliot Marshall. "Third Strike for NCI Breast Cancer Study." *Science.* 12/14/90.
7. Rennie, May/June 1993.
8. Rennie, May/June 1993.
9. Marshall, 12/14/90.
10. Susan Love and Karen Lindsey. *Dr. Susan Love's Breast Book.* New York: Addison-Wesley Publishing Company, 1990.
11. Personal interview with Ellen Hobbs.
12. N. F. Boyd, M. Cousins, G. Lockwood, et al. "The Feasibility of Testing Experimentally the Dietary Fat–Breast Cancer Hypothesis." *British Journal of Cancer.* 1990.
13. L. A. Cohen et al, 1993.
14. Personal interview with Larry Norton.
15. Wallis, 1/14/91.
16. Personal interview with Larry Norton.
17. W. Willett and M. Stampfer. "Dietary-Fat Intake and Breast-Cancer Risk." *Journal of the National Cancer Institute.* 9/20/89.
18. D. P. Rose, J. M. Connolly, and C. L. Meschter. "Effect of Dietary Fat on Human Breast-Cancer Growth and Lung Metastasis in Nude Mice." *Journal of the National Cancer Institute.* 10/16/91.
19. W. Willett et al., "Dietary Fat and Fiber in Relation to Risk of Breast Cancer: An 8-Year Follow-Up." *Journal of the American Medical Association.* 10/21/92.
20. Gina Kolata. "Big New Study Finds No Link Between Fat and Breast Cancer." *New York Times.* 10/21/92.
21. NCI statement, 10/21/92.
22. Dolores Kong. "Diet's Link to Breast Cancer is Downplayed." *Boston Globe.* 10/21/92.
23. "Cancer Risk Factor Challenged." *Washington Post.* 10/21/92.
24. Personal interview with David Rose.
25. Personal interview with David Rose.
26. Jane Brody. "Breast Cancer Weapons: Fruit, Vegetables and, Maybe, Olive Oil." *New York Times.* 1/18/95.
27. Women's Environment and Development Organization (WEDO) Public Hear-

ing of the Commission on the Status of Women. City Hall, New York City, 3/2/93.

28. H. Adlercreutz, T. Fotsis, C. Bannwart, et al. "Urinary Estrogen Profile Determination in Young Finnish Vegetarian and Omnivorous Women." *Journal of Steroid Biochemistry.* January 1986.

CHAPTER 7. HORMONAL HAZARDS

1. Judy Foreman. "The Cancer Risk in Delayed Pregnancy." *Boston Globe.* 9/27/93.
2. Women's Environment and Development Organization (WEDO) Public Hearing of the Commission on the Status of Women. City Hall, New York City, 3/2/93.
3. Rose Kushner. *Alternatives: New Developments in the War on Breast Cancer.* Cambridge, Mass.: Kensington Press, 1984.
4. Richard Theriault. "Estrogen Replacement Therapy in Younger Women with Breast Cancer." NCI conference, "Breast Cancer in Younger Women." Bethesda, MD. 1/28–29/93.
5. B. MacMahon and P. Cole. "The Ovarian Etiology of Human Breast Cancer." *Recent Results of Cancer Research.* Volume 39, pp. 185–92, 1972.
6. M. P. Osbourne, H. L. Bradlow, G. Y. C. Wong, and N. T. Telang. "Upregulation of Estradiol C16-Alpha-Hydroxylation in Human Breast Tissue: A Potential Biomarker of Breast Cancer Risk." *Journal of the National Cancer Institute.* 12/1/93.
7. D. W. Nebert. "Elevated Estrogen 16-Alpha-Hydroxylase Activity: Is This a Genotoxic or Nongenotoxic Biomarker in Human Breast Cancer Risk?" [Editorial]. *Journal of the National Cancer Institute.* 12/1/93.
8. Mats Lambe et al. "Transient Increase in the Risk of Breast Cancer after Giving Birth." *New England Journal of Medicine.* 7/7/94.
9. "Study Finds Pregnancy Lowers Risk of Breast Cancer Later On." *New York Times.* 4/7/94.
10. Thomas Maugh II. "Breast Cancer While Pregnant Raises Risk." *Los Angeles Times.* 6/24/94.
11. Maugh, 6/24/94.
12. "Intrauterine Influences, Mammary Gland Mass, and Breast Cancer Risk." President's Cancer Panel, Special Commission on Breast Cancer, 9/23/92.
13. Malcolm C. Pike. "The Prevention of Breast Cancer Through Reduced Ovarian Steroid Exposure." President's Cancer Panel, Special Commission on Breast Cancer, 11/12/92.
14. Personal interview with Mary Costanza.
15. Polly A. Newcomb, Barry E. Storer, Matthew P. Longnecker, et al. "Lactation and a Reduced Risk of Premenopausal Breast Cancer." *New England Journal of Medicine.* 1/13/94.
16. Jennifer L. Kelsey and Esther John. "Lactation and the Risk of Breast Cancer." *New England Journal of Medicine.* 1/13/94.
17. The Joan Hamburg Show. WOR Radio. 12/4/90.
18. J. R. Harris, M. E. Lippman, U. Veronesi, and W. Willett. "Breast Cancer (2)" and "Breast Cancer (3)." *New England Journal of Medicine.* 8/6/92 and 8/13/92.

19. David Alan Coia. "Having Abortion Increases Risk of Breast Cancer." *Washington Times.* 4/2/93.
20. Coia, 4/2/93.
21. Ruth A. Spear, ed. "Right Wing Asserts Early Abortion Causes Breast Cancer." *NABCO News, A Publication of the National Alliance of Breast Cancer Organizations.* January 1994.
22. M. C. Pike, B. E. Henderson, J. T. Casagrande, et al. "Oral Contraceptive Use and Early Abortion as Risk Factors for Breast Cancer in Young Women." *British Journal of Cancer.* January 1981.
23. Coia, 4/2/93.
24. H. L. Howe, R. T. Senie, H. Bzduch, et al. "Early Abortion and Breast Cancer Risk Among Women Under Age 40." *International Journal of Epidemiology.* June 1989.
25. J. R. Daling, K. E. Malone, L. F. Voight, et al. "Risk of Breast Cancer Among Young Women: Relationship to Induced Abortion." *Journal of the National Cancer Institute.* 11/2/94.
26. L. Rosenberg, J. R. Palmer, D. W. Kaufman, et al. "Breast Cancer in Relation to the Occurrence and Time of Induced and Spontaneous Abortion." *American Journal of Epidemiology.* May 1988.
27. Coia, 4/2/93.
28. Spear, January 1994.
29. J. L. Kelscy, J. Gammon, et al. "Reproductive Factors and Breast Cancer." *Epidemiological Review.* 1993.
30. Lawrence K. Altman. "New Study Links Abortions and Increase in Breast Cancer Risk." *New York Times.* 10/27/94.
31. Daling et al, 11/2/94.
32. Altman, 10/27/94.
33. Lynn Rosenberg. "Induced Abortion and Breast Cancer: More Scientific Data Are Needed." *Journal of the National Cancer Institute.* 11/2/94.
34. Altman, 10/27/94.
35. Centers for Disease Control and Prevention, 1990.
36. United States General Accounting Office.
37. Daniel Q. Haney. "No Menopause Harm Found in Estrogen." *Los Angeles Times.* 11/29/92.
38. Jane Brody. "Hormone Replacement Study Answers Questions, but Not All." *New York Times.* 1/18/95.
39. Jane E. Brody. "Personal Health: Estrogens After Menopause." *New York Times.* 10/12/89.
40. M. A. Cobleigh, R. F. Berris, T. B. Bush, et al. "Estrogen Replacement Therapy in Breast Cancer Survivors: A Time for a Change." *Journal of the American Medical Association.* 8/17/94.
41. Richard Theriault. "Estrogen Replacement Therapy in Younger Women with Breast Cancer." NCI Conference, "Breast Cancer in Younger Women." Bethesda, Maryland. 1/28–29/93.
42. Rena V. Sellin. "A Randomized, Prospective Trial of Estrogen Replacement Therapy in Women with a History of Breast Cancer." NCI Conference, "Breast Cancer in Younger Women." Bethesda, Maryland. 1/28–29/93.
43. Ridgely Ochs. "Estrogen Link to Cancer Eyed." *Newsday.* 8/16/94.

44. Cobleigh, et al, 8/17/94.
45. Richard Love. "Effects of Tamoxifen on Bone Mineral Density in Postmenopausal Women with Breast Cancer." *New England Journal of Medicine.* 3/26/92.
46. Alan Guttmacher Institute.
47. NCI conference, "Breast Cancer in Younger Women." Bethesda, Maryland. 1/28–29/93.
48. NCI Conference, 1/28–29/93.
49. E. White, K. E. Malone, N. S. Weiss, et al. "Breast Cancer Among Young U.S. Women in Relation to Contraceptive Use." *Journal of the National Cancer Institute.* 4/6/94.
50. "Oral Contraceptives and Breast Cancer." National Cancer Institute Fact Sheet. 4/20/94.
51. "Oral Contraceptives and Breast Cancer." 4/20/94.
52. "Oral Contraceptives and Breast Cancer." 4/20/94.
53. "Oral Contraceptives and Breast Cancer." 4/20/94.
54. D. R. Miller, L. Rosenberg, D. W. Kaufman, et al. "Breast Cancer Before Age 45 and Oral Contraceptive Uses: New Findings." *American Journal of Epidemiology.* February 1989.
55. C. Chilvers, K. McPherson, M. C. Pike, et al. (U.K. National Case-Control Study Group). "Oral Contraceptives and Breast Cancer." *National Cancer Institute.* 4/20/94.
56. H. Olsson, T. R. Moller, and J. Ranstam. "Early Oral Contraceptive Use and Breast Cancer Among Premenopausal Women: Final Report from a Study in Southern Sweden." *Journal of the National Cancer Institute.* 7/5/89.
57. Janet R. Daling. "Risk Factors for Breast Cancer in Younger Women." NCI conference, "Breast Cancer in Younger Women." 1/28–29/93.
58. S. Harlap. "Oral Contraceptives and Breast Cancer: Cause and Effect?" *Journal of Reproductive Medicine.* May 1991.
59. W. Hawley, J. Nuovo, C. P. DeNeef, et al. "Do Oral Contraceptive Agents Affect the Risk of Breast Cancer? A Meta-Analysis of the Case-Control Reports." *Journal of the American Board of Family Practice.* March/April 1993.
60. Personal interview with Susan Love.
61. NCI Conference, "Breast Cancer in Younger Women." Bethesda, Maryland. 1/28–29/93.

CHAPTER 8. ENVIRONMENTAL ENEMIES

1. Personal interview with Rita Arditti.
2. Personal interview with Alison Estabrook.
3. Personal interview with Sharon Green.
4. Women's Environment and Development Organization (WEDO) Public Hearing of the Commission on the Status of Women. City Hall, New York City, 3/2/93.
5. Roy E. Shore. "Radiation & Breast Cancer Risk." President's Cancer Panel, Special Commission on Breast Cancer. 9/23/92.
6. David Ozonoff at the conference "Breast Cancer and the Environment: Our Health at Risk." Massachusetts Breast Cancer Coalition. 10/28–29/94.

7. Joan D'Argo at the conference "Breast Cancer and the Environment: Our Health at Risk." Massachusetts Breast Cancer Coalition. 10/28–29/94.
8. WEDO, 3/2/93.
9. WEDO, 3/2/93.
10. Samuel Epstein at WEDO, 3/2/93.
11. Epstein at WEDO, 3/2/93.
12. Ana Soto, at the conference "Breast Cancer and the Environment: Our Health at Risk." Massachusetts Breast Cancer Coalition. 10/28–29/94.
13. Ruby Senie. "Pesticides and Obesity: Potential Link with Breast Cancer." WEDO, 3/2/93.
14. F. Falck, A. Ricci, M. Wolff, et al. "Pesticides and Polychlorinated Biphenyl Residues in Human Breast Lipids and Their Relation to Breast Cancer." *Archives of Environmental Health.* March/April 1992.
15. WEDO, 3/2/93.
16. Personal interview with Alison Estabrook.
17. WEDO, 3/2/93.
18. WEDO, 3/2/93.
19. Mary S. Wolff, Paolo G. Toniolo, Eric W. Lee, et al. "Blood Levels of Organochlorine Residues and Risk of Breast Cancer." *Journal of the National Cancer Institute.* 4/21/93.
20. President's Cancer Panel, 9/23/92.
21. WEDO, 3/2/93.
22. Hearing before the House Energy and Commerce Subcommittee on Health and the Environment, 10/21/93.
23. A. M. Soto, R. M. Silvia, and C. Sonnenschein. "A Plasma-Borne Specific Inhibitor of the Proliferation of Human Estrogen-Sensitive Breast Tumor Cells (Estrocolyone-I)." *Journal of Steroid Biochemistry and Molecular Biology.* December 1992.
24. WEDO, 3/2/93.
25. Jerome B. Westin and Elihu Richter. "The Israeli Breast Cancer Anomaly." In Devra Lee Davis and David Hoel, eds., *Trends in Cancer Mortality in Industrialized Countries.* New York: New York Academy of Sciences, 1990.
26. D. L. Davis, H. L. Bradlow, M. Wolff, et al. "Medical Hypothesis: Xenoestrogens as Preventable Causes of Breast Cancer." *Environmental Health Perspectives.* 1993.
27. N. Krieger, M. S. Wolff, R. A. Hiatt, et al. "Breast Cancer and Serum Organochlorines: A Prospective Study Among White, Black, and Asian Women." *Journal of the National Cancer Institute.* 4/20/94.
28. Thomas H. Maugh II. "Breast Cancer Study Clears DDT, PCBs." *Los Angeles Times.* 4/20/94.
29. Brian MacMahon. "Pesticide Residues and Breast Cancer?" *Journal of the National Cancer Institute.* 4/20/94.
30. Linda Anderson. "DDT and Breast Cancer: The Verdict Isn't In." *Journal of the National Cancer Institute.* 4/20/94.
31. New York State Department of Health, Division of Occupational Health and Environmental Epidemiology. "Residence Near Industries and High Traffic Areas and the Risk of Breast Cancer on Long Island." April 1994.

32. Michelle Slatalla. "Breast Cancer Follow-Up." *Newsday.* 4/14/94.
33. Diana Jean Schemo. "L.I. Breast Cancer Is Possibly Linked to Chemical Sites." *New York Times.* 4/13/94.
34. Schemo, 4/13/94.
35. Natalie S. Larsen. "Researchers to Comb Long Island for Potential Cancer Factors." *Journal of the National Cancer Institute.* 1/19/94.
36. Larsen, 1/19/94.
37. "Studies Under Way to Assess Environmental Exposures and Risk of Breast Cancer." National Cancer Institute fact sheet, 4/21/93.
38. NCI, 4/21/93.
39. NCI, 4/21/93.
40. NCI, 4/21/93.
41. I. MacKenzie. "Breast Cancer Following Multiple Fluoroscopies." *British Journal of Cancer.* January 1965.
42. A. B. Miller, G. R. Howe, G. J. Sherman, et al. "Mortality from Breast Cancer After Irradiation During Fluoroscopic Examinations in Patients Being Treated for Tuberculosis." *New England Journal of Medicine.* 11/9/89.
43. Kushner. *Alternatives.*
44. N. G. Hildreth, R. E. Shore, and P. M. Dvoretsky. "The Risk of Breast Cancer After Irradiation of the Thymus in Infancy." *New England Journal of Medicine.* 11/9/89.
45. Hildreth et al, 11/9/89.
46. A. Mattson, B. I. Ruden, P. Hall, et al. "Radiation-Induced Breast Cancer: Long-Term Follow-Up of Radiation Therapy for Benign Breast Disease." *Journal of the National Cancer Institute.* 10/20/93.
47. John Boice, et al. "Cancer in the Contralateral Breast After Radiotherapy for Breast Cancer." *New England Journal of Medicine.* 3/19/92.
48. WEDO, 3/2/93.
49. Ellen Mendelson. "Breast Imaging in Younger Women." NCI conference, "Breast Cancer in Younger Women." 1/28/93.
50. WEDO, 3/2/93.
51. WEDO, 3/2/93.
52. WEDO, 3/2/93.
53. Patricia Coogan, "Power Frequency Electromagnetic Fields and Breast Cancer Risk" at the conference "Breast Cancer and the Environment: Our Health at Risk." Massachusetts Breast Cancer Coalition. 10/28–29/94.
54. E. Lindgren and G. Pershagen. "Ionizing Radiation, Magnetic Fields and Cancer in Children." *Lakartidningen.* 12/9/92. Article is published in Swedish.
55. D. P. Loomis, D. A. Savitz, and C. V. Ananth. "Breast Cancer Mortality Among Female Electrical Workers in the United States." *Journal of the National Cancer Institute.* 6/15/94.
56. Coogan, 10/28–29/94.
57. "A Clear Point of View: Patricia Buffler on EMFs." *University of California at Berkeley Wellness Letter.* November 1994.
58. William Broad. "Power Line Concern Is Called Needless." *New York Times.* 5/14/95.
59. Bill Richards. "Cancer Link to Electromagnetic Fields Recognized in Washington State Ruling." *Wall Street Journal.* 7/14/94.

CHAPTER 9. OTHER RISKS

1. Jane E. Brody. "Smokers Have Higher Breast Cancer Death Risk." *New York Times.* 5/25/94.
2. Natalie S. Larsen. "Study Suggests Mechanism for Alcohol-Breast Cancer Link. *Journal of the National Cancer Institute.* 5/5/93.
3. "Smoking Found to Escalate Risk of Breast Cancer Death." Los Angeles Times. 6/5/94.
4. Brody, 5/25/94.
5. Personal interview with Frederica Perera on not-yet-published results of study.
6. "Smoking Tied to High Risk of Breast Cancer." *Washington Post.* 6/4/94.
7. W. C. Willett, M. J. Stampfer, G. A. Colditz, et al. "Moderate Alcohol Consumption and the Risk of Breast Cancer." *New England Journal of Medicine.* 5/7/87.
8. A. Schatzkin, D. Y. Jones, R. N. Hoover, et al. "Alcohol Consumption and Breast Cancer in the Epidemiologic Follow-Up Study of the First National Health and Nutrition Examination Survey." *New England Journal of Medicine.* 5/7/87.
9. E. B. Harvey, C. Schairer, L. A. Brinton, et al. "Alcohol Consumption and Breast Cancer." *Journal of the National Cancer Institute.* April 1987.
10. Brian MacMahon. "The Quantification of Alcohol-Caused Morbidity and Mortality in Australia: A Critique." *Medical Journal of Australia.* 10/19/92.
11. MacMahon, 10/19/92.
12. J. M. Martin-Moreno, P. Boyle, L. Gorgojo, et al. "Alcoholic Beverage Consumption and the Risk of Breast Cancer in Spain." *Cancer Causes & Control.* July 1993.
13. W. C. Willet, et al, 5/7/87.
14. M. E. Reichmann, J. T. Judd, C. Longcope, et al. "Effects of Alcohol Consumption on Plasma and Urinary Hormone Concentrations in Premenopausal Women." *Journal of the National Cancer Institute.* 5/5/93.
15. Shari Roan. "Cancer and the 'Invisible Population.' " *Los Angeles Times.* 3/23/93.
16. NCI Public Inquiries memo, 2/9/93.
17. Roan, 3/23/93.
18. Presentation by Katherine O'Hanlan, National Institutes of Health: Scientific Conference on Recruitment and Retention of Women in Health Research, Stanford University Medical Center, Stanford, California, 7/13/93.
19. P. E. Stevens and J. M. Hall. "Stigma, Health Beliefs and Experiences with Health Care in Lesbian Women." *Image: Journal of Nursing Scholarship.* Volume 20, number 1988.
20. O'Hanlan, 7/13/93.
21. American Medical Women's Association. "Position Paper on Lesbian Health Issues." 1993.
22. Keith Schneider. "Despite Critics, Dairy Farmers Increase Use of a Growth Hormone in Cows." *New York Times.* 10/30/94.
23. Schneider, 10/30/94.
24. Samuel S. Epstein. "A Needless New Risk of Breast Cancer." *Los Angeles Times.* 3/20/94.

25. "Dietary IGF-1 and rbST." *FDA Talk Paper*. 3/16/94.

26. Centers for Disease Control and Prevention, 1993.

27. "Some Professionals Linked to Higher Breast-Cancer Death Rate." *Washington Times*. 9/14/93.

28. Judy Foreman. "The Cancer Risk in Delayed Pregnancy." *Boston Globe*. 9/27/93.

29. Philip J. Hilts. "Studies Confirm Potential Cancer Risk from Coated Breast Implants," *New York Times*. 9/25/94.

30. Hilts, 9/25/94.

CHAPTER 10. PREVENTION

1. Eliot Marshall. "The Politics of Breast Cancer." *Science*. January 1993.

2. Cathy Perlmutter and Maureen Sangiorgio. "Women's Health." *Prevention*. February 1993.

3. Personal interview with Maryann Napoli.

4. Sandra Boodman. "Gambling on Radical Surgery." *Washington Post*. 1/5/93.

5. Elena Neumann. "Cancer: The Issue Feminists Forgot." *Washington Times Magazine*. 2/9/92.

6. Susan Love. "Breast Cancer." *Journal of the American Medical Association*. 5/12/93.

7. Rose Kushner testifying at "Progress in Controlling Breast Cancer." Hearing before the House Select Committee on Aging Subcommittee on Health and Long-Term Care. Chaired by Claude Pepper. 98th Congress. 6/28/84.

8. WEDO, 3/2/93.

9. Jerry E. Bishop. "ICI Cancer Drug's Planned Trials May Be Clouded." *Wall Street Journal*. 3/2/92.

10. "U.S. to Test Potential Breast Cancer Preventive in 16,000 Women." *Washington Post*. 4/30/92.

11. WEDO, 3/2/93.

12. Special hearing of the Committee on Government Operations Subcommittee on Human Resources and Intergovernmental Relations. 10/22/92.

13. Personal interview with Victor Vogel.

14. Richard Love. "Effects of Tamoxifen in Bone Mineral Density in Postmenopausal Women with Breast Cancer." *New England Journal of Medicine*. 3/26/92.

15. Perlmutter and Sangiorgio, February 1993.

16. Special Hearing of the House of Representatives Human Resources and Intergovernmental Relations subcommittee, 10/22/92.

17. Adriane Fugh-Berman. "Tamoxifen on Trial: The High Risks of Prevention." *Nation*. 12/21/92.

18. WEDO, 3/2/93.

19. WEDO, 3/2/93.

20. Personal interview with Ellen Hobbs.

21. Gina Kolata. "Data on Risks Create Debate About Drug to Prevent Breast Cancer." *New York Times*. 3/16/94.

22. Kolata, 3/16/94.

23. Kolata, 3/16/94.

24. Hearing before the House Committee on Energy and Commerce Subcommittee on Oversight and Investigations, 4/15/94.
25. Robin Herman. "Research Fraud Breaks Chain of Trust." *Washington Post.* 4/19/94.
26. Susan Jenks. "Congressional Hearing Delves into NSABP Fraud Issues." *Journal of the National Cancer Institute.* 5/4/94.
27. "Resumption of Study on Cancer Drug is Urged." *New York Times.* 6/8/94.
28. Sandra Boodman. "Gambling on Radical Surgery." *Washington Post.* 1/5/93.
29. Boodman, 1/5/93.
30. Boodman, 1/5/93.
31. Boodman, 1/5/93.
32. Personal interview with Mary Jo Kahn.
33. Personal interview with Susan Love.
34. Adrianne Rogers. "Diet-Related Studies of Breast Cancer in Laboratory Animals; Fat, Selenium, and Retinoids." President's Cancer Panel, Special Commission on Breast Cancer, 9/23/92.
35. Clifford Welsch. "Dietary Fat, Calories, Exercise, and Fiber in Mammary Cancer Development in Laboratory Animals." President's Cancer Panel, Special Commission on Breast Cancer, 9/23/92.
36. Hong Liu, Mark Wormke, Stephen H. Safe, and Leonard F. Bjeldanes. "Indolo[3,2-B]carbazole: a Dietary-Derived Factor That Exhibits Both Anti-estrogenic and Estrogenic Activity." *Journal of the National Cancer Society.* 12/7/94.
37. Barry R. Goldin. "Nonsteroidal Estrogens and Estrogen Antagonists: Mechanism of Action and Health Implications." *Journal of the National Cancer Society.* 12/7/94.
38. Jane Brody. "Breast Cancer Weapons: Fruit, Vegetables and, Maybe, Olive Oil." *New York Times.* 1/18/95.
39. Stephen Barnes, Clinton Grubbs, Kenneth Setchell, and James Carlson. "Soybeans Inhibit Mammary Tumors in Models of Breast Cancer." *Mutagens and Carcinogens in the Diet.* Wiley-Liss, 1990.
40. H. P. Lee, L. Gourley, S. W. Duffy, et. al. "Dietary Effects on Breast-Cancer Risk in Singapore." *Lancet.* 5/18/91.
41. Jan Ziegler. "Soybeans Show Promise in Cancer Prevention." *Journal of the National Cancer Institute.* 11/16/94.
42. Leslie Bernstein, Brian E. Henderson, Rosemarie Hanisch, et. al. "Physical Exercise and Reduced Risk of Breast Cancer in Young Women." *Journal of the National Cancer Institute.* 9/21/94.
43. Jane E. Brody. "Regimen of Moderate Exercise Tied to Drop in Breast Cancer." *New York Times.* 9/21/94.
44. Sheryl Stolberg. "Breast Cancer Risk Reduced by Exercise." *Los Angeles Times.* 9/21/94.
45. Stolberg, 9/21/94.
46. Stolberg, 9/21/94.

PART III. MAMMOGRAPHY: MIRACLE OR MYTH?

CHAPTER 11. THE REVEALING PHOTO

1. Personal interview with Susan Love.
2. Congressional hearing, 1992. Dusharme Carter was crowned Miss Oklahoma on October 1, 1992.
3. Charles R. Smart. "The Role of Mammography in the Prevention of Mortality from Breast Cancer." *Cancer Prevention.* June 1990.
4. Smart, June 1990.
5. Smart, June 1990.
6. M. L. Brown, et al. "Is the Supply of Mammography Machines Outstripping Need and Demand? An Economic Analysis." *Annals of Internal Medicine.* 10/1/90.
7. M. L. Brown, et al, 10/1/90.
8. Gina Kolata. "Insuring Women Receive Effective Mammograms." *New York Times.* 2/21/93.
9. Personal interview with Annette Brown.
10. Personal interview with Mary Katzke.
11. Susan Cahill. "Taking Control of Treatment." *Washington Post.* 4/19/94.
12. Alisa Solomon. "The Politics of Breast Cancer." *Village Voice.* 5/14/91.
13. Judith Brady, ed. *1 in 3: Women with Cancer Confront an Epidemic.* Pittsburgh: Cleis Press, 1991.
14. Personal interview with Susan Love.
15. Geoffrey Cowley. "The Politics of Breast Cancer." *Newsweek.* 12/10/90.
16. Personal interview with Larry Norton.
17. Nancy Wartik and Julie Felner. "Is Breast Self-Exam Out of Touch?" *Ms.* November/December 1994.
18. Victoria Champion. "The Role of Breast Self-Examination in Breast Cancer Screening." *Cancer.* 4/1/92.
19. Wartik and Felner, November/December 1994.
20. Cornelia J. Baines. "Breast Self-Examination." *Cancer.* 4/1/92.
21. Wartik and Felner, November/December 1994.
22. G. Costanza, J. Annas, M. L. Brown, et al. "Supporting Statements and Rationale." *Journals of Gerontology.* November 1992.
23. Wartik and Felner, November/December 1994.
24. Wartik and Felner, November/December 1994.
25. Susan M. Love and Karen Lindsey. *Dr. Susan Love's Breast Book.* Cambridge, Mass.: Addison-Wesley, 1990.
26. Champion, 4/1/92.
27. Marlene Cimons. "Federal Panel Withholds OK of Breast Exam Device." *Los Angeles Times.* 9/2/94.
28. Cimons, 9/2/94.
29. Brent Bowers. "How a Device to Aid in Breast Self-Exams Is Kept Off the Market." *Wall Street Journal.* 4/12/94.
30. Mary Lu Carnevale. "Ultrasensitive, Cheap Test Sought for Breast Cancer." *Wall Street Journal.* 8/2/94.
31. "FDA Seeks More Testing of a Device to Detect Breast Cancer." *New York Times.* 9/4/94.

32. "FDA Seeks More Testing," 9/4/94.
33. Associated Press. "F.D.A. Accepts Use of Product in Breast Exams." *New York Times.* 12/25/95.

CHAPTER 12. WHO GETS IT

1. Delia Marshall. "Mammograms Under 50?" *Working Woman.* October 1994.
2. Nancy Breen and Larry Kessler. "Changes in the Use of Screening Mammography: Evidence from the 1987 and 1990 National Health Interview Surveys." *American Journal of Public Health.* January 1994.
3. Breen and Kessler, 1994.
4. National Cancer Institute, 1990.
5. M. Romans, D. J. Marchant, W. H. Pearse, et al. "Utilization of Screening Mammography, 1990." *Women's Health Issues.* 1991.
6. J. Horton, M. Romans, and D. Cruess. "Mammography Attitudes and Usage Study, 1992." *Women's Health Issues.* Winter 1992.
7. Martha Romans. "Utilization of Mammo, Social and Behavioral Trends." *Cancer.* 8/15/93.
8. Romans, 8/15/93.
9. Personal interview with Fran Visco.
10. "Breast Cancer: Winning the Battles, Losing the War." Joint hearing before the House Select Committee on Aging Subcommittee on Health and Long-Term Care. Chaired by Mary Rose Oakar. 10/1/92.
11. "Breast Cancer: Race for the Cure." Hearing before the House Select Committee on Aging Subcommittee on Health and Long-Term Care. 5/16/90.
12. J. A. Horton, M. C. Romans, and D. F. Cruess. "Mammography Attitudes and Usage Study, 1992." *Women's Health Issues.* Volume 2, pp. 180–186. 1992.
13. American Cancer Society, 1986.
14. R. S. Hopkins and K. Hensley. "Breast Cancer Screening in Florida. Opportunities for Prevention." *Journal of the Florida Medical Association.* March 1993.
15. "Mammograms on Rise, Federal Study Finds." *New York Times.* 4/29/92.
16. Women's Leadership Summit on Mammography, Washington, D.C., 9/20/89.
17. ACS conference, Boston. 8/26/93.
18. Personal interview with Mary E. Costanza.
19. Mary E. Costanza. "Breast Cancer Screening in Older Women." *Cancer Supplement.* 4/1/92.
20. Betsy Lehman. "Mammogram Use Found to Be Spotty in Older Women." *Boston Globe.* 2/27/93.
21. "Older Women and Mammography: Experiences and Knowledge of Medicare Benefit." *Modern Maturity.* 10/91.
22. "Cost of Mammogram Deters Some Women." *New York Times.* 4/27/95.
23. Personal interview with Sandy Warshaw.
24. "Summary of Enacted Breast Cancer Legislation by Category as of September 1994." National Cancer Institute: State Cancer Legislative Database. Bethesda, Md. October 1994.

CHAPTER 13. BUT DOES IT SAVE LIVES?

1. Gina Kolata. "Studies Say Mammograms Fail to Help Many Women." *New York Times.* 2/26/93.

2. S. Shapiro, P. Strax, and L. Venet. "Periodic Breast Cancer Screening: The First Two Years of Screening." *Archives of Environmental Health*. November 1967. (The "HIP" study.)

3. "Mammography for Younger Women: Hardsell, No Benefit." *Health Facts*. June 1992.

4. John C. Bailar III. "Mammography: A Contrary View." *Annals of Internal Medicine*. January 1976.

5. Samuel Epstein, at the Women's Environment and Development Organization (WEDO) public hearing at City Hall, New York City. 3/2/93.

6. Samuel Epstein. "Evaluation of the National Cancer Program and Proposed Reforms." *American Journal of Industrial Medicine*. 7/24/93.

7. Epstein, at WEDO hearing. 3/2/93.

8. C. Smart, W. Hartmann, O. Beahrs, and L. Garfinkle. "Insights into Breast Cancer Screening." *Cancer*. 8/15/93.

9. K. C. Chu, C. R. Smart, and R. E. Tarone. "Analysis of Breast Cancer Mortality and Stage Distribution by Age for the Health Insurance Plan Clinical Trial." *Journal of the National Cancer Institute*. 9/21/88.

10. Napoli, June 1992.

11. "Role of Mammography in Prevention of Mortality from Breast Cancer." *Cancer Prevention*. 1988.

12. Kathy S. Albain. "Predictors of Outcome in Younger Women with Breast Cancer." Presented at the NCI conference "Breast Cancer in Younger Women," 1/28/93.

13. Personal interview with Annette Brown.

14. A. B. Miller, C. J. Baines, T. To, and C. Wall. "The Canadian National Breast Screening Study: 1. Breast Cancer Detection and Death Rates Among Women Aged 40 to 49 Years." *Canadian Medical Association Journal*. 5/5/92.

15. A. B. Miller, C. J. Baines, T. To, and C. Wall. "The Canadian National Breast Screening Study: 2. Breast Cancer Detection and Death Rates Among Women Aged 50 to 59 Years." *Canadian Medical Association Journal*. 11/15/92.

16. Napoli, June 1992.

17. Napoli, June 1992.

18. Napoli, June 1992.

19. Personal interview with Annette Brown.

20. Gina Kolata. "Early Mammogram Gets Endorsement." *New York Times*. 2/3/93.

21. Gina Kolata. "Studies Say Mammograms Fail to Help Many Women." *New York Times*. 2/26/93.

22. Walter Lawrence, Jr. "Conference Summary." Presented at the American Cancer Society workshop, "Breast Cancer Detection in Younger Women: A Current Assessment." 2/2/93.

23. Gerald D. Dodd. "ACS Guidelines from Past to Present." Presented at the ACS workshop, 2/1/93.

24. Laszlo Tabar. "New Swedish Breast Cancer Detection Results." Presented at the ACS Workshop, 2/1/93.

25. Kara Smigel. "Late News: International Workshop Assesses Evidence for Breast Screening." *Journal of the National Cancer Institute*. 3/17/93.

26. Personal interview with Victor Vogel.

27. National Cancer Institute conference. "Cancer Statistics Review 1973–1987, NCI, DCPC, NIH, HHS." Bethesda, Md., May 1990.
28. C. R. Smart, R. E. Hendrick, J. H. Rugledge, R. A. Smith. "Benefit of Mammography Screening in Women Ages 40 to 49 Years." *Cancer.* 4/1/95.
29. Kolata, 2/26/93.
30. Daniel Kopans at ACS workshop, 2/1/93.
31. Earl Eubell. "Stepping up the Fight Against Breast Cancer." *Washington Post/ Parade.* 9/11/94.
32. D. M. Eddy, V. Hasselblad, W. McGivney, and W. Hendee. "The Value of Mammography Screening in Women Under Age 50 Years." *Journal of the American Medical Association.* March 1988.

CHAPTER 14. THE GUIDELINES GUESSING GAME

1. NCI conference, "Breast Cancer in Younger Women." 1/29/93.
2. G. Marie Swanson. "May We Agree to Disagree, or How Do We Develop Guidelines for Breast Cancer Screening in Women?" *Journal of the National Cancer Institute.* 6/15/94.
3. National Cancer Institute. "Consensus Development Meeting on Breast Cancer Screening." U.S. Department of Health, Education, and Welfare, Public Health Service, National Cancer Institute (NIH). September 1977.
4. American Cancer Society. "Guidelines for the Cancer-related Checkup: Recommendations and Rationale." *Cancer.* 1980.
5. American Cancer Society. "Mammography Guidelines 1983: Background Statement and Update of Cancer-related Checkup Guidelines for Breast Cancer Detection in Asymptomatic Women Age 40–49." *Cancer.* 1983.
6. Gerald D. Dodd. "American Cancer Society Guidelines on Screening for Breast Cancer: An Overview." *Cancer.* 4/1/92.
7. Personal interview with Susan Love.
8. Kara Smigel. "Survey Shows: American Women Favor Mammography" [News]. *Journal of the National Cancer Institute.* 3/17/93.
9. Ellen Mendelson. "Breast Imaging in Younger Women." Presented at the NCI conference, "Breast Cancer in Younger Women," 1/28/93.
10. Personal interview with Larry Norton.
11. Cori Vanchieri. "Europeans Say Screen Only Women Age 50 and Older." *Journal of the National Cancer Institute.* 3/3/93.
12. Elisabeth Rosenthal. "Study Revives Debate on Need for Mammos Before 50." *New York Times.* 5/13/92.
13. Mary Costanza. "Older Women Underutilize Breast Cancer Screening." *Cancer Supplement.* 4/1/92.
14. Personal interview with Mary Jo Kahn.
15. Vanchieri, 3/3/93.
16. "NCAB asks NCI to Abandon Promulgation of Guidelines." *Cancer Letter.* 3/4/94.
17. Hearing before the House Subcommittee on Health and the Environment, 1/26/94.
18. Hearing before the House Subcommittee on Human Resources and Intergovernmental Relations of the Committee on Government Operations, 3/8/94.

19. Hearing before the House, 3/8/94.
20. Susan M. Love. "Truth Behind Mammogram Dispute." *Los Angeles Times.* 3/16/94.
21. Hearing before the House Subcommittee on Health and the Environment, 1/26/94.
22. Hearing before the House Subcommittee on Health and the Environment, 1/26/94.
23. Russell Harris. "Breast Cancer Among Women in Their Forties: Toward a Reasonable Research Agenda" [Editorial]. *Journal of the National Cancer Institute.* 3/16/94.
24. Hearing before the House, 3/8/94, and before the Subcommittee on Aging of the Senate Committee on Labor and Human Services, 3/9/94.
25. Hearing before the House, 1/26/94.
26. "House Committee Report Says NCI Ignored Data, Procedure in Making Guideline Change." *Cancer Letter.* 1/14/94.
27. "Cancer Institute Criticized for Mammography Shift." *Science & Government Report.* 12/1/94.

· CHAPTER 15. QUALITY CONTROL

1. Susan Love. "Truth Behind Mammogram Dispute." *Los Angeles Times.* 3/16/94.
2. Associated Press. "Most Clinics Meet Standard on Breast Test." *New York Times.* 10/1/94.
3. Hearing before the House Subcommittee on Human Resources and Intergovernmental Relations of the Committee on Government Operations, 3/8/94.
4. Kathleen Kelleher. "Mammography—Vital but Not Foolproof." *Los Angeles Times.* 3/29/92.
5. J. G. Elmore, C. K. Wells, C. H. Lee, et al. "Variability in Radiologists' Interpretations of Mammograms." *New England Journal of Medicine.* 12/1/94.
6. Kelleher, 3/29/92.
7. Personal interview with Betsy Lambert.
8. Jane Brody. "Mammography Interpretation Is Questioned." *New York Times.* 12/2/94.
9. Marian Segal. "Mammography Facilities Must Meet Quality Standards." *FDA Consumer.* March 1994.
10. Rose Kushner. *Alternatives: New Developments in the War on Breast Cancer.* New York: Kensington Press, 1984.
11. Segal, March 1994.
12. Segal, March 1994.
13. Ferris Hall. "Screening Mammography: Potential Problems on the Horizon." *New England Journal of Medicine.* 1/2/86.
14. Jonathan Rabinovitz. "Mammograms Called Faulty in Nassau." *New York Times.* 2/17/93.
15. Jonathan Rabinovitz. "Doctor Fined for Violations in LI Practice." *New York Times.* 3/17/93.
16. Rabinovitz, 2/17/93.
17. Rabinovitz, 2/17/93.
18. Rabinovitz, 2/17/93.

19. Patrick Borgen, at Memorial Sloan-Kettering Cancer Center conference. May 1993.
20. Borgen, May 1993.
21. "Breast Cancer: Race for the Cure." Hearing before the House Subcommittee on Health and Long-Term Care of the Select Committee on Aging. Chaired by Edward R. Roybal. 5/16/90.
22. Senate hearing on quality standards for mammography. 11/1/91.
23. "Summary of Enacted Breast Cancer Legislation by Category as of September 1994." National Cancer Institute: State Cancer Legislative Database. Bethesda, Md. October 1994.
24. "Mammography Quality Deadline: October 1, 1994." *FDA Talk Paper.* 9/29/94.
25. Associated Press. "Most Clinics Meet Standard on Breast Test." *New York Times.* 10/1/94.
26. Corrina Nelson. "More and Stiffer Mammography Clinic Regulations on the Way." *Journal of the National Cancer Institute.* 11/16/94.
27. Nelson, 11/16/94.
28. Nelson, 11/16/94.

CHAPTER 16. FUTURE PROJECTIONS

1. Peggy Eastman. "Technology Lends Itself to Breast Imaging." *Journal of the National Cancer Institute.* 11/16/94.
2. Beth Deutch, "Breast Magnetic Resonance Imaging." Delivered at Memorial Sloan-Kettering Cancer Center conference. 6/23/93.
3. George De Lama. "Breast Cancer Detection May Employ 'Star Wars' Technology." *Chicago Tribune.* 11/28/93.
4. Deutch, 6/23/93.
5. Sally Squires. "Doctors' Views of the Disease." *Washington Post.* 4/19/94.
6. "RFA Available: Cooperative Group for Breast Cancer MRI." *Cancer Letter.* 4/14/95.
7. Cheri Vogt. "New Technologies Proving Useful for Breast Cancer Diagnosis." *Journal of the National Cancer Institute.* 1/20/93.
8. De Lama, 11/28/93.
9. Eastman, 11/16/94.
10. "Mammogram-Reading Computer Helps to Find Elusive Tumors." *New York Times.* 4/2/95.
11. De Lama, 11/28/93.
12. I. Khalkhali, I. Mena, and L. Diggles. "Review of Imaging Techniques for the Diagnosis of Breast Cancer: A New Role of Prone Scintimammography Using Technetium-99m Sestamibi." *European Journal of Nuclear Medicine.* April 1994.
13. Natalie Angier. "A Tracer Improves Mammograms." *New York Times.* 12/30/94.
14. Sonia L. Nazario. "Breast-Cancer Researchers Try New Technique." *Wall Street Journal.* 7/31/92.
15. Vogt, 1/20/93.

16. Mary Lu Carnevale. "Ultrasensitive, Cheap Test Sought for Breast Cancer." *Wall Street Journal.* 8/2/94.

PART IV. TREATMENT: SLASH, BURN, AND POISON

CHAPTER 17. IN THE BEGINNING

1. "Progress in Controlling Breast Cancer." Hearing before the Subcommittee on Health and Long-Term Care of the House Select Committee on Aging. Chaired by Claude Pepper. 98th Congress. 6/28/84.
2. The source of the information in this chapter is taken from many sources, most notably from Daniel De Moulin's book *A Short History of Breast Cancer.* Hingham, Mass.: Martinus Nijhoff Publishers, 1983.

CHAPTER 18. SURGERY

1. Gina Kolata. "Why Do So Many Women Have Breasts Removed Needlessly?" *New York Times.* 5/5/93.
2. Leslie Laurence. "The Breast Cancer Epidemic: Women Aren't Just Scared, We're Mad." *McCall's.* November 1993.
3. Personal interview with Susan Love.
4. Susan Love, at the Breast Cancer Rally in Washington, D.C., 5/2/93.
5. Personal interview with Maryann Napoli.
6. Personal interview with Larry Norton.
7. Alice Garrard. "News About Breast Cancer: For You and Your Doctor." *Ms.* March 1975.
8. Rose Kushner testifying at "Progress in Controlling Breast Cancer." Hearing before the Subcommittee on Health and Long-Term Care of the House Select Committee on Aging. Chaired by Claude Pepper. 98th Congress. 6/28/84.
9. Maureen R. Michelson. "There Are Alternatives to Mastectomy." *Ms.* January 1979.
10. Michelson, January 1979.
11. Michelson, January 1979.
12. Michelson, January 1979.
13. Personal interview with Lee Miller.
14. Umberto Veronesi, Italy, at Memorial Sloan-Kettering Cancer Center conference. May 1993.
15. Veronesi, May 1993.
16. Veronesi, May 1993.
17. B. Fisher, C. Redmond, E. R. Fisher, et al. "Ten-Year Results of a Randomized Clinical Trial Comparing Radical Mastectomy and Total Mastectomy with or without Radiation in the Treatment of Breast Cancer." *New England Journal of Medicine.* 3/14/85.
18. B. Fisher, C. Redmond, R. Poisson, et al. "Five-Year Results of a Randomized Clinical Trial Comparing Total Mastectomy and Segmental Mastectomy with or without Radiation in the Treatment of Breast Cancer." *New England Journal of Medicine.* 3/14/85.
19. B. Fisher, C. Redmond, R. Poisson, et al. "Eight-Year Results of a Randomized

Clinical Trial Comparing Total Mastectomy and Lumpectomy with or without Irradiation in the Treatment of Breast Cancer." *New England Journal of Medicine.* 3/30/89.

20. J. A. Jacobson, D. N. Danforth, K. H. Cowan, et al. "Ten-Year Results of a Comparison of Conservation with Mastectomy in the Treatment of Stage I and II Breast Cancer." *New England Journal of Medicine.* 4/6/95.

21. "Federal Cancer Experts Endorse Less-Radical Breast Surgery Form." *New York Times.* 6/23/90.

22. "Excision Held Effective for Breast Cancer." *Boston Globe.* 3/30/89.

23. "Study Finds 2d Thoughts Concerning Mastectomy." *New York Times.* 6/27/89.

24. "Breast-Conserving Surgery Now 'Preferable' for Early-stage Cancer." *Ob.-Gyn. News.* 8/14/90.

25. Personal interview with Robert Osteen, cochair, Department of Surgery, Brigham & Women's Hospital.

26. Personal interview with Robert Osteen.

27. October 1990 recommendation from NIH for breast conservation therapy.

28. S. Hellman. "Dogma and Inquisition in Medicine: Breast Cancer as a Case Study." *Cancer.* 4/1/93.

29. A. E. Baue. "Breast-Conservation Operations for Treatment of Cancer of the Breast" [Editorial]. *Journal of the American Medical Association.* 4/20/94.

30. Kolata. *New York Times.* 5/5/93.

31. Marlene Cimons. "New Choices for the Best Years." *Los Angeles Times.* 10/90.

32. Kolata, 5/5/93.

33. Kolata, 5/5/93.

34. Jeanne A. Petrek, assistant attending surgeon, assistant professor of surgery, Cornell University Medical College, New York, New York, at Memorial Sloan-Kettering Cancer Center conference. May 1993.

35. Cimons, 10/90.

36. Personal interview with Ethyl Feldmeyer.

37. Cori Vanchieri. "Radiation After Quadrantectomy Questioned for Older Women" [News]. *Journal of the National Cancer Institute.* 6/16/93.

38. Kolata, 5/5/93.

39. Personal interview with Larry Norton.

40. J. R. Harris, S. Hellman, I. C. Henderson, D. W. Kinne, eds. *Breast Diseases.* Philadelphia: J.B. Lippincott, 1991.

41. Personal interview with Susan Pringle.

42. M. Swain. "In Situ or Localized Breast Cancer: How Much Treatment Is Needed?" [Editorial; Comment]. *New England Journal of Medicine.* 6/3/93.

43. Personal interview with Susan Pringle.

44. Rosenthal, 6/4/93.

45. Personal interview with Larry Norton.

CHAPTER 19. NSABP DATAGATE

1. Jean Seligman. "How Safe Is Lumpectomy?" *Newsweek.* 3/28/94.

2. "NIH Takes a Beating at Dingells Cancer Hearing." *Science & Government Report.* 4/15/94.

3. Samuel Broder, NCI director, before the House Committee on Energy and Commerce Subcommittee on Oversight and Investigations, 4/13/94.
4. "NCI Issues Information on Falsified Data in NSABP Trials." *Journal of the National Cancer Institute.* 4/6/94.
5. "NCI Issues . . ." 4/6/94.
6. NCI Press Office. "Independent Analysis Reaffirms Results of Breast Cancer Study." 4/12/94.
7. "NCI Issues . . ." 4/6/94.
8. Lawrence K. Altman. "Federal Officials to Review Documents in Breast Cancer Study with Falsified Data." *New York Times.* 3/27/94.
9. "LSU and Tulane Suspended from NSABP Studies." *Journal of the National Cancer Institute.* 5/18/94.
10. John Crewdson. "U.S. Assails Breast Cancer Group." *Chicago Tribune.* 4/4/94.
11. Susan Jenks. "Congressional Hearing Delves into NSABP Fraud Issues." *Journal of the National Cancer Institute.* 5/4/94.
12. Lawrence Altman. "Health Officials Apologize for Problems with Falsified Data in Cancer Study." *New York Times.* 4/14/94.
13. Altman, 4/14/94.
14. Robin Herman. "Research Fraud Breaks Chain of Trust." *Washington Post.* 4/19/94.
15. Altman, 4/14/94.
16. Jenks, 5/4/94.
17. Bernard Fisher. "Fraud in Breast Cancer Trials." *New England Journal of Medicine.* 5/19/94.
18. Marcia Angell and Jerome Krasner. "Setting the Record Straight in the Breast-Cancer Trials." *New England Journal of Medicine.* 5/19/94.
19. NCI Press Office. "Independent Analysis Reaffirms Results of Breast Cancer Study." 4/12/94.
20. "NCI to Take Pittsburgh Project Bids." *Washington Post.* 6/14/94.
21. Jeffrey Abrams and Timothy Chen. "Survival After Breast-Sparing Surgery Versus Mastectomy." *Journal of the National Cancer Institute.* 11/16/94.
22. "ORI Begins Investigation Related to NSABP of Possible Misconduct in Science." *Journal of the National Cancer Institute.* 11/16/94.
23. M. C. Christian, M. S. McCabe, et al. "The National Cancer Institute Audit of the National Surgical Adjuvant Breast and Bowel Project Protocol B-06." *New England Journal of Medicine.* 11/30/95.

CHAPTER 20. ADJUVANT THERAPY

1. Personal interview with Maryann Napoli.
2. Personal interview with Larry Norton.
3. B. Fisher, C. Redmond, R. Poisson, et al. "Five-Year Results of a Randomized Clinical Trial Comparing Total Mastectomy and Segmental Mastectomy with or without Radiation in the Treatment of Breast Cancer." *New England Journal of Medicine.* 3/14/85.
4. Jan Ziegler. "Swedish Study Helps Usher in a New Treatment Era." *Journal of the National Cancer Institute.* 5/4/94.
5. Ziegler, 5/4/94.

6. Ziegler, 5/4/94.
7. Rose Kushner. *Alternatives: New Developments in the War on Breast Cancer.* Cambridge, Mass.: Kensington Press, 1984.
8. V. Craig Jordan. "Targeted Hormone Therapy for Breast Cancer." *Hospital Practice.* 3/15/93.
9. Peter Waldman. "Breast Cancer Study Backs Hormone Use." *Wall Street Journal.* 1/3/92.
10. Umberto Veronesi, at Memorial Sloan-Kettering Cancer Center conference. May 1993.
11. Veronesi, May 1993.
12. G. Bonadonna, P. Valagussa, A. Moliterni, et al. "Adjuvant Cyclophosphamide, Methotrexate, and Fluorouracil in Node-Positive Breast Cancer." *New England Journal of Medicine.* 4/6/95.
13. Lawrence K. Altman. "Study on Breast Cancer Finds Therapy Is Effective for Years." *New York Times.* 1/3/92.
14. B. Fisher, C. Redmond, N. V. Dimitrov, et al. "A Randomized Clinical Trial Evaluating Sequential Methotrexate and Fluorouracil in the Treatment of Patients with Node-Negative Breast Cancer Who Have Estrogen-Receptor-Negative Tumors." *New England Journal of Medicine.* 2/23/89. B. Fisher, J. Constantino, C. Redmond, et al. "A Randomized Clinical Trial Evaluating Tamoxifen in the Treatment of Patients with Node-Negative Breast Cancer Who Have Estrogen Receptor-Positive Tumors. *New England Journal of Medicine.* 2/23/89. E. G. Mansour, R. Gray, A. H. Shatila, et. al. "Efficacy of Adjuvant Chemotherapy in High-Risk Node-Negative Breast Cancer: An Intergroup Study." *New England Journal of Medicine.* 2/23/89.
15. David Brown. "Breast Cancer Drugs Surprise Doctors." *Washington Post.* 1/3/92.
16. Altman, 1/3/92.
17. Brown, 1/3/92.
18. Brown, 1/3/92.
19. J. Harris, M. Lippman, U. Veronesi, and W. Willett. "Medical Practice: Breast Cancer, Part III." *New England Journal of Medicine.* 8/13/92.
20. "Chemotherapy for Node-Negative Breast Cancer: Evaluating the Prognostic Factors." *Oncology Times.* January 1992.
21. William L. McGuire and Gary M. Clark. "Prognostic Factors and Treatment Decisions in Axillary-Node-Negative Breast Cancer." *New England Journal of Medicine.* 6/23/92.
22. McGuire and Clark, 6/23/92.
23. McGuire and Clark, 6/23/92.
24. Susan Love and Dixie Mills. "Breast Cancer in the 1990s: Treatment Options and Controversies." Faulkner Breast Centre, West Roxbury, Mass. April 1992.
25. Personal interview with Larry Norton.
26. SHARE conference in New York City, 6/6/94.
27. Jordan, 3/15/93.
28. Office of Cancer Communications, "NCI Issues Clinical Announcement About Long-Term Use of Tamoxifen in Breast Cancer Treatment." NCI. 11/30/95.

CHAPTER 21. HIGH DOSE/HIGH TECH/HIGH COST CHEMOTHERAPY

1. Personal interview with Ellen Hobbs.
2. Personal interview with Beverly Zakarian.
3. Personal interview with Kimberly Calder.
4. Personal interview with George Raptis.
5. Bruce Cheson. "Autologous Bone Marrow Transplantation as a Treatment for Breast Cancer." Statement before the Subcommittee on Compensation and Employee Benefits on Post Office and Civil Service. 8/11/94.
6. William P. Peters, "Controversies in the Management of Breast Cancer" conference, Waldorf Astoria Hotel, New York, March 6–7, 1992.
7. Peters, March 6–7, 1992.
8. Personal interview with George Raptis.
9. Don Colburn. "Bone Marrow Transplants: A Tough Choice." *Washington Post.* 4/19/94.
10. W. C. Wood, D. R. Budman, A. H. Korzun, et al. "Dose and Dose Intensity of Adjuvant Chemotherapy for Stage II, Node-positive Breast Carcinoma." *New England Journal of Medicine.* 5/5/94.
11. Gina Kolata. "Increasing Chemotherapy May Prove Ineffective." *New York Times.* 5/17/94.
12. Kolata, 5/17/94.
13. David M. Eddy. "High Dose Chemotherapy with Autologous Bone Marrow Transplantation for the Treatment of Metastatic Breast Cancer." *Journal of Clinical Oncology.* April 1992.
14. Colburn, 4/19/94.
15. Cheson, 8/11/94.
16. Personal interview with Terry MacKinon.
17. Personal interview with George Raptis.
18. Harris Meyer. "Breast Study Woes Preview Reform Barriers." *American Medical News.* 3/8/93.
19. Meyer, 3/8/93.
20. Office of Cancer Communications. "Update." NCI. October 1994.
21. Meyer, 3/8/93.
22. Meyer, 3/8/93.
23. Personal interview with Ellen Hobbs.
24. Personal interview with Ricky Stouch.
25. Laura A. Kiernan. "N.H. Women Sue to Get Coverage of Cancer Treatment." *Boston Globe.* 10/6/91.
26. Spear, ed. *NABCO Newsletter.*
27. Doris Sue Wong. "Private Ordeal Led to Public Campaign." *Boston Globe.* 1/25/94.
28. William P. Peters and Mark C. Rogers. "Variation in Approval by Insurance Companies of Coverage for Autologous Bone Marrow Transplantation for Breast Cancer." *New England Journal of Medicine.* 2/17/94.
29. Peters and Rogers, 2/17/94.
30. Gina Kolata. "Patients' Lawyers Lead Insurers to Pay for Unproven Treatments." *New York Times.* 3/28/94.
31. Peters and Rogers, 2/17/94.

32. Ruth Larson. "Gap in Cancer Coverage Denounced." *Washington Times.* 8/12/94.
33. Peggy Eastman. "Does the Federal Health Benefits Plan Shortchange Breast Cancer Patients?" *Oncology Times.* October 1994.
34. Eastman, October 1994.
35. Eastman, October 1994.
36. Cheson, 8/11/94.
37. Eastman, October 1994.
38. Personal interview with Kimberly Calder.
39. Kiernan, 10/6/91.
40. Personal interview with Larry Norton.
41. Personal interview with Susan Love.
42. Eastman, October 1994.
43. Kiernan, 10/6/91.
44. Personal interview with Sharon Green.
45. Cori Vanchieri. "European Medical Oncologists Debate Benefits of Intensive Chemotherapy Regimens" [News]. *Journal of the National Cancer Institute.* 12/16/92.
46. Kiernan, 10/6/91.
47. Personal interview with George Raptis.

CHAPTER 22. ALTERNATIVE TREATMENTS

1. Michael Lerner. "The Role of Autonomous Cancer Self-Help Groups as a 'Third Force' in the Development of New Perspectives on Health Promotion, Conventional Cancer Treatments and Complementary Systems of Cancer Therapy and Self-Care." Paper presented at the World Health Organization Conference on Health Promotion and Chronic Illness, Bad Honnef, Germany. June 1987.
2. Ralph Moss, editor. *The Cancer Chronicles: Serious Consideration of Alternative Ideas.* March 1994.
3. Mary Talbot. "Is There an Alternative Practitioner in the House?" *Daily News.* 2/28/94.
4. *Unconventional Cancer Treatments.* Congressional Office of Technology Assessment (OTA) report. Washington, D.C.: U.S. Government Printing Office. 1990.
5. "Antineoplastons/Dr. Stanislaw Burzynski." NCI Cancer Facts. 4/8/94.
6. Ruth SoRelle. "Controversial Doctor Placed on Probation." *Houston Chronicle.* 8/21/94.
7. *Unconventional Cancer Treatments.*
8. "Cancell." NCI Cancer Facts. 4/29/92.
9. *Unconventional Cancer Treatments.*
10. *Unconventional Cancer Treatments.*
11. *Unconventional Cancer Treatments.*
12. *Unconventional Cancer Treatments.*
13. Ralph Moss. *The Cancer Industry: The Classic Exposé on the Cancer Establishment.* New York: Paragon House, 1989.
14. *Unconventional Cancer Treatments.*
15. *Unconventional Cancer Treatments.*

16. "Sharks Do Get Cancer." *Scientific American*. October 1993.
17. James Mathews. "Media Feeds Frenzy Over Shark Cartilage as Cancer Treatment." *Journal of the National Cancer Institute*. 8/4/93.
18. Mathews, 8/4/93.
19. Moss, 1994.
20. Moss, 1994.
21. Natalie Angier. "U.S. Head of Alternative Medicine Quits." *New York Times*. 8/1/94.
22. Mary Talbot. "Is There an Alternative Practitioner in the House?" *Daily News*. 2/28/94.

CHAPTER 23. MIND MATTERS

1. Personal interview with Loretta Fields.
2. David Spiegel. "Psychosocial Intervention in Cancer." *Journal of the National Cancer Institute*. 8/3/93.
3. Personal interview with Jan Kutschinski.
4. Roberta Altman and Michael J. Sarg. *The Cancer Dictionary*. New York: Facts on File, 1992.
5. Personal interview with Roz Kleban.
6. Personal interview with Sandy Warshaw.
7. Surgeon General's Conference on Self-help, in Washington, D.C. 1987.
8. "Breast Cancer: Winning the Battles, Losing the War." 10/1/92. Joint hearing before the House Subcommittee on Health and Long-Term Care and the Select Committee on Aging.
9. Personal interview with Julia Rowland.
10. Spiegel, 8/3/93.
11. Spiegel, 8/3/93.
12. Spiegel, 8/3/93.
13. Personal interview with Julia Rowland.
14. British Medical Journal, 5/92.
15. "Drugs, Diet Figure in Breast Cancer Debate." *Modern Maturity*. November 1993.
16. Daniel Goldman. "Support Groups May Do More in Cancer than Relieve the Mind." *New York Times*. 10/18/90.
17. Goldman, 10/18/90.
18. Spiegel, 8/3/93.
19. Sandra Evans. "Counseling: A Crucial Aspect of Care." *Washington Post*. 4/19/94.
20. Evans, 4/19/94.
21. Evans, 4/19/94.
22. Personal interview with Donna Sauer.
23. Bob Kirsch. "MD Counseling Improves BMT Outcome." *Oncology Times*. October 1994.
24. Kirsch, October 1994.
25. Kirsch, October 1994.
26. Kirsch, October 1994.

CHAPTER 24. DOCTOR/PATIENT RELATIONSHIPS

1. Personal interview with Betty Reed.
2. Personal interview with Pat Skowronski.
3. Personal interview with Mary Katzke.
4. Personal interview with Kimberly Calder.
5. Personal interview with Julia Rowland.
6. Personal interview with Ester Johnson.
7. Personal interview with Ruth Mendoza.
8. Personal interview with Marlene Kessler.
9. Personal interview with Lois Joy Thomi.
10. Personal interview with Lana Jensen.
11. "Cancer and Poverty: Double Jeopardy for Women." *Sojourner: The Women's Forum.* December 1992.
12. Personal interview with Larry Norton.

PART V. PSYCHOSOCIAL IMPACT

CHAPTER 25. SEXUALITY

1. "Cancer Aid Vital, Women Say." *Washington Times.* 10/19/92.
2. Personal interview with Ann Marcou.
3. Philip Strax. *Early Detection.* New York: Harper & Row, 1974.
4. Mildred Hope Witkin. "Sex Therapy and Mastectomy." *Journal of Sex and Marital Therapy.* Summer 1975.
5. Naomi Wolf. *The Beauty Myth.* New York: William Morrow, 1991.
6. Allan Mazur. "U.S. Trends in Feminine Beauty and Overadaptation." *Journal of Sex Research.* August 1986.
7. Arnold E. Andersen and Lisa DiDomenico. "Diet vs. Shape Content of Popular Male and Female Magazines: A Dose-Response Relationship to the Incidence of Eating Disorders?" *International Journal of Eating Disorders.* 1992.
8. Lorna Zabach. "Breast Reconstruction." *Healthsharing.* Summer 1987.
9. Rose Kushner. *Alternatives: New Developments in the War on Breast Cancer.* Cambridge, Mass.: Kensington Press, 1984.
10. Personal interview with Janet Perkins.
11. Christopher C. Gates. "The 'Most Significant Other' in the Care of the Breast Cancer Patient." *CA: A Cancer Journal for Clinicians.* May/June 1988.
12. Linda Dackman. *Up Front: Sex and the Post-Mastectomy Woman.* New York: Viking, 1990. Paperback ed. Viking Penguin, 1991.
13. E. Clifford, M. Clifford, and N. G. Georgiade. "The Meaning of Concepts Related to Breast Reconstruction." *Annals of Plastic Surgery.* July 1984.
14. Victoria Mock. "Body Image in Women Treated for Breast Cancer." *Nursing and Research.* May/June 1993.
15. Lena Williams. "Women Who Lose Breasts Define Their Own Femininity." *New York Times.* 12/25/91.
16. Personal interview with Julia Rowland.
17. Richard Theriault. "Estrogen Replacement Therapy in Younger Women with

Breast Cancer." At NCI conference, "Breast Cancer in Younger Women: Strategies for Future Research." 1/29/93.

18. Elizabeth J. Shakin Kunkel. "Healing the Hidden Scars: Sex After Breast Cancer." *Health*. July/August 1993.

19. Elaine Blume. "Sex After Chemo: A Neglected Issue." *Journal of the National Cancer Institute*. 5/19/93.

CHAPTER 26. RECONSTRUCTION OR DECONSTRUCTION?

1. Felicity Barringer. "First Steps Taken in Revived Use of Breast Implants." *New York Times*. 5/3/92.

2. Jane Gross. "What Now? Many Ask After Implant Decision." *New York Times*. 1/8/92.

3. Thomas M. Burton. "Breast Implants Raise More Safety Issues." *Wall Street Journal*. 2/4/93.

4. The Food and Drug Administration.

5. Virginia Postrel. "Science and Vanity. Implants: Medicine, Feminism and Freedom." *Washington Post*. 1/26/92.

6. The Food and Drug Administration. "Breast Implants for Reconstruction: Points to Discuss with Your Doctor." 1993.

7. Leonore Miller. "What Health Professionals Can Learn from Breast Cancer Patients." Surgeon General's Workshop on Self-Help. September 1987.

8. Judy Foreman. "Women and Silicone: A History of Risk." *Boston Globe*. 1/19/92.

9. Foreman, 1/19/92.

10. Foreman, 1/19/92.

11. Philip J. Hilts. "Makers of Implants Balked at Tests, Its Records Show." *New York Times*. 1/13/92.

12. Wendy S. Schain. "Breast Reconstruction: Update of Psychosocial and Pragmatic Concerns." *Cancer: A Journal of the American Cancer Society*. 9/1/91.

13. Schain, 9/1/91.

14. Schain, 9/1/91.

15. Personal interview with Julia Rowland.

16. Schain, 9/1/91.

17. Sharon Green. "A Woman's Right to Choose Breast Implants." *Wall Street Journal*. 1/20/92.

18. Schain, 9/1/91.

19. Personal interview with Diane Zarafonetis.

20. Personal interview with Rebecca Packer.

21. Personal interview with Mary Katzke.

22. Personal interview with Ann Marcou.

23. Personal interview with Jody Rogers.

24. Personal interview with Virginia Soffa.

25. "How Safe Are Breast Implants?" *Good Housekeeping*. April 1989.

26. Ruth B. Merkatz, Grant P. Bagley, and E. Jane McCarthy. "A Qualitative Analysis of Self-Reported Experiences Among Women Encountering Difficulties with Silicone Breast Implants." *Journal of Women's Health*. Volume 2, number 2, 1993.

27. Merkatz, et al., 1993.

28. Merkatz, et al., 1993.
29. B. F. Uretsky, J. J. O'Brien, E. H. Cortiss, and M. D. Becker. "Augmentation Mammoplasty Associated with a Severe Systemic Illness." *Annals of Plastic Surgery*. November 1979.
30. S. R. Weiner and H. E. Paulus. "Chronic Arthropathy Occurring After Augmentation Mammoplasty." *Journal of Plastic and Reconstructive Surgery*. February 1986.
31. Foreman, 1/19/92.
32. Joan E. Rigdon. "Informed Consent? Plastic Surgeons Had Warnings on Safety of Silicone Implants." *Wall Street Journal*. 3/12/92.
33. Rigdon, 3/12/92.
34. Bruce Ingersoll. "Industry Lobbying Drive Gives Voice to Women Favoring Breast Implants." *Wall Street Journal*. 1/14/92.
35. Marian Segal. "Silicone Breast Implants." *FDA Consumer*. June 1992.
36. Kim Painter. "Emotions Flood Implant Hearings." *USA Today*. 2/20/92.
37. Painter, 2/20/92.
38. Painter, 2/20/92.
39. Marlene Cimons. "FDA Panel Votes Implant Limits." *Los Angeles Times*. 2/21/92.
40. Malcolm Gladwell. "Silicone Breast Implants: After a Decade of Controversy, Key Questions Are Unanswered and the Future of the Device Is Unresolved." *Washington Post*. 3/3/92.
41. Scott McMurray. "FDA Group Votes to Allow Use of Implants." *Wall Street Journal*. 2/21/92.
42. Philip J. Hilts. "Studies See Greater Implant Danger." *New York Times*. 2/19/92.
43. Hilts, 2/19/92.
44. Hilts, 2/19/92.
45. McMurray, 2/21/92.
46. Gladwell, 3/3/92.
47. Green, 1/20/92.
48. Gladwell, 3/3/92.
49. Gladwell, 3/3/92.
50. Marcia Angell. "Breast Implants: Protectionism or Paternalism?" [Editorial; Comment]. *New England Journal of Medicine*. 6/18/92.
51. David A. Kessler. "The Basis of the FDA's Decision on Breast Implants." *New England Journal of Medicine*. 6/18/92.
52. Green, 1/20/92.
53. Edith H. Robinson. Letter to the editor. *Wall Street Journal*. 1/31/92.
54. "Medical Journal Assails Curbs on Breast Implants." *New York Times*. 6/18/92.
55. Philip J. Hilts. "AMA Urges Full Availability of Breast Implants." *New York Times*. 12/1/93.
56. Rigdon, 3/12/92.
57. Kim Painter. "FDA Reported as Lax on Implants." *USA Today*. 1/7/93.
58. Painter, 1/7/93.
59. Judy Foreman. "Long-Term Safety Was Concern of Researchers for Implant Makers." *Boston Globe*. 1/19/92.
60. Judy Foreman, "Women and Silicone: A History of Risk." *Boston Globe*. 1/19/92.

61. Foreman, 1/19/92. "Women and Silicone . . ."
62. Dow Corning sales memo. 5/12/75.
63. Foreman, 1/19/92. "Long-Term Safety . . ."
64. Hilts, 1/13/92.
65. Foreman, 1/19/92.
66. Foreman, 1/19/92. "Long-Term Safety . . ."
67. C. H. Dahl, et al. "A Silicone Gel Inflatable Mammary Prosthesis." D. L. Weiner. "A New, Soft, Round Silicone Gel Breast Implant." *Plastic and Reconstructive Surgery.* February 1974.
68. Boyce Rensberger. "Breast Implant Study Findings Misrepresented." *Washington Post.* 1/16/92.
69. Rensberger, 1/16/92.
70. Rensberger, 1/16/92.
71. Leia Zenderman's case is reported by Foreman, 1/19/92.
72. F. L. Ashley, S. Braley, T. D. Rees, et al. "The Present Status of Silicone Fluid in Soft Tissue Augmentation." *Plastic and Reconstructive Surgery.* April 1967.
73. Philip J. Hilts. "Two Studies Link Breast Implants and Antibodies." *New York Times.* 3/20/93.
74. Hilts, 3/20/93.
75. Hilts, 3/20/93.
76. Boyce Rensberger. "1975 Study on Breast Implants Indicated Immune System Harm." *Washington Post.* 4/8/94.
77. Sandra Blakeslee. "Dow Found Silicone Danger in 1975 Study, Lawyers Say." *New York Times.* 4/7/94.
78. Blakeslee, 4/7/94.
79. Blakeslee, 4/7/94.
80. Burton, 2/4/93.
81. Burton, 2/4/93.
82. Burton, 2/4/93.
83. H. Berkel, D. C. Birdsell, and H. Jenkins. "Breast Augmentation: A Risk for Breast Cancer?" *New England Journal of Medicine.* 6/18/92.
84. "Breast Implants Linked with Lower Risk of Cancer." *Washington Post.* 6/17/92.
85. Shari Roan. "Women Caught in Middle of Breast-Implant Debate." *Los Angeles Times.* 3/8/94.
86. Roan, 3/8/94.
87. Gina Kolata. "Study Finds No Implant-Disease Links." *New York Times.* 6/16/94.
88. Gina Kolata. "Tissue Illness and Implants: No Tie Is Seen." *New York Times.* 5/29/94.
89. Kolata, 5/29/94.
90. Kolata, 5/29/94.
91. Kolata, 5/29/94.
92. "Mixed Views on Breast Implants." Excerpts from the *Los Angeles Times. New York Newsday.* 4/3/94.
93. S. E. Gabriel, W. M. O'Fallon, L. T. Kurland, et al. "Risk of Connective-Tissue Diseases and Other Disorders After Breast Implantation." *New England Journal of Medicine.* 6/16/94.

94. Marcia Angell. "Do Breast Implants Cause Systemic Disease? Science in the Courtroom" [Editorial]. *New England Journal of Medicine.* 6/16/94.
95. Kolata, 6/16/94.
96. John Schwartz. "Breast Implant Study Finds No Link to Disease." *Washington Post.* 6/16/94.
97. Schwartz, 6/16/94.
98. Kim Painter. "Implant Fear May Be Unjustified." *USA Today.* 6/16/94.
99. Associated Press. "Breast Implant Study Finds No Disease Links." *Washington Times.* 6/16/94.
100. Schwartz, 6/16/94.
101. Linda F. Anderson. "Scientists Grapple with Silicone, Breast Implant Research." *Journal of the National Cancer Institute.* 5/3/95.
102. Gina Kolata. "Fund Proposed for Settling Suits over Breast Implants." *New York Times.* 9/10/93.
103. "Judge Accepts Terms of Implant Settlement." *New York Times.* 4/3/94.
104. "Judge Accepts Terms of Implant Settlement."
105. John Schwartz. "$4.25 Billion Settlement in Breast Implant Suit." *Washington Post.* 9/2/94.
106. Barry Meier. "3 Implant Companies Offer New Settlement." *New York Times.* 10/3/95.
107. Vicki L. Westbrook, Associate Implant Information Center at Dow Corning Corporation. Letter to author. 10/17/95.
108. *Journal of the American Medical Association,* October 1992.
109. Marilyn Elias. "Saline Implants Called Safe." *USA Today.* 4/19/93.
110. Elias, 4/19/93.
111. Marlene Cimons. "FDA Begins Inquiry into Saline Breast Implants." *Los Angeles Times.* 6/3/94.
112. Cimons, 6/3/94.
113. Cimons, 6/3/94.
114. Cimons, 6/3/94.
115. Kim Painter. "Saline Implant Makers Seek Time Before Review." *USA Today.* 6/3/94.
116. "Further U.S. Ban of Breast Implants Urged." *New York Times.* 8/5/94.
117. Joan E. Rigdon. "Swiss Company Gets FDA Approval to Test Soybean-Oil Breast Implants." *Wall Street Journal.* 8/2/94.

CHAPTER 27. MULTICULTURAL ISSUES

1. Personal interview with Harold Freeman.
2. Personal interview with Karen Schmidt.
3. Personal interview with Julia Rowland.
4. Personal interview with Amy Langer.
5. Alisa Solomon. "The Politics of Breast Cancer." *Village Voice.* 5/14/91.
6. Personal interview with Harold Freeman.
7. Delores M. Esparazza. "The Influence of Ethnic Patient Values on Cancer Nursing." In Lovell A. Jones, editor, *Minorities and Cancer.* New York: Springer-Verlag, 1989.
8. Personal interview with Jody Rogers.

9. Sheryl Stolberg. "Latinos' *Fatalismo* May Hinder Treatment of Cancer." *Los Angeles Times*. 1/7/93.
10. Personal interview with Ruth Mendoza.
11. Personal interview with Alison Estabrook.
12. Personal interview with Roz Kleban.
13. Personal interview with Karen Schmidt.
14. C. P. Hunter, C. K. Redmond, Vivien Chen, et al. "Breast Cancer: Factors Associated with Stage at Diagnosis in Black and White Women." *Journal of the National Cancer Institute*. 7/21/93.
15. *CA: Cancer Journal for Clinicians*. March/April 1995.
16. Corinna Nelson. "Cancer Screening, Clinical Trials for African Americans Still Problematic." *Journal of the National Cancer Institute*. 12/7/94.
17. Nelson, 12/7/94.
18. Dr. Marion Lee, at President's Cancer Panel Meeting: "Cancer and the Cultures of America," in San Francisco. 11/30/94.
19. Stephen McPhee, at President's Cancer Panel Meeting: "Cancer and the Cultures of America," in San Francisco. 11/30/94.

CHAPTER 28. DISCRIMINATION AND LITIGATION

1. Personal interview with Barbara Balaban.
2. Personal interview with Kimberly Calder.
3. Personal interview; name has been changed.
4. Personal interview with Ellen Stovall.
5. J. Z. Ayanian, B. A. Kohler, T. Abe, and A. M. Epstein. "The Relation Between Health Insurance Coverage and Clinical Outcomes Among Women with Breast Cancer." *New England Journal of Medicine*. 7/29/93.
6. "Insurance Linked to Early Diagnosis." *New York Times*. 7/29/93.
7. Ayanian et al., 7/29/93.
8. Personal interview with Mary Katzke.
9. Fitzhugh Mullan, M.D., Barbara J. D. Hoffman, editors. *Charting the Journey: An Almanac of Practical Resources for Cancer Survivors*. Consumer Reports Books, 1990.
10. Personal interview with Zora Brown.
11. Personal interview with Zora Brown.
12. Personal interview with Irene Card.
13. Personal interview with Nancy Cardwell.
14. Mullan and Hoffman, 1990.
15. Barbara Hoffman. "Working It Out: Your Employment Rights as a Cancer Survivor." NCCS. 1993.
16. Sandy Rovner. "Discrimination on the Job." *Washington Post*. 12/3/91.
17. Personal interview with Joyce Salzburg.
18. Hoffman, 1990.
19. Hoffman, 1990.
20. Hoffman, 1990.
21. Hoffman, 1990.

PART VI. FIGHTING BACK

CHAPTER 29. SETTING THE STAGE

1. Personal interview with Harvey Kushner.
2. At Washington, D.C. rally, 5/2/93.
3. Personal interview with Amy Langer.
4. Personal interview with Beverly Zakarian.
5. Personal interview with Ellen Hobbs.
6. Personal interview with Susan Claymon.
7. Jane Gross. "Turning Disease into a Cause: Breast Cancer Follows AIDS." *New York Times.* 1/7/91.
8. Personal interview with Diane Zarafonetis.
9. Rose Kushner. *Alternatives: New Developments in the War on Breast Cancer.* Cambridge, Mass.: Kensington Press, 1984.
10. Kushner, 1984.
11. Personal interview with Helen, a Reach to Recovery volunteer.
12. "The Other Epidemic." Produced by Linda Ellerbee, Lucky Duck Productions, PBS, WNET, New York, Channel 13 show, 10/15/93.
13. "Breast Cancer: Race for the Cure." 5/16/90. Hearing before the House Subcommittee on Health and Long-Term Care of the Select Committee on Aging.
14. Personal interview with Ann Marcou.
15. "Protestors Assail Refusal of Saks to Hire Woman After Mastectomy." *New York Times.* 3/25/77.
16. Personal interview with Lee Miller.
17. "Protestors Assail Refusal of Saks. . . ." 3/25/77.
18. Personal interview with Lee Miller.
19. Personal interview with Doris Erickson.
20. Personal interview with Terri Castagno.
21. Personal interview with Sandy Warshaw.
22. Personal interview with Mary Jo Kahn.
23. Personal interview with Ann Marcou.
24. Personal interview with Mary Jo Kahn.
25. Personal interview with Lee Miller.
26. Personal interview with Joanne Rathgeb.
27. Personal interview with Susan Claymon.
28. Personal interview with Mary Jo Kahn.
29. Susan Shapiro. "Cancer as a Feminist Issue." *Sojourner.* September 1989.
30. Personal interview with Rita Arditti.
31. Personal interview with Sheila Swanson.
32. Sheila Swanson. Letter to the editor. *San Jose Mercury News.* September 1991.
33. Sheila Swanson. Letter to the editor. *Coping.* January 1992.
34. Personal interview with Sheila Swanson.
35. Personal interview with Ellen Hobbs.
36. Personal interview with Ellen Hobbs.
37. Personal interview with Ellen Hobbs.
38. Personal interview with Barbara Balaban.

39. Personal interview with Barbara Balaban.
40. New York State Department of Health. "The Long Island Breast Cancer Study." Report Number 1, completed June 1988, released 1990.
41. Centers for Disease Control and Prevention, "Breast Cancer on Long Island, New York." 12/17/92.
42. Women's Environment and Development Organization (WEDO) Public Hearing of the Commission on the Status of Women. City Hall, New York City, 3/2/93.
43. Jimmy Breslin. "Women in the Fight of Their Lives." *New York Newsday.* 5/10/92.
44. Personal interview with Ann Marcou.
45. Kushner, 1984.
46. Toni Locy. "Bay State Declares Breast Cancer Rate at Epidemic Level." *Boston Globe.* 5/21/92.
47. Melinda Beck, et al. "The Politics of Breast Cancer." *Newsweek.* 12/10/90.

CHAPTER 30. A NATIONAL MOVEMENT

1. Personal interview with Fran Visco.
2. Judy Foreman. "Breast Cancer: A Special Terror." *Boston Globe.* 11/11/91.
3. Secretary's Conference to Establish a National Action Plan on Breast Cancer. Bethesda, Md. 3/14–15/94.
4. Fact sheet from the Komen Foundation.
5. Roxanne Roberts. "Nancy Brinker and Her Running Obsession." *Washington Post.* 6/12/91.
6. Personal interview with Harvey Kushner.
7. Personal interview with Amy Langer.
8. Memo supplied by Amy Langer.
9. Press release from Amy Langer.
10. Letter supplied by Amy Langer.
11. Personal interview with Mary Jo Kahn.
12. Personal interview with Fran Visco.
13. Hearings Summary and Conclusions of the Breast Cancer Coalition Research Task Force, March 1992.
14. Personal interview with Mary Rose Oakar.
15. Breast cancer rally in Washington, D.C. 10/18/93.
16. "IOM Advises Defense Dept. to Fund Research, Training, Infrastructure." *Cancer Letter.* 5/31/93.
17. Personal interview with Mary Rose Oakar.
18. Jocelyn Kaiser. "Army Doles Out Its First $210 Million." *Science.* 10/14/94.
19. Francis X. Mahaney. "Army Awards Breast Cancer Grants." *Journal of the National Cancer Institute.* 12/7/94.
20. Corinna Nelson."Breast Cancer Grants Spur New Research Programs." *Journal of the National Cancer Institute.* 10/5/94.
21. Gina Kolata. "Weighing Spending on Breast Cancer." *New York Times.* 10/20/93.
22. Kolata, 10/20/93.
23. Anna Quindlen. "Competitive Cancer." *New York Times.* 10/31/94.

24. Foreman, 11/11/91.
25. Breast cancer rally in Washington, D.C. 10/18/93.
26. Personal interview with Barbara Vucanovich.
27. "Progress in Controlling Breast Cancer." Hearing before the House Select Committee on Aging Subcommittee on Health and Long-Term Care. Chaired by Claude Pepper. 6/28/84.
28. Personal interview with Harvey Kushner.
29. Personal interview with Susan Love.
30. Breast cancer rally in Washington, D.C. 10/18/93.
31. Personal interview with Kimberly Calder.
32. Breast cancer rally in Washington, D.C. 10/18/93.
33. Personal interview with Larry Norton.
34. Eliot Marshall. "The Politics of Breast Cancer." *Science.* 1/29/93.
35. Personal interview with Mary Rose Oakar.
36. Personal interview with Susan Love.
37. Conference to Establish a National Action Plan on Breast Cancer, Bethesda, Md. 12/14/93.
38. "National Action Plan on Breast Cancer: Progress Report." Department of Health and Human Services. 12/19/94.
39. National Cancer Advisory Board. "Executive Summary of the President's Cancer Panel Special Commission on Breast Cancer." *Cancer at a Crossroads: A Report to Congress for the Nation.* September 1994.
40. "Breast Cancer Action Plan Issues RFA for Small Grants; Other Initiatives Coming Soon." *Cancer Letter.* 4/14/95.
41. Personal interview with Mary Rose Oakar.
42. "Progress in Controlling Breast Cancer." Hearing before the House Select Committee on Aging Subcommittee on Health and Long-Term Care. Chaired by Claude Pepper. 6/28/84.
43. Personal interview with Sharon Green.
44. President's Cancer Panel: Special Commission on Breast Cancer (NCI). *Breast Cancer: A National Strategy — A Report to the Nation.* October 1993.
45. Personal interview with Sharon Green.
46. Personal interview with Ellen Hobbs.
47. Personal interview with Virginia Soffa.
48. Breast Cancer Action Group news release, 10/1/93.

EPILOGUE

1. Peter Marks. "Breast Cancer as a Political Issue." *New York Times.* 11/4/94.
2. Personal interview with Harold Freeman.
3. Personal interview with Joyce Ford.
4. David Spiegel. "Psychosocial Intervention in Cancer." *Journal of the National Cancer Institute.* 8/3/93.

Bibliography

Altman, Roberta, and Sarg, Michael, M.D., *The Cancer Dictionary*. New York: Facts on File, 1992.

Boston Women's Health Collective. *The New Our Bodies Ourselves: A Book by and for Women*. New York: Simon and Schuster, 1992.

Brady, Judy, ed. *1 in 3 Women with Cancer Confront an Epidemic*. Pittsburgh: Cleis Press, 1991.

Bruning, Nancy. *Breast Implants: Everything You Need to Know*. Alameda, Calif.: Hunter House, 1995.

———. *Coping with Chemotherapy*. New York: Ballantine Books, 1993.

Cooper, Gary L., ed. *Stress and Breast Cancer*. New York: John Wiley and Sons, 1988.

Costello, Cynthia, and Anne J. Stone, eds. *The American Woman 1994–95: Where We Stand*. New York: W. W. Norton, 1994.

Dackman, Linda. *Up Front: Sex and the Post-Mastectomy Woman*. New York: Viking, 1990. Paperback ed. Viking Penguin, 1991.

De Moulin, Daniel. *A Short History of Breast Cancer*. Hingham, Mass.: Martinus Nijhoff Publishers, 1983.

Fink, John M. *Third Opinion: An International Directory to Alternative Therapy Centers for the Treatment and Prevention of Cancer and Other Degenerative Diseases*. Garden City Park, N.Y.: Avery Publishing Company, 1988.

Greenberg, Mimi. *Invisible Scars: A Guide to Coping with the Emotional Impact of Cancer*. New York: St. Martin's Press, 1989.

Greenspan, Ezra M., M.D. *The Breast Cancer Epidemic in the United States*. New York: Chemotherapy Foundation, 1993.

Gross, Amy, and Ito, Dee. *Women Talk About Breast Surgery*. New York: Random House, 1990.

Harpham, Wendy Schlessel, M.D. *Diagnosis Cancer: Your Guide Through the First Few Months*. New York: W. W. Norton, 1992.

Herter, Frederic P., et al., eds. *Human and Ethical Issues in the Surgical Care of Patients with Life-Threatening Disease*. Springfield, Ill.: Charles C. Thomas, 1986.

Johnson, Judi, and Klein, Linda. *I Can Cope: Staying Healthy with Cancer*. Wayzata, Minn.: DCI Publishing, 1994.

Jones, Lovell A., ed., *Minorities and Cancer.* New York: Springer-Verlag, 1989.

Kahane, Deborah Hobler. *No Less a Woman: Ten Women Shatter the Myths About Breast Cancer.* New York: Simon and Schuster, 1993.

Kaye, Ronnie. *Spinning Straw into Gold: Your Emotional Recovery from Breast Cancer.* New York: Simon and Schuster, 1991.

Kemeny, M. Margaret, M.D., and Dranov, Paula. *Breast Cancer and Ovarian Cancer: Beating the Odds.* Reading, Mass.: Addison-Wesley, 1992.

Komarnicky, Lydia, M.D., and Rosenberg, Anne, M.D., with Betancourt, Marian. *What to Do If You Get Breast Cancer.* Boston, Mass.: Little, Brown, 1995.

Kushner, Rose. *Alternatives: New Developments in the War on Breast Cancer.* Cambridge, Mass.: Kensington Press, 1984.

Kushner, Rose. *If You've Thought About Breast Cancer.* Kensington, Maryland: Women's Breast Cancer Advisory Center, 1989.

LaTour, Kathy. *The Breast Cancer Companion.* New York: William Morrow, 1994.

Laurence, Leslie, and Weinhouse, Beth. *Outrageous Practices: The Alarming Truth About How Medicine Mistreats Women.* New York: Ballantine Books, 1994.

Lerner, Michael. *Choices in Healing: Integrating the Best of Conventional and Complementary Approaches to Cancer.* Cambridge: MIT Press, 1994.

Lorde, Audre. *The Cancer Journals.* San Francisco: Aunt Lute Books, 1980.

Love, Susan M., M.D., with Lindsey, Karen. *Dr. Susan Love's Breast Book.* Reading, Mass.: Addison-Wesley, 1990.

Morra, Marion, and Potts, Eve. *Choices.* New York: Avon Books, 1994.

Moss, Ralph W., Ph.D. *Cancer Therapy: The Independent Consumers Guide to Nontoxic Treatment and Prevention.* New York: Equinox Press, 1992.

Moss, Ralph. *The Cancer Industry: The Classic Exposé on the Cancer Establishment.* New York: Paragon House, 1991.

Mullan, Fitzhugh, M.D., Hoffman, Barbara, J. D., eds. *Charting the Journey: An Almanac of Practical Resources for Cancer Survivors.* Consumer Reports Books, 1990.

Nechas, Eileen, and Foley, Denise. *Unequal Treatment: What You Don't Know About How Women are Mistreated by the Medical Community.* New York: Simon and Schuster, 1994.

Nessim, Susan, and Ellis, Judith. *Cancervive: The Challenge of Life After Cancer.* Boston: Houghton Mifflin, 1992.

Office of Technology Assessment. *Unconventional Cancer Treatments.* Washington, D.C.: U.S. Government Printing Office, 1990.

Payer, Lynn. *Medicine and Culture.* New York: Penguin Books, 1988.

Randall-David, Elizabeth, Ph.D. *Strategies for Working with Culturally Diverse Communities and Clients.* Washington, D.C.: Association for the Care of Children's Health, 1989.

Royak-Schaler, Renee, Ph.D., and Benderly, Beryl Lieff. *Challenging the Breast Cancer Legacy: A Program of Emotional Support and Medical Care for Women at Risk.* New York: HarperCollins, 1992.

Soffa, Virginia. *The Journey Beyond Breast Cancer.* Rochester, Vermont: Healing Arts Press, 1994.

Stewart, Susan K. *Bone Marrow Transplants: A Book of Basics for Patients.* Highland Park, Ill.: BMT Newsletter, 1992.

Stocker, Midge, ed. *Confronting Cancer, Constructing Change: New Perspectives on Women and Cancer*. Chicago: Third Side Press, 1993.

Strax, Philip. *Make Sure You Do Not Have Breast Cancer*. New York: St. Martin's Press, 1991.

Swirsky, Joan, and Balaban, Barbara. *The Breast Cancer Handbook: Taking Control After You've Found a Lump*. New York: HarperCollins, 1994.

Walters, Richard. *Options: The Alternative Cancer Therapy Book*. Honesdale, Pa.: Paragon Press, 1993.

Wolf, Naomi. *The Beauty Myth*. New York: Doubleday, 1991.

Index